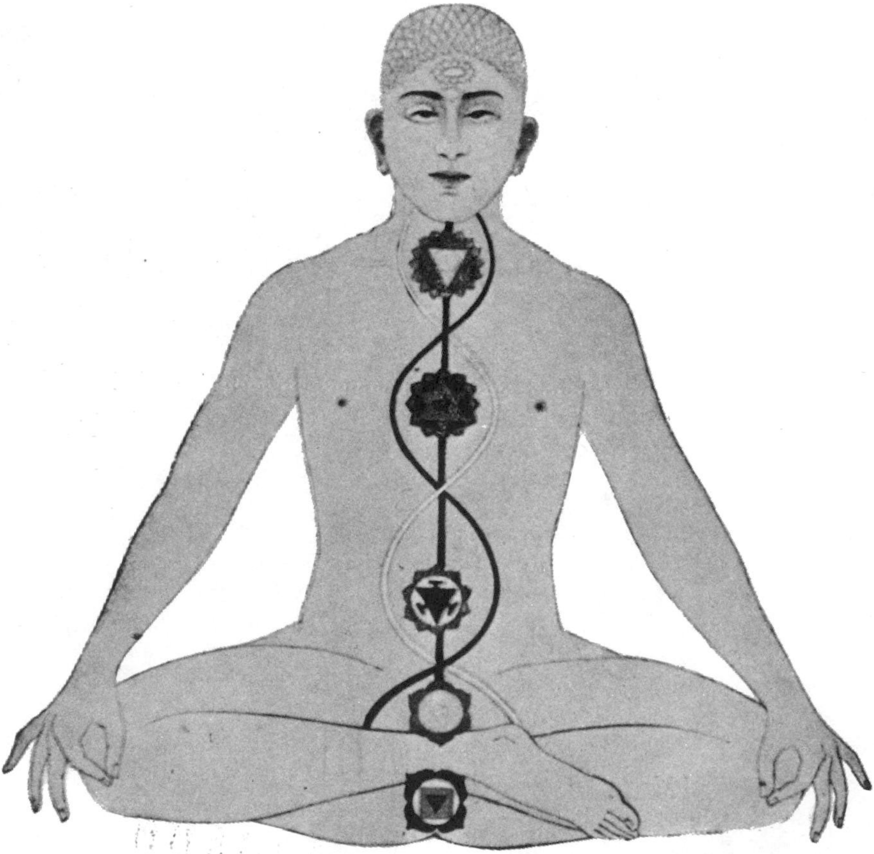

Plate I] The Centres or Lotuses [*Frontispiece*

THE SERPENT POWER

BEING THE

ṢAṬ-CAKRA-NIRŪPAṆA AND
PĀDUKĀ-PAÑCAKA

TWO WORKS ON LAYA-YOGA, TRANSLATED FROM THE SANSKRIT, WITH INTRODUCTION AND COMMENTARY

BY

ARTHUR AVALON
(SIR JOHN WOODROFFE)

DOVER PUBLICATIONS, INC.
NEW YORK

This Dover edition, first published in 1974, is a republication of the seventh edition of the work as published by Ganesh & Co. (Madras) Private Ltd., Madras, India, in 1964 (the first edition was published by Luzac & Co., London, in 1919).

In the present edition, which is published by special arrangement with Ganesh & Co., the Sanskrit text that was included with the seventh edition has been omitted, and Plates I through VIII, originally in color, appear in black and white.

International Standard Book Number: 0-486-23058-9
Library of Congress Catalog Card Number: 74-75259

Manufactured in the United States of America
Dover Publications, Inc.
180 Varick Street
New York, N.Y. 10014

PUBLISHERS' NOTE TO SIXTH EDITION

THE growing interest evinced by the public to understand rightly the literature of Tantra Śāstra and more especially the Yoga of Kuṇḍalinī Śakti has encouraged us to bring out this new edition of the almost unique original work on the subject.

The opportunity has been availed of to add a transliteration of all the Sanskrit verses and provide indexes in English for half-verses, authors, citations, words, etc.

June 1958

PUBLISHERS' NOTE TO FIFTH EDITION

WITHIN the last three years most of the Works of Sir John Woodroffe have been published by us after they had been out of print for nearly twenty years. It is gratifying to note that the public have appreciated the valuable nature of these books and their new, uniform get-up. The last Edition of SERPENT POWER was exactly the same as its predecessor but in the present one, to make reference to the Sanskrit portion easier and more convenient to critical students, indexes have been included for the verses, authors, citations, bibliography and important words at the end of the book. It is hoped that these additions would prove useful to at least some of the readers.

November 1953

PREFACE TO THIRD EDITION

This edition to which some additions have been made and in which some errors have been corrected has been revised throughout. Since the issue of the second edition several new volumes have appeared in the series of "Tāntrik Texts". In connection with this book the reader is specially referred to the *Kāmakalāvilāsa*, one of such Texts, as also to the essay on "Creation in the Tantras" which with other new material is printed in *Śakti and Śākta.* The publishers have published a volume called *Mahāmāya* by Professor Pramatha Nātha Mukhyopādhyāya and myself in which comparison is made of the concept of Māyā as held by the Śāktas and Māyāvādins respectively. I repeat that it is not possible to understand this Yoga without having been first well grounded in its philosophy. I say 'understand' only because the question of the reality and value of this form of Yoga is not one with which this book is concerned.

Since the publication of the second edition, there has been issued a monograph on the Cakras by the well-known Theosophist, the Right Reverend C. W. Leadbeater, which includes matter published by him in 1910. The volume contains plates of the Cakras as said to have been seen clairvoyantly as also a plate of the Cakras according to Johann Georg Gichtel, a pupil of Jakob Boehme taken from his *Theosophia Practica* originally issued in 1696 and reprinted in 1897 (Chacornac, Paris. See also Plates at the end of Dr. Law's edition of the translation into English of Behmen).

Dr. Rele has also published a book entitled *The Mysterious Kuṇḍalinī* (Taraporewalla, Bombay) to which I have written an Introduction.

OXFORD A. A.

September 11, 1928

PREFACE TO SECOND EDITION

Considering the recondite nature of the subject, the first edition published by Messrs. Luzac & Co., London, has had a more rapid sale than was expected, and a call for a second edition has enabled me to revise the whole work and to make several corrections and additions both in the Introduction and Text. To this second edition has been added the Sanskrit Text of the works here translated which formerly appeared as Vol. 2 of the Tāntrik Texts and which has since gone out of print. This edition also contains in addition to the original coloured plates of the Cakras, a number of half-tone plates taken from Life, showing some positions in Kuṇḍalinī-Yoga.

The Introduction deals in a general way with the subject-matter of the Texts translated. I take however this opportunity to say again that it has not been possible to give here a full explanation of such matters, and refer my reader to my other works dealing with the Tantras and their Ritual, namely, *Principles of Tantra*, a work of peculiar value in that it is a translation of the work of a Bengali Paṇḍit, himself a Śākta unacquainted with the English language but an inheritor of the old traditions; as also my *Śakti and Śākta* dealing with ritual, published since the date of my first Preface. The *Studies in Mantra-Śāstra* referred to therein has also recently been published under the title of *Garland of Letters*. All such technical terms as Bindu, Nāda and the like used in the works translated have been fully explained therein as also the general principles of Mantra. It is necessary also to know with accuracy the exact meaning of the terms Consciousness, Mind, Life, Matter and so forth as used in Vedānta and these have been given in the series of little works under the general caption *The World as Power*.[1] It is not possible to understand the rationale of Yoga without an accurate understanding of these fundamental terms. It has been rightly said that "the practical portion of all Yoga, specially of Rāja Yoga, is concerned with mental practices. It is therefore absolutely necessary that the student of Yoga should know what his mind is and how it works" (*Rāja Yoga*, by Swāmī Dayānand, p. 9). I have given a short account of Sarvānanda and his life in the *Hindusthan Review*. Other works by me on the Śāstra are noted in the advertisement sheet at the end of the book.

LES ANDELYS EURE A. AVALON

October, *1922*

[1] Since republished in one volume (1957).

PREFACE

"We pray to the Paradevatā united with Śiva, whose substance is the pure nectar of bliss, red like unto vermilion, the young flower of the hibiscus, and the sunset sky; who, having cleft Her way through the mass of sound issuing from the clashing and the dashing of the two winds in the midst af Suṣuṁṇā, rises to that brilliant Energy which glitters with the lustre of ten million lightnings. May She, Kuṇḍalinī, who quickly goes to and returns from Śiva, grant us the fruit of Yoga! She being awakened is the Cow of Plenty to Kaulas and the Kalpa Creeper of all things desired for those who worship Her."

—Śāradā-Tilaka, xxxv, 70

In my work *Śakti and Śākta* I outlined for the first time the principles of "Kuṇḍali-Yoga" so much discussed in some quarters, but of which so little was known.

This work is a description and explanation in fuller detail of the Serpent Power (Kuṇḍali-Śakti), and the Yoga effected through it, a subject occupying a pre-eminent place in the Tantra-Śāstra. It consists of a translation of two Sanskrit works published some years ago in the second volume of my series of Tāntrik Texts, but hitherto untranslated. The first, entitled "Ṣaṭcakra-nirūpaṇa" ("Description of and Investigation into the Six Bodily Centres"), has as its author the celebrated Tāntrik Pūrṇānanda-Svāmī, a short note on whose life is given later. It forms the sixth chapter of his extensive and unpublished work on Tāntrik Ritual entitled "Śrī-tattva-cintāmaṇī". This has been the subject of commentaries by among others Śaṁkara and Viśvanātha cited in Volume II of the Tāntrik Texts, and used in the making of the present translation. The commentary here translated from the Sanskrit is by Kālīcaraṇa.

The second text, called " Pādukā-Pañcaka " (" Five-fold Footstool of the Guru ") deals with one of the Lotuses described in the larger work. To it is appended a translation from the Sanskrit of a commentary by Kālīcaraṇa. To the translation of both works I have added some further explanatory notes of my own. As the works translated are of a highly recondite character, and by themselves unintelligible to the English reader, I have prefaced the translation by a general Introduction in which I have endeavoured to give (within the limits both of a work of this kind and my knowledge) a description and explanation of this form of Yoga. I have also included some plates of the Centres, which have been drawn and painted according to the description of them as given in the first of these Sanskrit Texts.

It has not been possible in the Introduction to do more than give a general and summary statement of the principles upon which Yoga, and this particular form of it, rests. Those who wish to pursue the subject in greater detail are referred to my other published books on the Tantra Śāstra. In *Principles of Tantra* will be found general Introductions to the Śāstra and (in connection with the present subject) valuable chapters on Śakti and Mantras. In my recent work, *Śakti and Śākta* (the second edition of which is as I write reprinting), I have shortly summarised the teaching of the Śākta Tantras and their rituals. In my *Studies in the Mantra-Śāstra*, the first three parts of which have been reprinted from the " Vedānta Kesarī," in which they first appeared, will be found more detailed descriptions of such technical terms as Tattva, Causal Śaktis, Kalā, Nāda, Bindu, and so forth, which are referred to in the present book. Other works published by me on the

Tantra, including the *Wave of Bliss*, will be found in the page of advertisements.

The following account of Pūrṇānanda, the celebrated Tāntrika Sādhaka of Bengal, and author of the "Ṣaṭ-cakra-nirūpaṇa," has been collected from the descendants of his eldest son, two of whom are connected with the work of the Varendra Research Society, Rajshahi, to whose Director, Sj. Akṣaya-Kumāra-Maitra, and Secretary, Sj. Rādha-Govinda-Baisāk, I am indebted for the following details:

Pūrṇānanda was a Rahri Brāhmaṇa of the Kāśyapa Gotra, whose ancestors belonged to the village of Pakrashi, which has not as yet been identified. His seventh ancestor Anantācārya is said to have migrated from Baranagora, in the district of Murshidabad, to Kaitali, in the district of Mymensingh. In his family were born two celebrated Tāntrika-Sādhakas—namely, Sarvānanda and Pūrṇānanda. The descendants of Sarvānanda reside at Mehar, while those of Pūrṇānanda reside mostly in the district of Mymensingh. Little is known about the worldly life of Pūrṇānanda, except that he bore the name of Jagadānanda, and copied a manuscript of the Viṣṇupurāṇam in the Śāka year 1448 (A.D. 1526). This manuscript, now in the possession of one of his descendants named Paṇḍit Hari-Kishore-Bhattācārya, of Kaitali, is still in a fair state of preservation. It was brought for inspection by Paṇḍit Satis-Candra-Siddhāntabhūṣaṇa of the Varendra Research Society. The colophon states that Jagadānanda Śarma wrote the Purāṇa in the Śāka year 1448.

This Jagadānanda assumed the name of Pūrṇānanda when he obtained his Dīkṣā (Initiation) from Brahmānanda and went to Kāmarūpa (Assam), in which province he is believed to have obtained his "Siddhi" or state of spiritual perfection in the Āśrama, which still goes by the name of Vaśiṣṭhāśrama, situated at a distance of about seven miles from the town of Gauhati (Assam). Pūrṇānanda never returned home, but led the life of a Paramahamsa and compiled several Tāntrik works, of which the Śrī-tattva-cintāmaṇi, composed in the Śāka year 1499 (A.D. 1577), Śyāmārahasya, Śākta-krama, Tattvānanda-taraṅgiṇī, and Yoga-sāra are known. His commentary on the Kālīkakārakūta hymn is well known. The Ṣaṭ-cakra-nirūpaṇa, here translated, is not, however an independent work, but a part of the sixth Paṭala of the Śrī-tattva-cintāmaṇī. According to a genealogical table of the family of this Tāntrika-Ācārya and Virācāra-Sādhaka, given by one of his descendants, Pūrṇānanda is removed from his present descendants by about ten generations.

This work has been on hand some five years, but both the difficulties of the subject and those created by the war have delayed its publication. I had hoped to include some other plates of original paintings and drawings in my possession bearing on the subject, but present conditions do not allow of this, and I have therefore thought it better to publish the book as it stands rather than risk further delay.

ARTHUR AVALON

RANCHI

September 20, 1918

CONTENTS

ILLUSTRATIONS (CAKRAS)

ILLUSTRATIONS (YOGĀSANAS)

THE SIX CENTRES AND THE SERPENT POWER

I

INTRODUCTION

THE two Sanskrit works here translated—Ṣat-cakra-nirūpaṇa ("Description of the Six Centres, or Cakras") and Pādukā-pañcaka ("Fivefold footstool")—deal with a particular form of Tāntrik Yoga named Kuṇḍalinī-Yoga or, as some works call it, Bhūta-śuddhi. These names refer to the Kuṇḍalinī-Śakti, or Supreme Power in the human body by the arousing of which the Yoga is achieved, and to the purification of the Elements of the body (Bhūta-śuddhi) which takes place upon that event. This Yoga is effected by a process technically known as Ṣat-cakra-bheda, or piercing of the Six Centres or Regions (Cakra) or Lotuses (Padma) of the body (which the work describes) by the agency of Kuṇḍalinī-Śakti, which, in order to give it an English name, I have here called the Serpent Power.[1] Kuṇḍala means coiled. The power is the Goddess (Devī) Kuṇḍalinī, or that which is coiled; for Her form is that of a coiled and sleeping serpent in the lowest bodily centre, at the base of the spinal column, until by the means described She is aroused in that Yoga which is named after Her. Kuṇḍalinī is the Divine Cosmic Energy in bodies

[1] One of the names of this Devī is Bhujaṅgī, or the Serpent.

(*v. post*). The Saptabhūmi, or seven regions (Lokas),[1] are, as popularly understood, an exoteric presentment of the inner Tāntrik teaching regarding the seven centres.[2]

The Yoga is called Tāntrik for a twofold reason. It will be found mentioned in the Yoga-Upaniṣads which refer to the Centres, or Cakras, and in some of the Purāṇas. The treatises on Haṭhayoga also deal with the subject. We find even similar notions in systems other than the Indian, from which possibly in some cases they have been borrowed. Thus, in the Risala-i-haq-numa, by Prince Mahomed Dara Shikoh,[3] a description is given of the three centres " Mother of Brain," or " Spherical heart " (Dil-i-muddawar); the " Cedar heart " (Dil-i-sanowbari); and the Dil-i-nilofari, or " Lily heart ".[4] Other references may be found in the works of the Mahomedan Sufis. So some of the Sufi fraternities (as the Naqshbandi) are said [5] to have devised, or rather borrowed, from the Indian Yogīs [6] the Kuṇḍalinī method as a means to realization.[7] I am told that correspondences are discoverable

[1] The seven " worlds " Bhūh, Bhuvah, Suvah, Mahah, Janah, Tapah, Satya. See my " Wave of Bliss " (Comm. to v. 35). Lokas are what are seen (lokyante)—that is, attained—and are hence the fruits of Karma in the form of particular re-birth. Satyānanda's " Comm. on Īśa Up.," Mantra 2. See p. 258.

[2] That is, the six Cakras and the upper cerebral centre, or Sahasrāra. As to Upaniṣads and Purāṇas, see *post*.

[3] " The Compass of Truth." The author was the eldest son of the Emperor Shah-i-Jehan, and died in A.D. 1659. Its teaching is alleged to be that of the secret doctrine of the " Apostle of God."

[4] Chapter I on Alam-i-nasut: the physical plane, or what the Hindus call the Jāgrat state. Ed. Rai Bahadur Srisha-Candra-Vasu.

[5] See " The Development of Metaphysics in Persia," by Shaikh Muhammed Iqbal, p. 110.

[6] Al-Biruni is said to have translated Patañjali's works, as also the Sāmkhya-Sūtras, into Arabic at the beginning of the eleventh century.

[7] The author cited, however, says: " Such methods of contemplation are quite unislamic in character, and the higher Sufis do not attach any importance to them."

between the Indian (Asiatic) Śāstra and the American-Indian Māyā Scripture of the Zunis called the Popul Vuh.[1] My informant tells me that their "air-tube" is the Suṣumnā; their "twofold air-tube" the Nāḍīs Idā and Piṅgalā. "Hurakan," or lightning, is Kuṇḍalinī, and the centres are depicted by animal glyphs. Similar notions have been reported to me as being held in the secret teaching of other communities. That the doctrine and practice should be widespread, we might expect, if it has a foundation on fact. This form of Yoga is, however, in particular associated with the Tantras or Āgamas, firstly, because these Scriptures are largely concerned therewith. In fact, such orderly descriptions in practical full detail as have been written are to be found chiefly in the Haṭhayoga works and Tantras which are the manuals, not only of Hindu worship, but of its occultism. Next, Yoga through action on the lowest centre seems characteristic of the Tāntrik system, the adepts of which are the custodians of the practical knowledge whereby the general directions in the books may be practically applied. The system is of a Tāntrik character also in respect of its selection of the chief centre of consciousness. Various people have in antiquity assigned to various parts of the body the seat of the "soul" or life, such as the blood,[2] the heart and the breath. Generally the brain was not so regarded. The Vaidik system posits the heart as the chief centre of Consciousness—a relic of which notion we also still preserve in such as "take it to heart" and to "learn by heart". Sādhaka, which is one of the five functions of Pitta,[3] and which is situated in the heart.

[1] A translation was, I am told, begun and not finished by the occultist James Pryse in *Lucifer*, the old Theosophical journal, which I have not seen.

[2] *Cf.* the Biblical saying, "The blood is the life".

[3] See p. 12 of the Introduction to the third volume of my Tāntrik Texts (Prapañcasāra-Tantra).

indirectly assists in the performance of cognitive functions by keeping up the rhythmic cardiac contractions, and it has been suggested [1] that it was perhaps this view of the heart's construction which predisposed Indian physiologists to hold it to be the seat of cognition. According to the Tantras, however, the chief centres of consciousness are to be found in the Cakras of the cerebro-spinal system and in the upper brain (Sahaśrāra), which they describe, though the heart is also recognized as a seat of the Jīvātmā, or embodied spirit, in its aspect as vital principle or Prāṇa.[2] It is for the reasons mentioned that the first verse of the Ṣat-cakra-nirūpaṇa here translated speaks of the Yoga which is to be achieved "*according to the Tantras*" (Tantrānusāreṃa)—that is, as Kālīcaraṇa, its Commentator, says, "following the authority of the Tantras".

Recently some attention has been given to the subject in Western literature of an occult kind. Generally its authors and others have purported to give what they understood to be the Hindu theory of the matter, but with considerable inaccuracies. These are not limited to works of the character mentioned. Thus, to take but two instances of these respective classes, we find in a well-known Sanskrit dictionary [3] that the Cakras are defined to be "circles or depressions (*sic*) of the body for mystical or chiromantic purposes," and their location has in almost every particular been wrongly given. The

---

[1] Kavirāja-Kuñjalāla-Bhiṣagaratna in his edition of the Suśruta-Saṁhitā. Another explanation, however, may be given—namely, that during man's history the importance of the various perceptive centres has in fact varied.

[2] According to some Indian views, the brain is the centre of the mind and senses, and the heart that of life. Caraka says that the heart is the root from which spring all other parts of the body, and is the centre of some of the functions or organs. According to Suśruta, the heart is the seat of sensations.

[3] Professor Monier Williams' Sanskrit Dictionary, *sub voce* "Cakra".

Mūlādhāra is inaccurately described as being "above the pubis". Nor is the Svādhiṣṭhāna the umbilical region. Anāhata is not the root of the nose, but is the spinal centre in the region of the heart; Viśuddha is not "the hollow between the frontal sinuses," but is the spinal centre in the region of the throat. Ājñā is not the fontanelle or union of the coronal and sagittal sutures, which are said to be the Brahma-randhra,[1] but is in the position allotted to the third cyc, or Jñāna-cakṣu. Othcrs, avoiding such gross crrors, are not free from lesser inaccuracies. Thus, an author who, I am informed, had considerable knowledge of things occult, speaks of the Suṣumnā as a "force" which "cannot be energised until Idā and Piṅgalā have preceded it," which "passes to the accompaniment of violent shock through each section of the spinal marrow," and which, on the awakening of the sacral plexus, passes along the spinal cord and impinges on the brain, with the result that the neophyte finds "himself to be an unembodied soul alone in the black abyss of empty space, struggling against dread and terror unutterable". He also writes that the "current" of Kuṇḍalinī is called Nāḍī; that the Suṣumnā extends as a nerve to the Brahma-randhra; that the Tattvas are seven in number; and other matters which are inaccurate. The Suṣumnā is not a "force," [2] and does not pass and impinge upon anything, but is the outer of the three Nāḍīs, which form the conduit for the force which is the arousing of the Devī called Kuṇḍalinī, the Cosmic Power in bodies, which force is not itself a Nāḍī, but passes through the innermost, of Citriṇī-Nāḍī, which terminates at the twelve-petalled lotus below the Sahasrāra, from which ascent is made to the Brahma-randhra. It would be easy to

[1] A term which is also employed to denote the Brahma-nāḍī, in that the latter is the passage whereby the Brahma-randhra in the cerebrum is attained.

[2] Except in the sense that everything is a manifestation of power.

point out other mistakes in writers who have referred to the subject. It will be more profitable if I make as correct a statement as my knowledge admits of this mode of Yoga. But I desire to add that some modern Indian writers have also helped to diffuse erroneous notions about the Cakras by describing them from what is merely a materialistic or physiological standpoint. To do so is not merely to misrepresent the case, but to give it away; for physiology does not know the Cakras as they exist in themselves—that is, as centres of consciousness—and of the activity of Sūkṣma-Prāṇa-vāyu or subtle vital force; though it does deal with the gross body which is related to them. Those who appeal to physiology only are likely to return non-suited.

We may here notice the account of a well-known "Theosophical" author[1] regarding what he calls the "Force centres" and the "Serpent Fire," of which he writes that he has had personal experience. Though its author also refers to the Yoga-Śāstra, it may perhaps exclude error if we here point out that his account does not profess to be a representation of the teaching of the Indian Yogīs (whose competence for their own Yoga the author somewhat disparages), but that it is put forward as the Author's own original explanation (fortified, as he conceives, by certain portions of Indian teaching) of the personal experience which (he writes) he himself has had. This experience appears to consist in the conscious arousing of the "Serpent Fire,"[2] with the enhanced "astral" and mental vision which he

[1] "The Inner Life," by C. W. Leadbeater, pp. 443-478, First Series.

[2] This and the following notes compare his and the Indian theory. The Devī or Goddess is called Bhujaṅgī or Serpent because at the lowest centre (Mūlādhāra) She lies "coiled" round the Liṅga. "Coiled"=at rest. The Cosmic Power in bodies is here at rest; when roused it is felt as intense heat.

believes has shown him what he tells us.[1] The centres, or Cakras, of the human body are described to be vortices of "etheric" matter[2] into which rush from the "astral"[3] world, and at right angles to the plane of the whirling disc, the sevenfold force of the Logos bringing "divine life" into the physical body. Though all these seven forces operate on all the centres, in each of them one form of the force is greatly predominant. These inrushing forces are alleged to set up on the surface of the "etheric double"[4] secondary forces at right angles to themselves. The primary force on entrance into the vortex radiates again in straight lines, but at right angles. The number of these radiations of the primal force is said to determine the number of "petals"[5] (as the Hindus call them) which the "Lotus" or vortex exhibits. The secondary force rushing round the vortex produces, it is said, the appearance of the petals of a flower, or, "perhaps more accurately, saucers or shallow vases of wavy iridescent glass". In this way—that is, by the supposition of an etheric vortex subject to an incoming force of the Logos—both the "Lotuses" described in the Hindu books and the number of their petals is accounted for by the author, who substitutes for the Svādhiṣṭāna centre a six-petalled lotus at the spleen,[4] and corrects the number of petals of the lotus in the head, which he says is not a thousand, as the books of this Yoga say, "but exactly 960".[6] The "etheric" centre which keeps alive the physical vehicle

---

[1] Certain Siddhis or occult powers are acquired at each centre as the practitioner works his way upwards.

[2] The petals of the lotus are Prāṇa-śakti manifested by Prāṇa-vāyu or vital force. Each lotus is a centre of a different form of "matter" (Bhūta) there predominant.—A.A.

[3] This is a Western term.—A.A.

[4] Not mentioned in the account here given.—A.A.

[5] See note 2, above.

[6] So little attention seems to be given to exactitude in this matter that one of the letters is dropped in order to make 1,000 petals—that is 50×20. "Thousand" is, here, only symbolic of magnitude.—A.A.

is said to correspond with an "astral" centre of four dimensions, but between them is a closely woven sheath or web composed of a single compressed layer of physical atoms, which prevents a premature opening up of communication between the planes. There is a way, it is said, in which these may be properly opened or developed so as to bring more through this channel from the higher planes than ordinarily passes thereby. Each of these "astral" centres has certain functions; at the navel, a simple power of feeling; at the spleen, "conscious travel" in the astral body; at the heart, "a power to comprehend and sympathise with the vibrations of other astral entities"; at the throat, power of hearing on the astral plane; between the eyebrows, "astral sight"; at the "top of the head," perfection of all faculties of the astral life.[1] These centres are therefore said to take the place to some extent of sense organs for the astral body. In the first centre, "at the base of the spine," is the "Serpent Fire," or Kuṇḍalinī, which exists in seven layers or seven degrees of force.[2] This is the manifestation in etheric matter, on the physical plane, of one of the great world forces, one of the powers of the Logos of which vitality and electricity are examples. It is not, it is said, the same as Prāṇa or vitality.[3] The "etheric centres" when fully aroused by the "Serpent Fire" bring down, it is alleged, into physical consciousness whatever may be the quality inherent in the astral centre which corresponds to it. When vivified by the "Serpent Fire" they become gates of connection between the

[1] Certain Siddhis are said to be gained at each centre. But the top of the head is far beyond the "astral" life. There Sāmādhi, or union with the Supreme Consciousness, is had.—A.A.

[2] Para-śabda which is Kuṇḍalinī in Her aspect as cause of all sound has seven aspects from Kuṇḍalī to Biṅdu—A.A.

[3] Kuṇḍalī is Śabda-brahman or the "Word (Vāk)" in bodies, and is in Her own form (Svarūpa) Pure Consciousness, and is all Powers (Sarva-śaktimayī). Kuṇḍalinī is in fact the cosmic energy in bodies and as such the cause of all and though manifesting as, is not confined to, any of Her products.—A.A.

physical and "astral" bodies. When the astral awakening of these centres first took place, this was not known to the physical consciousness. But the sense body can now "be brought to share all these advantages by repeating that process of awakening with the etheric centres". This is done by the arousing through will-force of the "Serpent Fire," which exists clothed in "etheric matter in the physical plane, and sleeps [1] in the corresponding etheric centre—that at the base of the spine". When this is done, it vivifies the higher centres, with the effect that it brings into the physical consciousness the powers which were aroused by the development of their corresponding astral centres. In short, one begins to live on the astral plane, which is not altogether an advantage, were it not that entry into the heaven world is said to be achieved at the close of life on this plane.[2] Thus, at the second centre, one is conscious in the physical body "of all kinds of astral influences, vaguely feeling that some of them are friendly and some hostile without in the least knowing why". At the third centre one is enabled to remember "only partially" vague astral journeys, with sometimes half-remembrance of a blissful sensation of flying through the air. At the fourth centre man is instinctively aware of the joys and sorrows of others, sometimes reproducing in himself their physical aches and pains. At the arousing of the fifth centre he hears voices "which make all kinds of suggestions to him". Sometimes he hears music "or other less pleasant sounds".[3] Full development secures

[1] Kuṇḍalinī is called the Serpent (Bhujaṅgī). She sleeps in the Mūlādhāra. As to what She is, see last note. She sleeps because She is at rest. Then man's consciousness is awake to the world, Her creation, in which She is immanent. When She awakes and Yoga is completed man sleeps to the world and enjoys super-worldly experience.

[2] The end of Kuṇḍalī-Yoga is beyond all Heaven worlds. No Yogī seeks "Heaven" but union with that which is the source of all worlds.

[3] According to the text translated, the sound of the Śabda-brahman is heard at the Anāhata, or fourth centre.—A.A.

clairaudience in the "astral" plane. The arousing of the sixth centre secures results which are at first of a trivial character, such as "half seeing landscapes and clouds of colour," but subsequently amount to clairvoyance. Here it is said there is a power of magnification by means of an "etheric" flexible tube which resembles "the microscopic snake on the head-dress of the Pharaohs". The Power to expand or control the eye of this "microscopic snake" is stated to be the meaning of the statement, in ancient books, of the capacity to make oneself large or small at will.[1] When the pituitary body is brought into working order, it forms a link with the astral vehicle, and when the Fire reaches the sixth centre, and fully vivifies it, the voice of the "Master" (which in this case means the higher Self in its various stages) is heard.[2] The awakening of the seventh centre enables one to leave the body in full consciousness. "When the fire has thus passed through all these centres in a certain order (which varies for different types of people), the consciousness becomes continuous up to the entry into the heaven world[3] at the end of the life on the astral plane."

There are some resemblances between this account and the teaching of the Yoga-Śāstra, with which in a general way the author cited appears to have some acquaintance, and which may have suggested to him some features of his account. There are firstly seven centres, which with one exception correspond with the Cakras described. The author says that there are three other lower centres, but that concentration on them is full of danger. What these are is not stated. There is no centre lower, that I am aware of, than

[1] There is no mention of such a "snake". The Siddhis—Animā, etc., do not depend on it. It is consciousness which identifies itself with the small or the great.—A.A.

[2] As the text here translated says, the Ājñā is so called because here is received the command of the Guru from above.—A.A.

[3] See note 2, page 9 *ante*.

the Mūlādhāra (as the name " root-centre " itself implies), and the only centre near to it which is excluded, in the above-mentioned account, is the Apas Tattva centre, or Svādhiṣṭāna. Next there is the Force, " the Serpent Fire," which the Hindus call Kuṇḍalinī, in the lowest centre, the Mūlādhāra. Lastly, the effect of the rousing of this force, which is accomplished by will power (Yoga-bala),[1] is said to exalt the physical consciousness through the ascending planes to the " heaven world ". To use the Hindu expression, the object and aim of Ṣat-cakra-bheda is Yoga. This is ultimately union with the Supreme Self or Paramātmā; but it is obvious that, as the body in its natural state is already, though unconsciously, in Yoga, otherwise it would not exist, each conscious step upwards is Yoga, and there are many stages of such before complete or Kaivalya Mukti is attained. This and, indeed, many of the preceding stages are far beyond the " heaven world " of which the author speaks. Yogīs are not concerned with the " heaven world," but seek to surpass it; otherwise they are not Yogīs at all. What, according to this theory, manifested force apparently does is this: it enhances the mental and moral qualities of the self-operator as they existed at the time of its discovery. But if this be so, such enhancement may be as little desirable as the original state. Apart from the necessity for the possession of health and strength, the thought, will and morality, which it is proposed to subject to its influence must be first purified and strengthened before they are intensified by the vivifying influence of the aroused force. Further, as I have elsewhere pointed out,[2] the Yogīs say that the piercing of the Brahma-granthi or " knot "[3]

---

[1] With the aid of bodily purification, certain Āsanas and Mudrās (*v. post*).

[2] See p. 137, " Introduction to Tantra-Śāstra ".

[3] There are three " knots " which have to be pierced or centres where the force of Māyā is particularly strong.

sometimes involves considerable pain, physical disorder, and even disease, as is not unlikely to follow from concentration on such a centre as the navel (Nābhipadma).

To use Hindu terms, the Sādhaka must be competent (Adhikārī), a matter to be determined by his Guru, from whom alone the actual method of Yoga can be learned. The incidental dangers, however, stated by the author, go beyond any mentioned to me by Indians themselves, who seem to be in general unaware of the subject of "phallic sorcery," to which reference is made by the author, who speaks of Schools of (apparently Western) "Black Magic" which are said to use Kuṇḍalinī for the purpose of stimulating the sexual centre. Another author says: [1] "The mere dabbler in the pseudo-occult will only degrade his intellect with the puerilities of psychism, become the prey of the evil influence of the phantasmal world, or ruin his soul by the foul practices of phallic sorcery—as thousands of misguided people are doing even in this age." Is this so? It is possible that perverse or misguided concentration on sexual and connected centres may have the effect alluded to. And it may be that the Commentator Lakṣmīdhara alludes to this when he speaks of Uttara-Kaulas who arouse Kuṇḍalinī in the Mūlādhāra to satisfy their desire for world-enjoyment and do not attempt to lead Her upwards to the Highest Centre which is the object of Yoga seeking super-worldly bliss. Of such, a Sanskrit verse runs "they are the true prostitutes". I have, however, never heard Indians refer to this matter, probably because it does not belong to Yoga in its ordinary sense, as also by reason of the antecedent discipline required of those who would undertake this Yoga, the nature of their practice, and the aim they have in view, such a possibility does not come under consideration. The Indian who practises this or any other

[1] "The Apocalypse Unsealed," p. 62.

kind of spiritual Yoga ordinarily does so not on account of a curious interest in occultism or with a desire to gain " astral " or similar experiences.[1] His attitude in this as in all other matters is essentially a religious one, based on a firm faith in Brahman (Sthiraniṣthā) and inspired by a desire for union with It, which is Liberation.

What is competency for Tantra (Tantra-śāstrādhikāra) is described in the second chapter of the Gandharva-Tantra as follows: The aspirant must be intelligent (Dakṣa) with senses controlled (Jitendriya), abstaining from injury to all beings (Sarva-himsā-vinirmukta), ever doing good to all (Sarva-prāṇi-hite ratah), pure (Śuci); a believer in Veda (Āstika), whose faith and refuge is in Brahman (Brahmiṣṭah, Brahmavādī, Brāhmī, Brahmaparāyaṇa), and who is a non-dualist (Dvaita-hīna). " Such an one is competent in this Scripture, otherwise he is no Sādhakah ". (Sossmin śāstre-s dhikārī syāt tadanyatra na sādhakah.) With such an attitude it is possible that, as pointed out by an Indian writer (Ch. VII *post*), concentration on the lower centres associated with the passions may, so far from rousing, quiet them. It is quite possible, on the other hand, that another attitude, practice, and purpose, may produce another result. To speak, however, of concentration on the sexual centre is itself misleading, for the Cakras are not in the gross body, and concentration is done upon the subtle centre, with its presiding Consciousness, even though such centres may have ultimate relation with gross physical function. Doubtless, also, there is a relationship and correspondence between the Śaktis of the mental and sexual centres, and the force

[1] Those who do practise magic of the kind mentioned work only in the lowest centre, have recourse to the Prayoga, which leads to Nāyikā-Siddhi, whereby commerce is had with female spirits and the like. The process in this work described is one upon the path of Liberation and has nothing to do with sexual black magic.

of the latter, if directed upwards, extraordinarily heightens all mental and physical functioning.[1] In fact those who are "centred" know how to make all their forces converge upon the object of their will, and train and then use all such forces and neglect none. The experienced followers of this method, however, as I have stated, allow that this method is liable to be accompanied by certain inconveniences or dangers, and it is therefore considered inadvisable except for the fully competent (Adhikārī).

There are, on the other hand, many substantial points of difference between the account which has been summarized and the theory which underlies the form of Yoga with which this work deals. The terminology and classification adopted by that account may be termed "Theosophical"[2]; and though it may be possible for those who are familiar both with this and the Indian terminology to establish points of correspondence between the two systems, it must by no means be assumed that the connotation even in such cases is always exactly the same. For though "Theosophical" teaching is largely inspired by Indian ideas, the meaning which it attributes to the Indian terms which it employs is not always that given to these terms by Indians themselves. This is sometimes confusing and misleading, a result which would have been avoided had the writers of this school adopted in all cases their own nomenclature and

---

[1] Mind, Breath and Sexual function are interconnected. The aim of the Yogī is to carry "his seed high" to be Ūrdhva-retās as it is called. For this purpose the Niparīta-Mudrās are designed.

[2] I am aware that the Theosophical Society has no official doctrine. What I call "Theosophical" are the theories put forward by its leading exponents and largely accepted by its members. I put the word in inverted commas to denote doctrine so taught and held by this Society, with which doctrines, Theosophy, in its general sense, is not necessarily wholly identified.

definitions.[1] Though for the visualization of our conceptions the term "planes" is a convenient one, and may be so employed, the division by "principles" more nearly adumbrates the truth. It is not easy for me to correlate with complete accuracy the Indian and Theosophical theories as to man's principles. It has, however, been stated [2] that the physical body has two divisions, the "dense" and "etheric" body; that these correspond to the Annamaya and Prāṇa-maya-Kośas, and that the "astral" body corresponds to the Kāmik or desire side of the Manomaya-Kośa or mental sheath. Assuming for argument the alleged correspondence, then the "etheric centres" or Cakras, according to this account, appear to be centres of energy of the Prāṇa-vāyu or Vital Force. The lotuses are also this and centres of the universal consciousness. Kuṇḍalinī is the static form of the creative energy in bodies which is the source of all energies, including Prāṇa. According to this author's theory, Kuṇḍalinī is some force which is distinct from Prāṇa, understanding this term to mean vitality or the life-principle, which on entrance into the body shows itself in various manifestations of life which are the minor Prāṇas, of which inspiration is called by the general name of the force itself (Prāṇa). Verses 10 and 11 say of Kuṇḍalinī: "It is She who maintains all the beings (that is, Jīva, Jīvātmā) of the world by means of inspiration and expiration." She is thus the Prāṇa Devatā, but, as She is (Comm., vv. 10 and 11) Sṛṣti-sthiti-layātmikā, *all*

---

[1] Thus, the Theosophical Sanskritist Śrīśa-Candra-Vasu, in his "Introduction to Yoga Philosophy," calls the Liṅga-Śarīra "the ethereal duplicate" (p. 35). According to the ordinary Indian use of that term the Liṅga-Śarīra is the subtle body—that is, the Antahkaraṇa and Indriyas—vehicled by the Tanmātras, or according to another account, the five Prāṇas. Elsewhere (p. 51) it is called the "Astral" body, and some statements are made as to the Cakras which are not in accordance with the texts with which I am acquainted.

[2] "Ancient Wisdom," p. 176, by Dr. A. Besant.

forces therefore are in Her. She is, in fact, the Śabdabrahman or "Word" in bodies. The theory discussed appears to diverge from that of the Yogīs when we consider the nature of the Cakras and the question of their vivification. According to the English author's account, the Cakras are all vortices of "etheric matter," apparently of the same kind and subject to the same external influence of the inrushing sevenfold force of the "Logos" but differing in this, that in each of the Cakras one or other of their sevenfold forces is predominant. Again, if, as has been stated, the astral body corresponds with the Manomayakośa, then the vivification of the Cakras appears to be, according to this account, a rousing of the Kāmik side of the mental sheath. According to the Hindu doctrine, these Cakras are differing centres of consciousness, vitality and Tāttvik energy. Each of the five lower Cakras is the centre of energy of a gross Tattva—that is, of that form of Tāttvik activity or Tanmātra which manifests the Mahābhūta or sensible matter. The sixth is the centre of the subtle mental Tattva, and the Sahasrāra is not called a Cakra at all. Nor, as stated, is the splenic centre included among the six Cakras which are dealt with here.

In the Indian system the total number of the petals corresponds with the number of the letters of the Sanskrit Alphabet,[1] and the number of the petals of any specific lotus is determined by the disposition of the subtile "nerves" or Nāḍīs around it. These petals, further, bear subtile sound-powers, and are fifty [1] in number, as are the letters of the Sanskrit Alphabet.

This Sanskrit work also describes certain things which are gained by contemplation on each of the Cakras. Some of them are of a general character, such as long life, freedom from desire and sin, control of the senses, knowledge, power

[1] Which are sometimes given as 50 and sometimes as 51.

of speech and fame. Some of these and other qualities are results common to concentration on more than one Cakra. Others are stated in connection with the contemplation upon one centre only. Such statements seem to be made, not necessarily with the intention of accurately recording the specific result, if any, which follows upon concentration upon a particular centre, but by way of praise for increased self-control, or Stuti-Vāda; as where it is said in v. 21 that contemplation on the Nābhi-padma gains for the Yogī power to destroy and create the world.

It is also said that mastery of the centres may produce various Siddhis or powers in respect of the predominating elements there. And this is, in fact, alleged.[1] Paṇḍit Ananta-Kṛṣṇa-Śāstrī says: [2] " We can meet with several persons every day elbowing us in the streets or bazaars who in all sincerity attempted to reach the highest plane of bliss, but fell victims on the way to the illusions of the psychic world, and stopped at one or the other of the six Cakras. They are of varying degrees of attainment, and are seen to possess some power which is not found even in the best intellectuals of the ordinary run of mankind. That this school of practical psychology was working very well in India at one time is evident from these living instances (not to speak of the numberless treatises on the subject) of men roaming about in all parts of the country." The mere rousing of the Serpent Power does not, from the spiritual Yoga standpoint, amount to much. Nothing, however, of real moment, from the higher Yogī's point of view, is achieved until the Ājñā Cakra is reached. Here, again, it is said that the Sādhaka whose Ātmā is nothing but a

---

[1] See Yogatattva-Upaniṣad, where contemplation on the Earth centre secures mastery over earth, etc. At the same time it points out that these " powers " are obstacles to Liberation.

[2] See p. 29, " Saundarya-Laharī," (1957), Ganesh & Co. (Madras) Private Ltd.

meditation on this lotus "becomes the creator, preserver and destroyer of the three worlds"; and yet, as the commentator points out (v. 34), "This is but the highest Praśaṃsā-vāda or Stuti-vāda, that is, compliment—which in Sanskrit literature is as often void of reality as it is in our ordinary life. Though much is here gained, it is not until the Tattvas of this centre are also absorbed, and complete knowledge [1] of the Sahasrāra is gained, that the Yogī attains that which is both his aim and the motive of his labour, cessation from rebirth which follows on the control and concentration of the Citta on the Śivāsthānam, the Abode of Bliss. It is not to be supposed that simply because the Serpent Fire has been aroused that one has thereby become a Yogī or achieved the end of Yoga. There are other points of difference which the reader will discover for himself, but into which I do not enter, as my object in comparing the two accounts has been to establish a general contrast between this modern account and that of the Indian schools. I may, however, add that the differences are not only as to details. The style of thought differs in a way not easy shortly to describe, but which will be quickly recognized by those who have some familiarity with the Indian Scriptures and mode of thought. The latter is ever disposed to interpret all processes and their results from a subjective standpoint, though for the purposes of Sādhana the objective aspect is not ignored. The Indian theory is highly philosophical. Thus, to take but one instance, whilst the Rt. Rev. Leadbeater attributes the

[1] This, it is obvious, comes only after long effort, and following on less complete experiences and results. According to Indian notions, success (Siddhi) in Yoga may be the fruit of experiences of many preceding lives. Kuṇḍalinī must be gradually raised from one centre to another until she reaches the Lotus in the cerebrum. The length of time required varies with the individual—it may be years ordinarily or in exceptional cases months.

power of becoming large or small at will (Aṇimā and Mahimā Siddhi) to a flexible tube or "microscopic snake" in the forehead, the Hindu says that all powers (Siddhi) are the attributes (Aiśvarya) of the Lord Īśvara, or Creative Consciousness, and that in the degree that the Jīva realizes that consciousness [1] he shares the powers inherent in the degree of his attainment.

That which is the general characteristic of the Indian systems, and that which constitutes their real profundity, is the paramount importance attached to Consciousness and its states. It is these states which create, sustain and destroy the worlds. Brahmā, Viṣṇu and Śiva are the names for functions of the one Universal Consciousness operating in ourselves. And whatever be the means employed, it is the transformation of the "lower" into "higher" states of consciousness which is the process and fruit of Yoga and the cause of all its experiences. In this and other matters, however, we must distinguish both practice and experience from theory. A similar experience may possibly be gained by various modes of practice, and an experience may be in fact a true one, though the theory which may be given to account for it is incorrect.

The following sections will enable the reader to pursue the comparison for himself.

As regards practice I am told that Kuṇḍalinī cannot be roused except in the Mūlādhāra and by the means here indicated, though this may take place by accident when by chance a person has hit upon the necessary positions and conditions, but not otherwise. Thus the story is told of a

---

[1] As this is by the Devī's grace, She is called "the giver of the eight Siddhis" (Īśitvādyāṣṭasiddhidā). See Triśatī, II. 47. She gives Aiśvarya.

man being found whose body was as cold as a corpse, though the top of the head was slightly warm. (This is the state in Kuṇḍalinī-yoga, Samādhi.) He was massaged with ghee (clarified butter), when the head got gradually warmer. The warmth descended to the neck, then the whole body regained its heat with a rush. The man came to consciousness, and then told the story of his condition. He said he had been going through some antics, imitating the posture of a Yogī, when suddenly "sleep" had come over him. It was surmised that his breath must have stopped, and that, being in the right position and conditions, he had unwittingly roused Kuṇḍalinī who had ascended to Her cerebral centre. Not, however, being a Yogī he could not bring her down again. This, further, can only be done when the Nāḍīs (*v. post*) are pure. I told the Paṇḍit (who gave me this story, who was learned in this Yoga, and whose brother practised it) of the case of a European friend of mine who was not acquainted with the Yoga processes here described, though he had read something about Kuṇḍalī in translation of Sanskrit works, and who, nevertheless, believed he had roused Kuṇḍalī by meditative processes alone. In fact, as he wrote me, it was useless for him as a European to go into the minutiæ of Eastern Yoga. He, however, saw the "nerves" Idā and Piṅgalā (*v. post*), and the "central fire" with a trembling aura of rosy light, and blue or azure light, and a white fire which rose up into the brain and flamed out in a winged radiance on either side of the head. Fire was seen flashing from centre to centre with such rapidity that he could see little of the vision, and movements of forces were seen in the bodies of others. The radiance or aura round Idā was seen as moonlike—that is, palest azure —and Piṅgalā red or rather pale rosy opalescence. Kuṇḍalī appeared in vision as of intense golden-like white fire rather curled spirally. Taking the centres, Suṣumnā, Idā and

Piṅgalā, to be symbolized by the Caduceus of Mercury,[1] the little ball at the top of the rod was identified with the Sahasrāra or pineal gland,[2] and the wings as the flaming of auras on each side of the centre when the fire strikes it. One night, being abnormally free from the infection of bodily desires, he felt the serpent uncoil, and it ran up, and he was "in a fountain of fire," and felt, as he said, "the flames spreading wingwise about my head and there was a musical clashing as of cymbals, whilst some of these flames, like emanations, seemed to expand and meet like gathered wings over my head. I felt a rocking motion. I really felt frightened, as the Power seemed somthing which could consume me." My friend wrote me that in his agitation he forgot to fix his mind on the Supreme, and so missed a divine adventure. Perhaps it was on this account that he said he did not regard the awakening of this power as a very high spiritual experience or on a level with other states of consciousness he experienced. The experience, however, convinced him that there was a real science and magic in the Indian books which treat of occult physiology.

The Paṇḍit's observations on this experience were as follows: If the breath is stopped and the mind is carried downwards, heat is felt. It is possible to "see" Kuṇḍalinī with the mental eye, and in this way to experience Her without actually arousing Her and bringing Her up, which can only be effected by the Yoga methods prescribed. Kuṇḍalinī may have thus been seen as Light in the basal centre (Mūlādhāra). It was the mind (Buddhi) (*v. post*) which perceived Her, but as the experiencer had not been taught the practice

[1] In which the rod is the central channel (Suṣumnā), which is interlaced by the Iḍā and Piṅgalā sympathetics, the points of section being at the centres. The two wings at the top are the two lobes or petals of the Ājñā-Cakra.

[2] Here I differ. The Sahasrāra is at the top of the skull or upper brain. The pineal gland is much lower in the region of Ājñā-Cakra.

he got confused. There is one simple test whether the Śakti is actually aroused. When she is aroused intense heat is felt at that spot but when she leaves a particular centre the part so left becomes as cold and apparently lifeless as a corpse. The progress upwards may thus be externally verified by others. When the Śakti (Power) has reached the upper brain (Sahasrāra) the whole body is cold and corpse-like; except the top of the skull, where some warmth is felt, this being the place where the static and kinetic aspects of Consciousness unite.

The present work is issued, not with the object of establishing the truth or expediency of the principles and methods of this form of Yoga, a matter which each will determine for himself, but as a first endeavour to supply, more particularly for those interested in occultism and mysticism, a fuller, more accurate and rational presentation of the subject.

An understanding of the recondite matters in the treatise here translated is, however, only possible if we first shortly summarize some of the philosophical and religious doctrines which underlie this work and a knowledge of which in his reader is assumed by its author.

The following sections, therefore, of this Introduction will deal firstly with the concepts of Consciousness[1] and of the unconscious, as Mind, Matter and Life and with their association in the embodied Spirit or Jīvātmā. Nextly the kinetic aspect of Spirit, or Śakti, is considered; its creative ideation and manifestation in the evolved Macrocosm and in the human body or Microcosm (Kṣudra-brahmāṇda), which is a replica on a small scale of the greater world. For as is said in the Viśvasāra-Tantra, "What is here is elsewhere.

---

[1] For the meaning of this term as here used, see my "Śakti and Śākta", "The World As Power" and "Mahāmāya".

What is not here is nowhere" (Yad ihāsti tad anyatra yannehāsti na tat kvacit). After an account of the "Word" and the letters of speech, I conclude with the method of involution or Yoga. The latter will not be understood unless the subject of the preceding sections has been mastered.

It is necessary to explain and understand the theory of world-evolution even in the practical matters with which this work is concerned. For as the Commentator says in v. 39, when dealing with the practice of Yoga, the rule is that things dissolve into that from which they originate, and the Yoga process here described is such dissolution (Laya). This return or dissolution process (Nivṛtti) in Yoga will not be understood unless the forward or creative (Pravṛtti) process is understood. Similar considerations apply to other matters here dealt with.

So also will a short analysis of the Śākta doctrine of Power be of value.

All that is manifest is Power (Śakti) as Mind, Life and Matter. Power implies a Power-Holder (Śaktimān). There is no Power-Holder without Power, or Power without Power-Holder. The Power-Holder is Śiva. Power is Śakti, the Great Mother of the Universe. There is no Śiva without Śakti, or Śakti without Śiva. The two as they are in themselves are one. They are each Being, Consciousness and Bliss. These three terms are chosen to denote ultimate Reality, because Being or 'Is-ness', as distinguished from particular forms of Being, cannot be thought away. 'To be' again is "to be conscious" and lastly perfect Being-Consciousness is the Whole, and unlimited unconstrained Being is Bliss. These three terms stand for the ultimate creative Reality as it is in itself. By the imposition upon these terms of Name (Nāma) and Form (Rūpa) or Mind and Matter, we have the limited Being-Consciousness and Bliss which is the Universe.

What then of Power when there is no Universe? It is then Power to Be, to self-conserve and resist change. In evolution it is Power to become and to change, and in its manifestation as forms it is as material cause, the changeful Becoming of Worlds. Becoming does not = God, for it is finite form and He is the formless infinite. But the essence of these forms is infinite Power which = infinite Power-Holder. It is He who puts forth Power and creates the Universe.

Rest implies Activity, and Activity implies Rest. Behind all activity there is a static background. Śiva represents the static aspect of Reality and Śakti the moving aspect. The two, as they are in themselves, are one.[1] All is Real, both Changeless and Changeful. Māyā is not in this system "illusion", but is in the concise words of the Śākta Sādhaka Kamalākānta 'the Form of the Formless' (Śūnyasya ākāra iti Māyā). The world is *its* form and these forms are therefore Real.

Man is then as to his essence the static Power-Holder, or Śiva who is pure Consciousness; and, as Mind and Body, he is the manifestation of Śiva's Power, or Śakti or Mother. He is thus Śiva-Śakti. He is as he stands an expression of Power. The object of Sādhana or Worship and Yoga is to raise this Power to its perfect expression, which is perfect in the sense of unlimited experience. One mode of so doing is the Yoga here described, whereby man exchanges his limited or worldly experience for that which is the unlimited Whole (Pūrṇa) or Perfect Bliss.

---

[1] See as to Power, Chhand. Up., 6-2-1; 6-3-4; 6-8-6; 7-26-1; 6-2-3. Taitt. Up. Śveta. Up., 1-3: 6-8. Ṛgveda S., 10-129-2; 10-129-5. Taitt. Br., 3-8; 17-3. Yajurveda, 7-3-14-1. Muṇd. Up., 1-9. Kūrma-Purāṇa, 1-12-28.

II

BODILESS CONSCIOUSNESS

THE bases of this Yoga are of a highly metaphysical and scientific character. For its understanding there is required a full acquaintance with Indian philosophy, religious doctrine, and ritual in general, and in particular with that presentment of these three matters which is given in the Śākta and Monistic (Advaita)[1] Śaiva-Tantras. It would need more than a bulky volume to describe and explain in any detail the nature and meaning of this Yoga, and the bases on which it rests. I must, therefore, assume in the reader either this general knowledge or a desire to acquire it, and confine myself to such an exposition of general principles and leading facts as will supply the key by which the doors leading to a theoretical knowledge of the subject may be opened by those desirous of passing through and beyond them, and as will thus facilitate the understanding of the difficult texts here translated. For on the practical side I can merely reproduce the directions given in the books together with such explanations of them as I have received orally. Those who wish to go farther, and to put into actual process this Yoga, must first satisfy themselves of the value and suitability of this Yoga and then learn directly of a Gurù who has himself been through it (Siddha). His experience alone will say whether the aspirant is capable of success. It is said that of those who

[1] As to the Advaita of Śākta-Tantra, see "Śakti and Śākta."

attempt it, one out of a thousand may have success. If the latter enters upon the path, the Guru alone can save him from attendant risks, moulding and guiding the practice as he will according to the particular capacities and needs of his disciple. Whilst, therefore, on this heading it is possible to explain some general principles, their application is dependent on the circumstances of each particular case.

The ultimate or irreducible reality is 'Spirit' in the sense of Pure Consciousness (Cit, Saṁvit) from out of which as and by its Power (Śakti), Mind and Matter proceed. Spirit[1] is one. There are no degrees or differences in Spirit. The Spirit which is in man is the one Spirit which is in everything and which, as the object of worship, is the Lord (Īśvara) or God. Mind and Matter are many and of many degrees and qualities. Ātmā or Spirit as such is the Whole (Pūrṇa) without section (Akhaṇḍa). Mind and Matter are parts in that Whole. They are the not-whole (Apūrṇa) and are the section (Khaṇḍa). Spirit is infinite (Aparicchinna) and formless (Arūpa). Mind and Matter are finite (Paricchinna) and with form (Rūpa). Ātmā is unchanged and inactive. Its Power (Śakti) is active and changes in the form of Mind and Matter. Pure Consciousness is Cit or Saṁvit. Matter as such is the unconscious. And Mind too is unconscious according to Vedānta. For all that is not the conscious self is the unconscious object. This does not mean that it is unconscious in itself. On the contrary all is essentially consciousness, but that it is unconscious because it is the object of the conscious self. For mind limits Consciousness so as to enable man to have finite experience. There is no Mind without consciousness as its background, though

---

[1] Spirit is Ātmā which manifests as the Self. Its vehicles are Mind or Antahkaraṇa working with Manas and the Senses or Indṛyas, and Matter, namely, the five kinds of Bhūta or sensible matter.

supreme Consciousness is Mindless (Amanah). Where there is no mind (Amanah), there is no limitation. Consciousness remaining in one aspect unchanged changes in its other aspect as active Power which manifests as Mind and Body. Man then is Pure Consciousness (Cit) vehicled by its Power as Mind and Body.

In Theology this Pure Consciousness is Śiva, and His Power (Śakti) who as She is in Her formless self is one with Him. She is the great Devī, the Mother of the Universe who as the Life-Force resides in man's body in its lowest centre at the base of the spine just as Śiva is realized in the highest brain centre, the cerebrum or Sahasrāra-Padma. Completed Yoga is the Union of Her and Him in the body of the Sādhaka. This is Laya or dissolution, the reverse of Sṛṣṭi or involution of Spirit in Mind and Matter.

Some worship predominantly the masculine or right side of the conjoint male and female figure (Ardhanārīśvara). Some, the Śāktas, predominantly worship the left, and call Her Mother, for She is the Great Mother (Magna Mater), the Mahādevī who conceives, bears, and nourishes the universe sprung from Her womb (Yoni). This is so because She is the active aspect [1] of Consciousness, imagining (Sṛṣṭi-kalpanā)[2] the world to be, according to the impressions

[1] The quiescent Śiva-aspect is by its definition inert. It is because of this that the Devī is in the Tantras symbolically represented as being above the body of Śiva, who lies under Her like a corpse (Śava). As the Kubjikā-Tantra, Ch. I, states, it is not Brahmā, Viṣṇu and Rudra, who create, maintain and destroy, but their Śaktis, Brahmāṇī, Vaiṣṇavī, Rudrāṇī. See Prāṇa-toṣiṇī, 9. Activity is the nature of Prakṛti (Sāṁkhya-Pravacana Sutra, III. 66). For the same reason the female form is represented in sexual union as being above (Viparīta) the male. When the Devī stands above Śiva, the symbolism also denotes (particularly in the case of Kālī) the liberating aspect of the Mother. See "Principles of Tantra."

[2] The world is called an imagination (Kalpanā), for it is creative ideation on the recalled memory of the past universe. As the Yoginī-hṛdaya-Tantra says, "The picture of the world is designed by her own will" (Svecchā-viśvamayollekha-khachitaṁ), "seeing which Bhagavān was very pleased."

(Saṁskāra) derived from enjoyment and suffering in former worlds. It is held natural to worship Her as Mother. The first Mantra into which all men are initiated is the word Mā (Mother). It is their first word and generally their last. The father is a mere helper (Sahakāri-mātra) of the Mother.[1] The whole world of the five elements also springs from the Active Consciousness or Śakti, and is Her manifestation (Pūrṇa-vikāsa). Therefore men worship the Mother,[2] than whom is none more tender,[3] saluting Her smiling beauty as the rosy Tripurasundarī, the source of the universe, and Her awe-inspiring grandeur as Kālī, who takes it back into Herself. Here we are concerned with Yoga which is the realization of the union of the Mother and Lord aspects in that state of consciousness which is the Absolute.

Veda says: "All this (that is, the manifold world) is (the one) Brahman" (Sarvaṁ khalvidaṁ Brahma).[4] How the many can be the one [5] is variously explained by the different schools. The interpretation here given is that contained

---

[1] The Supreme Father gives His illumination (Prakāśa). She, the Vimarśa-śakti, produces, but not alone. (Vimarśa-śakti prakāśaśātmanā paramaśivena sāmarasya-viśvaṁ sṛjati na tu kevalā—Yoginī-hṛdaya-Tantra).

[2] In Mātṛ-bhāva, according to the Sanskrit term. Philosophically also this is sound, for all that man knows (outside ecstasy of Samādhi) is the Mother in Her form as the world. The Supreme Śakti, who is not different from Śiva (Parāṣakti-śivāhbinnā), is embodied in every order of thing (Sarva-krama-śarīriṇī—Yoginī-hṛdaya-Tantra).

[3] It is said that "there is nothing more tender than Prakṛti," who serves Puruṣa in every way in His enjoyment, finally giving Mukti or Liberation by retiring from Him when He no longer serves Her.

[4] This, as the Mahānirvāṇa-Tantra says (VII. 98), is the end and aim of Tāntrik Kulācāra, the realization of which saying the Prapañcasāra-Tantra calls the fifth or supreme State (Ch. XIX, Prapañcasāra-Tantra).

[5] Thus it is said of Devī that She is in the form of one and many (Ekānekākṣarākṛtih). Ekaṁ=ekaṁ ajñānaṁ or Māyā. Anekāni=the several Ajñānas—that is, Avidyā. She is both as Upādhi of Īśvara and Jīva (Triśatī, II. 23).

in the Śākta-Tantras or Āgamas. In the first place, what is the one Reality which appears as many? What is the nature of Brahman as it is in itself (Svarūpa)? The answer is Sat-Cit-Ānanda—that is, Being-Consciousness-Bliss. Consciousness or feeling, as such (Cit or Saṁvit), is identical with Being as such. Though in ordinary experience the two are essentially bound up together, they still diverge or seem to diverge from each other. Man by his constitution inveterately believes in an objective existence beyond and independent of himself. And there is such objectivity as long as, being embodied Spirit (Jīvātmā), his consciousness is veiled or contracted [1] by Māyā. But in the ultimate basis of experience, which is the Supreme Spirit (Paramātmā), the divergence has gone, for in it lie, in undifferentiated mass, experiencer, experience, and the experienced. When, however, we speak of Cit as Feeling-Consciousness we must remember that what we know and observe as such is only a limited changing manifestation of Cit, which is in itself the infinite changeless principle, which is the background of all experience. This Being-Consciousness is absolute Bliss (Ānanda), which is defined as "resting in the self" (Svarūpa-viśrānti). It is Bliss because, being the infinite All (Pūrṇa), it can be in want of nothing. This blissful consciousness is the ultimate or irreducible nature or Svarūpa or own form of the one Reality which is both the Whole as the irreducible Real and Part as the reducible Real. Svarūpa is the nature of anything as it is in itself, as distinguished from what it may appear to be. Supreme Consciousness is the Supreme Śiva-Śakti (Paraśiva Paraśakti) which never changes, but eternally endures the same throughout all change effected in its creative aspect as Śiva-Śakti. All manifestation

[1] Saṁkoca. Fullness or wholeness is "veiled" in order that the part or particular may be experienced.

is associated with apparent unconsciousness. The mind is evidently not a pure, but a limited consciousness. What limits it must be something either in itself unconscious or, if conscious, capable of producing the appearance of consciousness.[1] In the phenomenal world there is nothing absolutely conscious nor absolutely unconscious. Consciousness and unconsciousness are always intermingled. Some things, however, appear to be more conscious, and some more unconscious than others. This is due to the fact that Cit, which is never absent in anything, yet manifests itself in various ways and degrees. The degree of this manifestation is determined by the nature and development of the mind and body in which it is enshrined. Spirit remains the same; the mind and body change. The manifestation of consciousness is more or less limited as ascent is made from the mineral to man. In the mineral world Cit manifests as the lowest form of sentiency evidenced by reflex response to stimuli, and that physical consciousness which is called in the West atomic memory. The sentiency of plants is more developed, though it is, as Cakrapāṇi says in the Bhānumatī, a dormant consciousness. This is further manifested in those micro-organisms which are intermediate stages between the vegetable and animal worlds, and have a psychic life of their own. In the animal world consciousness becomes more centralized and complex, reaching its fullest development in man, who possesses all the psychic functions such as cognition, perception, feeling and will. Behind all these particular changing forms of sentiency or consciousness is the one formless, changeless Cit as it is in itself (Svarūpa), that is, as distinguished from the particular forms of its manifestation.

---

[1] The alternative is given to meet the differing views of Māyā-vāda and Śakti-vāda.

As Cit throughout all these stages of life remains the same it is not in itself really developed. The appearance of development is due to the fact that it is now more and now less veiled or contracted by Mind and Matter. It is this veiling by the power of Consciousness (Śakti) which creates the world. What is it, then, which veils consciousness and thus produces world-experience?

The answer is Power or Śakti as Māyā. Māyā-Śakti is that which seemingly makes the Whole (Pūrṇa) into the not whole (Apūrṇa), the infinite into the finite, the formless into forms and the like. It is a power which thus cuts down, veils and negates. Negates what? Perfect consciousness. Is Śakti in itself the same as or different from Śiva or Cit? It must be the same, for otherwise all could not be one Brahman. But if it is the same it must be also Cit or Consciousness. Therefore it is Saccidānandamayī [1] and Cidrūpiṇī.[2]

And yet there is, at least in appearance, some distinction. Śakti, which comes from the root *Śak*, "to have power," "to be able," means power. As She is one with Śiva as Power-holder (Śaktimān), She as such Power is the power of Śiva or Consciousness. There is no difference between Śiva as the possessor of power (Śaktimān) and Power as It is in Itself. The power of Consciousness *is* Consciousness in its *active* aspect. Whilst, therefore, both Śiva and Śakti are Consciousness, the former is the changeless static aspect of Consciousness, and Śakti is the kinetic, active aspect of the same Consciousness. The particular power whereby the

---

[1] That is, its substance is Sat, Cit, Ānanda. The suffixes Mayī and Rūpiṇī indicate a subtle distinction—namely, that She is in Herself, Cit, and yet by appearance the effect of the Power, something different from it.

[2] In the form or nature of Cit. As the Kubjikā Tantra says, the Parama-Kalā is both Cit (Cidrūpa) and Nāda (Nādarūpa).

dualistic world is brought into being is Māyā-Śakti, which is both a veiling (Āvaraṇa) and projecting (Vikṣepa) Śakti. Consciousness veils itself to itself, and projects from the store of its previous experiences (Saṁskāra) the notion of a world in which it suffers and enjoys. The universe is thus the creative imagination (Sṛṣṭi-kalpanā, as it is called) of the Supreme World-thinker (Īśvara). Māyā is that power by which things are "measured"—that is, formed and made known (Mīyate anayā iti māyā). It is the sense of difference (Bhedabuddhi), or that which makes man see the world, and all things and persons therein, as different from himself, when in essence he and they are the one Self. It is that which establishes a dichotomy in what would otherwise be a unitary experience, and is the cause of the dualism inherent in all phenomenal experience. Śakti as action veils consciousness by negating in various degrees Herself as Consciousness.

Before the manifestation of the universe, infinite Being-Consciousness-Bliss alone was—that is, Śiva-Śakti as Cit and Cidrūpiṇī respectively.[1]

This is the Experience-whole (Pūrṇa) in which as the Upaniṣad says, "The Self knows and loves the Self." It is this Love which is Bliss or "resting in the self," for, as it is elsewhere said, "Supreme love is bliss" (Niratiśaya-premāspadatvaṁ ānandatvaṁ). This is Paraśiva, who in the scheme of the Thirty-six Tattvās,[2] is known as

[1] Ahaṁ prakṛti-rūpā cet cidānanda-parāyaṇa (Kulachūdāmaṇi-Nigama, Ch. I, vv. 16-24).

[2] Rāghava-Bhatta says: Yā anādirūpā caitanyādhyasena mahāpralaye sūkṣmā sthitā (Comm. on Śāradā-Tilaka, Ch. I).

See as to the Kashmir School, and its Philosophy of the Tattvas J. C. Chatterji's work on "Kashmir Śaivism".

This is Paramaśiva, or Nirguṇa (attributeless), or Niṣkala (devoid of manifested Śakti) Śiva or Parabrahman, as contrasted with Saguṇa (with attribute), or Sakala (with parts or Śakti), Śiva, or Śabda-brahman (Brahman as the source of "sound," *v. post*).

Para-saṁvit. This Monism posits a dual aspect of the single Consciousness—one the transcendental changeless aspect (Para-saṁvit), and the other the creative changing aspect, which is called Śiva-Śakti-Tattva. In Para-saṁvit the " I " (Ahaṁ) and the " This " (Idaṁ), or universe of objects, are indistinguishably mingled in the supreme unitary experience.[1]

In Śiva-Śakti-Tattva, Śakti, which is the negative aspect of the former, Her function being negation (Niṣedha-vyapāra-rūpā Śaktih), negates Herself as the object of experience, leaving the Śiva consciousness as a mere " I," " not looking towards another " (Ananyonmukhah ahaṁ-pratyayah). This is a state of mere subjective illumination (Prakāśa-mātra)[2] to which Śakti, who is called Vimarśa [3] again presents Herself, but now with a distinction of " I " and " This " as yet held together as part of one self. At this point, the first incipient stage of dualism, there is the first transformation of consciousness, known as Sadāśiva or Sadākhya-Tattva, which is followed by the second or Īshvara Tattva, and then by the third or Śuddha-vidyā-Tattva. In the first emphasis is laid on the " This ", in the second on the " I," and in the third on both equally. Then Māyā severs the united consciousness so that the object is seen as other than the self and then as split up into the multitudinous objects of the universe.

---

[1] As the Yoginīhṛdaya-Tantra says: The Parā Devī is Prakāśa-vimarśa-sāmarasyarūpiṇī. This is the Nirvikalpajñāna state in which there is no distinction of " This " and " That ", of " I " and " This ". In Vikalpa-jñāna there is subject and object.

[2] Paramaśiva has two aspects—Prakāśa and Vimarśa, or Kāmeśvara and Kameśvarī the Paraliṅga. Prakāśa=asphuṭasphūtīkara, or manifestation of what is not manifest.

[3] This word comes from the root *mrish*=to touch, to affect, to cogitate. It is that which is pounded or handled by thought, that is, object of reflective thought. Pradhāna and Prakṛti also involve the meaning " placing in front "; that which is so placed is object. All three terms denote the principle of objectivity.

In the Mantra side of the Tantra-Śāstra, dealing with Mantra and its origin, these two Tattvas emanating from Śakti are from the sound side known as Nāda and Bindu. Paraśiva and Parāśakti are motionless (Nih-spanda) and soundless (Nih-śabda).

Nāda is the first produced movement in the ideating cosmic consciousness leading up to the Sound-Brahman (Śabda-brahman), whence all ideas, the language in which they are expressed (Śabda), and the objects (Artha) which they denote, are derived.

Bindu literally means a point and the dot (Anusvāra), which denotes [1] in Sanskrit the nasal breathing (°). It is placed in the Candra-bindu nasal breathing above Nāda (°). In its technical Mantra sense it denotes that state of active Consciousness or Śakti in which the "I" or illuminating aspect of Consciousness identifies itself with the total "This". [2] It subjectifies the "This," thereby becoming a point (Bindu) of consciousness with it. When Consciousness apprehends an object as different from Itself, It sees that object as extended in space. But when that object is completely subjectified, it is experienced as an unextended point. This is the universe-experience of the Lord-experiencer as Bindu. [3]

Where does the Universe go at dissolution? It is withdrawn into that Śakti which projected it. It collapses, so to speak, into a mathematical point without any magnitude

---

[1] *Lit.* What goes (aṇu) with vowel sound (Svāra or Svara).

[2] For until the operation of Māyā at a later stage the "This" is still experienced as part of the "I". Therefore there is no manifestation or dualism.

[3] For the same reason Śakti is then said to be Ghanībhūtā, which is literally massive or condensed. It is that state of gathered-up power which immediately precedes the burgeoning forth (Sphuraṇa) of the universe.

whatever.[1] This is the Śiva-bindu, which again is withdrawn into the Śiva-Śakti-Tattva which produced it. It is conceived that round the Śiva-Bindu there is coiled Śakti, just as in the earth centre called Mūlādhāra-Cakra in the human body a serpent clings round the self-produced Phallus (Svayaṁbhu-liṅga). This coiled Śakti may be conceived as a mathematical line, also without magnitude, which, being everywhere in contact with the point round which it is coiled, is compressed together with it, and forms therefore also one and the same point. There is one indivisible unity of dual aspect which is figured also in the Tantras[2] as a grain of gram (Canaka), which has two seeds so closely joined as to look as one surrounded by an outer sheath.[3]

To revert to the former simile, the Śakti coiled round Śiva, making one point (Bindu) with it, is Kuṇḍalinī Śakti. This word comes from the word Kuṇḍala or " a coil," " a bangle ". She is spoken of as coiled; because She is likened to a serpent (Bhujaṅgī), which, when resting and sleeping, lies coiled; and because the nature of Her power is spiraline, manifesting itself as such in the worlds—the spheroids or " eggs of Brahmā " (Brahmāṇḍa), and in their circular or revolving orbits and in other ways. Thus the Tantras speak of the development of the straight line, (Riju-rekhā) from the point which, when it has gone its length as a point, is turned (Vakra-rekhā aṁkushākāra) by the force of the spiraline sack of Māyā in which it works so as to form a

[1] The imagery, like all of its kind, is necessarily imperfect; for such a point, though it has no magnitude, is assumed to have a position. Here there is none, or we are in spacelessness.

[2] See the Commentary, *post*.

[3] The two seeds are Śiva and Śakti, and the sheath is Māyā. When they come apart there is " creation ". Again the imagery is faulty in that there are two seeds, whereas Śiva and Śakti are the One with dual aspect.

figure of two dimensions, which again is turned upon itself, ascending as a straight line into the plane of the third dimension, thus forming the triangular or pyramidal figure called Śṛṅgātaka.[1] In other words, this Kuṇḍalī-Śakti is that which, when it moves to manifest itself, appears as the universe. To say that it is "coiled" is to say that it is *at rest*—that is, in the form of *static potential energy*. This Śakti coiled round the Supreme Śiva is called Mahā-kuṇḍalī ("The great coiled power"), to distinguish it from the same power which exists in individual bodies, and which is called Kuṇḍalinī.[2] It is with and through the last power that this Yoga is effected. When it is accomplished the individual Śakti (Kuṇḍalī) is united with the great cosmic Śakti (Mahā-Kuṇḍalī), and She with Śiva, with whom She is essentially one. Kuṇḍalinī is an aspect of the eternal Brahman (Brahmarūpa Sanātanī), and is both attributeless and with attribute (Nirguṇa and Saguṇa). In Her Nirguṇa aspect She is pure Consciousness (Caitanya-rūpiṇī) and Bliss itself (Ānandarūpiṇī, and in creation, Brahmānanda-prakāśinī). As Saguṇa She it is by whose power all creatures are displayed (Sarvabhūta-prakāśinī.[3] Kuṇḍalī-Śakti in individual bodies is *power at rest*, or the *static centre* round which every form of existence as moving power revolves. In the universe there is always in and behind every form of activity a static background. The one Consciousness is polarized into static (Śiva) and kinetic (Śakti) aspects for the purpose of "creation". This Yoga is the resolution of this duality into unity again.

---

[1] The shape of the Siṅgārā, water-nut, which grows freely in the lakes of Kashmir. Here I may observe that Yantras, though drawn on the flat, must be conceived of in the solid mass. The flat drawing is a mere suggestion of the three-dimensional figure which the Yantra is.

[2] Because She is thus bent, the Devī is called Kubjika (hunchback).

[3] Kubjikā-Tantra, Ch. I, Prāṇa-toṣiṇī, p. 8.

The Indian Scriptures say, in the words of Herbert Spencer in his "First Principles", that the universe is an unfoldment (Sṛṣṭī) from the homogeneous (Mūla-prakṛti) to the heterogeneous (Vikṛti), and back to the homogeneous again (Pralaya or Dissolution). There are thus alternate states of evolution and dissolution, manifestation taking place after a period of rest. So also Professor Huxley, in his "Evolution and Ethics," speaks of the manifestation of cosmic energy (Māyā-Śakti) alternating between phases of potentiality (Pralaya) and phases of explication (Sṛṣṭi). "It may be," he says, "as Kant suggests, every cosmic magma predestined to evolve into a new world has been the no less predestined end of a vanished predecessor." This the Indian Sāstra affirms in its doctrine that there is no such thing as an absolutely first creation, the present universe being but one of a series of worlds which are past and are yet to be.

At the time of Dissolution (Pralaya) there is in Consciousness as Mahā-kuṇḍalī, though undistinguishable from its general mass, the potentiality or seed of the universe to be. Māyā, as the world, potentially exists as Mahā-kuṇḍalī, who is Herself one with Consciousness or Śiva. This Māyā contains, and is in fact constituted by, the collective Samskāra or Vāsanā—that is, the mental impressions and tendencies produced by Karma accomplished in previously existing worlds. These constitute the mass of the potential ignorance (Avidyā) by which Consciousness veils itself. They were produced by desire for worldly enjoyment, and themselves produce such desire. The worlds exist because they, in their totality, will to exist. Each individual exists because his will desires worldly life. This seed is therefore the collective or cosmic will towards manifested life—that is the life of form and enjoyment. At the end of the period of rest, which is Dissolution, this seed ripens into Consciousness. Consciousness has thus a twin aspect; its liberation (Mukti) or formless aspect, in which it *is* as mere Consciousness-Bliss; and a universe or form aspect, in which it *becomes* the world of enjoyment (Bhukti). One of the cardinal principles of the Śākta-Tantra is to secure by its Sādhanā both Liberation (Mukti) and Enjoyment (Bhukti).[1] This is possible by the identification of the self when in enjoyment with the soul of the world. When this seed ripens, Śiva is said to put forth His Śakti. As this Śakti is Himself, it is He in His Śiva-Śakti aspect who comes forth (Prasarati) and endows Himself with all the forms of worldly life. In the pure, perfect, formless Consciousness there springs up the desire to manifest in the world of forms—the desire for enjoyment of and as form. This takes place as a limited stress in the unlimited unmoving surface of pure Consciousness, which is Niṣkala-Śiva, but without affecting the latter. There is thus change in changelessness and changelessness in change. Śiva in His transcendent aspect does not change but Śiva (Sakala) in His immanent aspect as Śakti does. As creative will arises, Śakti thrills as Nāda,[2] and assumes the form of Bindu, which is Īśvara-Tattva, whence all the worlds derive. It is for their creation that Kuṇḍalī uncoils. When Karma ripens, the Devī, in the words of the Nigama,[3] "becomes desirous of creation, and covers Herself with Her

---

[1] Bhogena mokṣaṁ-āpnoti bhogena kulasādhanaṁ

Tasmād yatnād bhogayukto bhaved vīravarah sudhīh.

(Kulārṇava-Saṁhitā, v. 219)

"By world-experience (Bhoga Bhukti) he gains Liberation or World experience is the means for the attainment of Kula. Therefore, the wise and good Vīra should carefully be united with world-experience."

[2] Literally "sound," that initial activity which is the first source of the subsequently manifested Śabda (sound) which is the Word to which corresponds the Artha or Object.

[3] "Kulacūdāmaṇi", Ch. I, vv. 16-24.

own Māyā". Again, the "Devī, joyful in the mad delight of Her union with the Supreme Akula,[1] becomes Vikāriṇī"[2] —that is, the Vikāras or Tattvas of Mind and Matter, which constitute the universe, appear.

The Śāstras have dealt with the stages of creation in great detail both from the subjective and objective viewpoints as changes in the limited consciousness or as movement (Spanda), form, and "sound" (Śabda). Both Śaivas and Śāktas equally accept the Thirty-Six categories or Tattvas, the Kalās, the Śaktis Unmanī and the rest in the Tattvas, the Ṣadadhvā, the Mantra concepts of Nāda, Bindu, Kāmakalā, and so forth.[3] Authors of the Northern Śaiva School, of which a leading Śāstra is the Mālinīvijaya-Tantra, have described with great profundity these Tattvas. General conclusions only are, however, here summarized. These thirty-six Tattvas are in the Tantras divided into three groups, called Ātma, Vidyā and Śiva Tattvas. The first group includes all the Tattvas, from the lowest Pṛthivi ("earth") to Prakṛti, which are known as the impure categories (Aśuddha-Tattva); the second includes Māyā, the Kañcukas,[4] and Puruṣa, called the pure-impure categories (Śuddha-aśuddha-Tattva); and

---

[1] Akula is a Tāntrik name for Śiva, Sakti being called Kula, which is Mātṛ, Māna, Meya. In the Yoginī-hṛdaya-Tantra it is said (Ch. I): Kulaṁ meya-māna-mātṛ-lakṣaṇaṁ, kaulastatsamastih. These three are: Knower, Knowing, Known, for that is Consciousness as Śakti.

[2] "Kulacūdāmaṇi", Ch. I, vv. 16-24.

[3] See as to these terms the author's "Garland of Letters".

[4] Forms of Śakti whereby the natural perfections of Consciousness are limited. Thus from all-knowing it becomes little-knowing; from being almighty, it becomes a little-doer, etc. See "Garland of Letters".

The term Saṁkoca (contraction) expresses the same idea. The Devī is Saṁkucadrūpā through Matṛ, Māna, and Meya, and therefore so also is Śiva as Jīva (tathā śivopi saṁkucadrūpah).—Yoginī-hṛdaya-Tantra.

the third includes the five highest Tattvas called the pure Tattvas (Śuddha-Tattva), from Śiva-Tattva to Śuddha-vidyā. As already stated, the supreme changeless state (Para-saṁvit)[1] is the unitary experience in which the "I" and "This" coalesce in unity.

In the kinetic or Śakti aspect, as presented by the pure categories, experience recognizes an "I" and "This," but the latter is regarded, not as something opposed to and outside the "I," but as part of a one self with two sides —an "I" (Ahaṁ) and "This" (Idaṁ). The emphasis varies from insistence on the "I" to insistence on the "This," and then to equality of emphasis on the "I" and "This" as a preparation for the dichotomy in consciousness which follows.

The pure-impure categories are intermediate between the pure and the impure. The essential characteristic of experience constituted by the impure categories is its dualism effected through Māyā—and its limitations—the result of the operation of the Kañcukas. Here the "This" is not seen as part of the Self, but as opposed to and without it as an object seen outside. Each consciousness thus becomes mutually exclusive the one of the other. The states thus described are threefold: a transcendent mingled "I" and "This" in which these elements of experience are as such not evolved; and a pure form of experience intermediate between the first and last, in which both the "I" and the "This" are experienced as part of the one self; and, thirdly, the state of manifestation proper, when there is a complete cleavage between the "I" and the "This," in which an outer object is presented to the consciousness of a knower which is other than the subject. This last stage is itself twofold. In the first the Puruṣa experiences a homogeneous universe, though different from himself

[1] This is not counted as a Tattva, being Tattvātītā.

as Prakṛti; in the second Prakṛti is split up into its effects (Vikṛti), which are Mind and Matter, and the multitudinous beings of the universe which these compose. Śakti as Prakṛti first evolves mind (Buddhi, Ahaṁkāra, Manas) and senses (Indṛya), and then sensible matter (Bhūta) of fivefold form ("ether," "air," "fire," "water," "earth")[1] derived from the supersensible generals of the sense-particulars called Tanmātra. When Śakti has entered the last and grossest Tattva ("earth")—that is, solid matter—there is nothing further for Her to do. Her creative activity then ceases, and *She rests.* She rests in Her last emanation, the "earth" principle. She is again coiled and sleeps. She is now Kuṇḍalī-Śakti, whose abode in the human body is the Earth centre or Mūlādhāra-Cakra. As in the supreme state She lay coiled as the Mahākuṇḍalī round the Supreme Śiva, so here She coils round the Svayaṁbhū-Liṅga in the Mūlādhāra. This last centre or Cakra and the four above it are centres of the five forms of Matter. The sixth centre is that of Mind. Consciousness and its processes through Śakti prior to the appearance of Māyā are realized in the seventh lotus (Sahasrāra-padma) and centres intermediate between it and the sixth or Ājñā Mind centre.

The mantra evolution, which must be known if the Text is to be understood, is set forth with great clarity in the Śāradā-Tilaka, wherein it is said that from the Sakala-Śiva (Śiva-Tattva), who is Sat-Cit-Ānanda, issued (Śakti-Tattva); from the latter Nāda (Sadākhya Tattva); and from Nāda evolved Bindu (Īśvara-Tattva),[2] which, to distinguish

[1] These terms have not the ordinary English meaning, but denote the ethereal, gaseous, igneous, liquid, and solid states of matter. In worship (Pūjā) they are symbolized by the following ingredients (Upacāra): Puṣpa (flower), ether; Dhūpa (incense), air; Dīpa (light), fire; Naivedya (food-offering), water; Candana (sandal), earth.

[2] Saccidānanda-vibhavāt sakalāt parameśvarāt
Āsīcchaktis tato nādo nādād bindu-samudbhavah. (Ch. I.)

it from the Bindu which follows, is called the Supreme Bindu (Para-Bindu). Nāda and Bindu are, like all else, aspects of Power, or Śakti, being those states of Her which are the proper conditions for Upayogā-vasthā) and in which She is prone to (Ucchūnāvasthā) "creation". In those Tattvas the germ of action (Kriyā-Śakti) sprouts towards its full manifestation.

The Tantras, in so far as they are Mantra-Śāstras, are concerned with Śabda or "Sound", a term later explained. Mantra is manifested Śabda. Nāda, which also literally means "sound," is the first of the produced intermediate causal bodies of manifested Śabda. Bindu, which has previously been explained, is described as the state of the letter "Ma" before manifestation, consisting of the Śiva-Śakti-Tattva enveloped by Māyā or Parama-Kuṇḍalinī. It implies both the void (Śūnya)—that is, the Brahman state (Brahmapada)—in the empty space within the circle of the Bindu; as also the Guṇas which are implicitly contained in it, since it is in indissoluble union with Śakti, in whom the Guṇas or factors constituting the material source of all things are contained.[1] The Para-bindu is called the Ghanāvasthā or massive state of Śakti. It is Cid-ghana or massive consciousness—that is, Cit associated with undifferentiated (that is, Cidrūpiṇī) Śakti, in which lie potentially in a mass (Ghana), though undistinguishable the one from the other, all the worlds and beings to be created. This is Parama-Śiva, in whom are all the Devatās. It is this Bindu who is the Lord (Īśvara) whom some Paurāṇikas call Mahāviṣṇu and others the Brahmapuruṣa.[2] As the Commentator says, it does not matter what

---

[1] See vv. 41-49, *post*; Todala-Tantra, Ch. IV; and Kāmakalāmālinī-Tantra, cited in v. 43.

[2] See v. 49, *post*.

He is called. He is the Lord (Īśvara) who is worshipped in secret by all Devas,[1] and is pointed to in different phases of the Bhandrabindu, or Nāda, Bindu, Śakti and Śānta of the Oṁ and other Bīja-Mantras. Its abode is Satyaloka, which within the human body exists in the pericarp of the thousand-petalled lotus (Sahasrāra) in the highest cerebral centre. The Śāradā[2] then says that this Para-bindu, whose substance is Supreme Śakti, divides itself into three—that is, appears under a threefold aspect. There are thus three Bindus, the first of which is called Bindu,[3] and the others Nāda and Bīja. Bindu is in the nature of Śiva and Bīja of Śakti.[4] Nāda is Śiva-Śakti—that is, their mutual relation or interaction (Mithah samavāyah)[5] or Yoga (union), as the Prayoga-sāra calls it.[6] The threefold Bindu (Tri-bindu) is supreme (Para), subtle

---

[1] See v. 41, *post.*

[2] Ch. I.

[3] Kārya, or produced, Bindu, to distinguish it from the causal (Kāraṇa) Bindu or Para-bindu.

[4] In the case of the Mantras, Bīja (according to the Kulacūdāmaṇi, v. 58) is the first letter of a Kūta or group and what follows is Śakti. Thus in the Mantra "Krīṁ," K is Bīja and R and I are Śakti. By the Bīja form is made (Bījena mūrti-kalpanā).

[5] Paraśaktimayah sākṣāt tridbāsau bhidyate punah
Bindur nādo bījaṁ iti tasya bhedāh samīritāh.
Binduh śivātmako bījaṁ śaktir nādas tayor mithah
Samavāyah samākhyātah sarvāgamaviśāradaih. (Ch. I).

"This (Bindu) which is both Śiva and Śakti divides itself again into three parts. Bindu, Nāda and Bīja are its three parts. Bindu is Śivātmaka (*i.e.*, Śiva), Bīja is Śakti and Nāda is said to be the mutual relation between them by all who are versed in the Āgamas."

The first word of the third line reads better as Bindu śivātmako than as Bindur nādātmako, as some MSS., such as that from which I quoted in Introduction to the Mahānirvāṇa. The Commentary to v. 40. *post,* also speaks of Bindu as being Nādātmaka, but explains that that means Śivātmaka. See also to the same effect Kriyā-sāra.

[6] See Rāghava-Bhatt's Comm. on Ch. I, v. 8 of Śāradā:

(Sūkṣma) and gross (Sthūla).[1] Nāda is thus the union of these two in creation. As the Text says (v. 40), it is by this division of Śiva and Śakti that there arises creative ideation (Sṛṣṭi-kalpanā). The causal Bindu is from the Śakti aspect undifferentiated Śakti (Abhedarūpā-Śakti) with all powers (Sarva-śaktimaya); from the Prakṛti aspect Triguṇamayi Mūla-prakṛti; from the Devatā aspect the unmanifest (Avyakta); from the Devī aspect Śāntā. The three Bindus separately indicate the operations of the three powers of Will (Icchā), Knowledge (Jñāna), and Action (Kriyā), and the three Guṇas (Rajas, Sattva, Tamas); also the manifestation of the three Devīs (Vāmā, Jyeṣṭhā,

---

Nirguṇah saguṇaś ceti śivo jñeyah sanātanah.
Nirguṇāccaiva samjātā bindavas traya eva ca
Brahmabindur viṣṇubindū rudrabindur maheśvari.

"The eternal Śiva is to be known both as Nirguṇa (without attributes) and Saguṇa (with attributes). From the attributeless (Nirguṇa), O Maheśvari, originated the three Bindus which are Brahma-bindu, Viṣṇu-bindu and Rudra-bindu."

The verse as cited in Prāṇa-toṣinī (p. 13) reads in the second line Nirguṇaśaiva; but this must be a mistake for Nirguṇāccaiva, for the Bindus themselves are not Nirguṇa but spring from it.

[1] Asmācca kāraṇabindoh sakāśāt krameṇa kāryabindus tato nādas tato bījaṁ iti trayaṁ utpannaṁ tad idaṁ parasūkṣmasthūla-padaih kathyate (Lalita-Sahasranāma, Comm.).

From this Causal (Kāraṇa) Bindu again there originated Kārya (Effect) Bindu, and thereafter Nāda and thereafter Bīja—these three. These are spoken of as Para (transcendent), Sūkṣma (subtle) and Sthūla (gross).

These represent the Cit, Cidacit, Acit aspects of nature. Cidaṁśah cidacinmiśrah acidaṁśahśca teṣāṁ rūpāṇi (Bhāskararāya: Comm. Lalitā).

Kālena bhidyamānastu sa bindur bhavati tridhā,
Sthūlakṣmaparatvena tasya traividhyamiṣyate,
Sa bindunādabījatva bhedena ca nigadyate.

Ete ca kāraṇabhindvādayaścātvāra ādhidaivataṁ avyakteśvara-hiraṇyagarbha-virātsvarūpāh śāntā-vāmā-jyeṣṭhā-raudrīrūpa ambikecchā-jñāna-kriyārūpāśca (ib.). Ādhibhūtaṁ tu kāmarūpa-pūrṇagiri-jālandhara-udyānapīṭharūpāh. Pīṭharūpā iti tu nityāhṛdaye spaṣṭaṁ (ib.). Citing Rahasyāgama.

Raudrī) and the three Devatās (Brahmā, Viṣṇu, Rudra) who spring from them.[1] It is said in the Prayoga-sāra and Śāradā that Raudrī issued from Bindu, Jyeṣṭhā from Nāda, and Vāmā from Bīja. From these came Rudra, Viṣṇu, Brahmā, which are in the nature of Jñāna, Kriyā, Icchā, and Moon, Sun and Fire.[2] The three Bindus are known as Sun (Ravi), Moon (Candra), and Fire (Agni), terms constantly appearing in the works here translated.

In Sun there are Fire and Moon.[3] It is known as Miśra-Bindu, and in the form of such is not different from Paramaśiva, and is Kāmakalā.[4] Kāmakalā is the Triangle

---

[1] Icchā, Rajas, Vāmā, Brahmā, Paśyantī-śabda.
Jñānā, Sattva, Jyeṣṭhā, Viṣṇu, Madhyamā-śabda,
Kriyā, Tamas, Raudrī Rudra, Vaikharī-śabda.

See Comm. 22 Śloka, "Kāmakalāvilāsa", Saṁkcta, 1, Yoginīhṛdaya-Tantra, and Saubhāgya-subhodaya, cited in Saṁketa 2 of the last Tantra. As the Rudra-Yāmala says (II. 2), the three Devas are aspects of the One.

Ekā mūrtistrayo devā brahmāviṣṇumaheśvarāh,
Mama vigrahasaṁkḷptā srijaty avati hanti ca.

But see next note.

[2] Cited in Prāṇa-toṣinī, p. 8.

Raudrī bindos tato nādāj jyeṣṭhā bījād ajāyata,
Vāmā tābhyah samutpannāh rudra-brahmā-ramādhipāh,
Te jnānecchā-kriyātmāno vahnīndvarka-svarūpiṇah.
Icchā kriyā tathā jnānaṁ gaurī brāhmitī vaiṣṇavi
Tridhā śaktih sthitā yatra tatparaṁ jyotir oṁ iti.

As the author of the Prāṇa-toṣiṇī (p. 9) says, the names are not to be read in the order of words (Pratiśabdaṁ), otherwise Jñāna would be associated with Vaiṣṇavī, but according to the facts (Yath-saṁbhavaṁ) as stated in the text. According to this account it would seem that Jñāna, Sattva, and Kriyā Tamas in note 1, should be transposed.

[3] It is Agnīsomamayah. See Tīkā, vv. 6, 7, of "Kāmakalāvilāsa". See my "Garland of Letters".

[4] That is, Kāmayuktā Kalā, Kalā with creative will (here its manifestation).

Mahā-bindu=Paramaśiva=Miśra-bindu=Ravi=Kāmakalā.
Ravī-paramaśivābhinnā miśra-bindurūpā Kāmakalā.

of Divine Desire formed by the three Bindus—that is, their collectivity (Samaṣti-rūpā).[1] This Kāmakalā is the root (Mūla) of all Mantra. Moon (Soma, Candra) is Śiva-Bindu, and white (Sita-Bindu); Fire (Agni) is Śakti-bindu, and red (Śoṇa-bindu); Sun is the mixture of the two. Fire, Moon and Sun are the Icchā, Jñāna, Kriyā-Śaktis (Will, Knowledge, Action). On the material plane the white Bindu assumes the form of semen (Śukrā), and the red Bindu of menstrual fluid (Rajasphala, Śoṇita). Mahā-bindu is the state before the manifestation of Prakṛti.[2] All three Bindus—that is, the Kāmakalā—are Śakti, though one may indicate predominantly the Śiva, the other the Śakti, aspect. Sometimes Miśra-Bindu is called Śakti-Tattva, to denote the supremacy of Śakti, and sometimes Śiva-Tattva, to denote the supremacy of the possessor of power (Śaktimān). It is of coupled form (Yāmala-rūpā). There is no Śiva without Śakti, nor Śakti without Śiva.[3] To separate[4] them is as impossible as to separate the moving wind from the steadfast ether in which it blows. In the one Śiva-Śakti there is a union (Maithuna),[5] the thrill of which is Nāda, whence Mahā-bindu is born, which itself becomes threefold

---

[1] As Ravi or Sūrya (Sun) Bindu is in the form of Para-śiva, and in it are the other two Bindus, it is the Samaṣti-rūpa of them, and is thus called Kāmakalā.

[2] This, which is O, becomes ईँईँ—that is, Candra, Ravi and Ra (fire).

[3] Tayor yad yāmalaṁ rūpaṁ sa saṁghatta iti smṛtah—

Ānanda-śaktih saivoktā yato viśvaṁ visṛjyati,
Na Śivah Śaktirahito na Śaktih Śivavarjitā.
(Tantrāloka-Āhnika, 3.)

"The coupled form of these two (Śivā-Śakti) is called junction. That is called the blissful Śakti from which creation arises. There is no Śiva without Śakti, nor Śakti without Śiva."

[4] *Ib.*, 3 Ahn.

[5] On the physical plane this word denotes sexual union.

(Tri-bindu), which is Kāmakalā.[1] It is said in the Śāradā-Tilaka that on the "bursting" or differentiation of the Supreme Bindu there was unmanifested "sound" (Śabda).[2] This unmanifested Śabda is through action (Kriyā-Śakti) the source of the manifested Śabda and Artha described later.[3] The Brahman as the source of language (Śabda) and ideas on one hand, and the objects (Artha) they denote on the other, is called Śabda-brahman, or, to use a Western term, the Logos.[4] From this differentiating Bindu in the form of Prakṛti are evolved the Tattvas of Mind and Matter in all their various forms, as also the Lords of the Tattvas (Tattveśa)—that is, their directing intelligences—Śaṁbhu,[5] the presiding Devatā

---

[1] In the Śrīcakra this is in the region of Baindava-Cakra, the highest, followed by the triangular Cakra, which is Kāmeśvarī, Bhagamālinī and Vajreśvarī. See further as to Kāmakālā, *post.*

[2] Bhidyamānāt parād bindor avyaktāma-ravoś bhavat,
Śabdabrahmetī taṁ prāhuh sarvāgamaviśāradāh.
(Śāradā-Tilaka, Ch. I.)

It will be observed that in this verse the first Bindu is called Para and to make this clear the author of the Prāṇa-toṣinī adds the following note:

Parādbindor ityanena śaktyavasthārupo yah prathamo bindus tasmāt (By Para-bindu is meant the first Bindu, which is a state of Śakti.) See "Garland of Letters".

[3] See Rāghava-Bhātta, Comm. Ch. I, v. 12. Śāradā, on the same.
Kriyāśaktipradhānāyāh śabda śabdārthakāraṇaṁ,
Prakṛter bindurupinyāh śabdabrahmā, bhavat paraṁ.

As the Kulārnava-Tantra (Khanda 5, Ullāsa I) says the one Brahman has twofold aspects as Paraṁbrahman (transcendent) and Śabdabrahman (immanent). Śabdabrahmaparaṁbrahmabhedena brahmaṇor dvaividhyaṁ uktaṁ. (And see also Śrīmad-Bhāgavata, 6 Skanda, 16 Ch.) Tena śabdārtharūpaviśiṣṭasya śabdabrahmatvaṁ avadāritaṁ (Prāṇa-toṣinī, 10).

[4] It is said in the Prāna-toṣinī, p. 22, that Shaṁbhu is the "associate of time" (Kālabandhu) because Kāla in the form of Nāda assists in giving birth to Him and the other Devatās.

[5] Atha bindvātmanah Śaṁbhoh kālabandhoh kalātmanah,
Ajāyata jagat-sākṣī sarva-vyāpī Sadāśivah.
Sadāśivāt bhaved Īśas tato Ruḍrasamudbhavah,
Tato Viṣṇu tato Brahmā teṣāṁ evaṁ samudbhavah.
(Śāradā, Ch. I, vv. 15, 16.)

over the Ājñā-Cakra, the centre of the mental faculties; and Sadāśiva, Īśa, Rudra, Viṣṇu, Brahmā, the Devatās of the five forms of Matter, concluding with Pṛthivī ("earth") in the Mūlādhāra centre, wherein the creative Śakti, having finished Her work, again rests, and is called Kuṇḍalinī.

Just as the atom consists of a static centre round which moving forces revolve, so in the human body Kuṇḍalinī in the "Earth-Cakra" is the static centre (Kendra) round which She in kinetic aspect as the forces of the body works. The whole body as Śakti is in ceaseless movement. Kuṇḍalinī Śakti is the immobile support of all these operations. When She is aroused and Herself moves upwards, She withdraws with and into Herself these moving Śaktis, and then unites with Śiva in the Sahasrāra Lotus. The process upward (evolution) is the reverse of the involution above described. The Worlds are dissolved (Laya) from time to time for all beings. The perfected Yogī dissolves the Universe for all time for himself. Yoga is thus Laya.

Before proceeding to a description of the Cakras it is, firstly necessary to describe more fully the constituents of the body—that is, Power manifest as the Tattvas mentioned, extending from Prakṛti to Pṛthivī. It is of these Tattvas that the Cakras are centres. Secondly, an explanation is required of the doctrine of "Sound" (Śabda), which exists in the body in the three inner states (Parā, Paśyantī, Madhyamā) and is expressed in uttered speech (Vaikharī). This will help the reader to an understanding of the meaning of Mantra or manifested Śabda, and of the "Garland of Letters" which is distributed throughout the six bodily centres.

Here they are mentioned in connection with the form creation (Artha-sṛṣṭi). The Prāṇa-toṣiṇī: Atra arthasṛṣṭau punah rudrādīnāṁ utpattiṣtu artha-rūpeṇa. Pūrvaṁ teṣāṁ utpattih śabda-rūpeṇa, ato na pāunaruktyaṁ iti kalā-māyā-tadātmanas tadutpannatvāt.

III

EMBODIED CONSCIOUSNESS (JĪVĀTMĀ)

CONSCIOUSNESS as one with dual aspect is Transcendent and Immanent. The Transcendental Consciousness is called the Paramātmā. The consciousness which is embodied in Mind and Matter is the Jīvātmā. In the first case Consciousness is formless and in the second it is with form. Form is derivable from Consciousness as Power (Śakti). One of these powers is Prakṛti-Śakti—that is, the immediate source of Mind and Matter. The corresponding static aspect is called Puruṣa. This term is sometimes applied to the Supreme, as in the name Brahma-puruṣa.[1] Here is meant a centre of limited consciousness—limited by the associated Prakṛti and its products of Mind and Matter. Popularly by Puruṣa, as by Jīva, is meant sentient being with body and senses—that is, organic life.[2] Man is a microcosm (Kṣudra-Brahmāṇḍa).[3] The world is the macrocosm (Brahmāṇḍa). There are numberless worlds, each of which is governed by its own Lords, though there is but one great Mother of all whom these Lords

---

[1] So it is said: Puruṣān na paraṁ kiṁcit sā kāṣṭha sā parā gatih.

[2] Dehendriyādiyuktah cetano jīvah. The Kulārṇava-Tantra, I. 7-9, describes the Jīvas as parts of Śiva enveloped in Māyā (which thus constitutes them as separate entities), like sparks issuing from fire—an old Vedāntic idea. As, however, Jīva in Māyāvāda Vedānta is really Brahman (Jīvo brahmaiva nāparah) there is according to such doctrine in reality no independent category called Jīva (Nahi jīvo nāma kaścit svatantrah padārthah.) Ātmā is called Jīva when with Upādhi—that is, body, etc. Philosophically, all Ātmā with Upādhi (attribute) is Jīva.

[3] "Little egg (spheroid) of Brahmā."

themselves worship, placing on their heads the dust of Her feet. In everything there is all that is in anything else. There is thus nothing in the universe which is not in the human body. There is no need to throw one's eyes into the heavens to find God. He is within, being known as the "Ruler within" (Antaryāmin) or "Inner self" (Antarātmā).[1] All else is His power as Mind and Matter. Whatever of Mind or Matter exists in the universe exists in some form or manner in the human body. So as already stated it is said in the Viśvasāra-Tantra: "What is here is there. What is not here is nowhere."[2] In the body there are the Supreme Śiva-Śakti who pervade all things. In the body is Prakṛti-Śakti and all Her products. In fact, the body is a vast magazine of Power (Śakti). The object of the Tāntrik rituals is to raise these various forms of power to their full expression. This is the work of Sādhana. The Tantras say that it is in the power of man to accomplish all he wishes if he centres his will thereon. And this must, according to their doctrine, be so, for man is in his essence one with the Supreme Lord (Īśvara) and Mother (Īśvarī) and the more he manifests Spirit the greater is he endowed with its powers. The centre and root of all his powers as Jīva is Kuṇḍalinī-Śakti. The centre in which the quiescent consciousness is realized is the upper brain or Sahasrāra, whence in the case of the Yogī, the Prāṇa escapes through the fissure called Brahmarandhra at death. (See Plate VIII). The Mind and Body are effects of Prakṛti.

---

[1] The Jñānārṇava-Tantra (XXI, 10) says that "antah" implies secret and subtle, for the Ātmā, fine like an atom, is within everything. This is the bird Hamsa which disports in the Lake of Ignorance. On dissolution, when it is Saṁhārarūpī, Ātmā is revealed. The Mother is the Antaryāmin of the Devatās also, such as the five Śivas, Brahmā, etc., for She is Parabrahmānandarūpā, Para-prakāśa-rūpā, Sadrūpā and Cidrūpā and thus directs them (Triśatī, II. 47).

[2] Yad ihāsti tad anyatra yan nehāsti na tat kvacit—an Indian version of the Hermetic maxim, "As above, so below".

Both having the same origin, each as such, whether as Mind or Matter, are "material" things—that is, they are of the nature of forces,[1] and limited instruments through which Spirit or Consciousness functions, and thus, though itself unlimited, appears to be limited. The light in a lantern is unaffected, but its manifestation to those without is affected by the material through which the light shines. Prakṛti, however, is not scientific Matter. The latter is only its grossest product, and has as such no lasting existence. Prakṛti is the ultimate "material" cause of both Mind and Matter, and the whole universe which they compose. It is the mysterious fructescent womb (Yoni) whence all is born.[2] What She is in Herself cannot be realized. She is only known by Her effects.[3] Though Mūla-prakṛti is the material cause

---

[1] So Herbert Spencer holds, in conformity with Indian doctrine, that the universe, whether physical or psychical, is a play of force which in the case of matter we as the self or mind experience as object. As to Mind and Matter see "The World As Power".

[2] The word has been said to be derived form *Kṛ* and the affix *ktin*, which is added to express *bhāva*, or the abstract idea, and sometimes the Karma, or object of the action, corresponding with the Greek affix *sis*. *Ktin* inflected in the nominative becomes *tih*, *tis*. Prakṛti therefore has been said to correspond with φυσις (nature) of the Greeks (Banerjee, "Dialogues on Hindu Philosophy," 24). It is also called Pradhāna. Pra+dhā+anat=Pradhatte sarvaṁ ātmani, or that which contains all things in itself, the source and receptacle of all matter and form. Pradhānā also literally means "chief" (substance), for according to Sāṁkhya it is the real creator.

[3] See the splendid Hymn to Prakṛti in Prapañcasāra-Tantra. What can be seen by the eyes can be defined, but not She. "It cannot be seen by the eyes." Kena Up., 1-6: "Yat cakṣuṣā na paśyati." She is beyond the senses. Hence the Triśatī addressess the Devī (II. 44) as Īdṛgityavinirdeśyā (who is not to be particularly pointed out as being this or that). See Śāradā-Tilāka, Vāmakeśvara, and Viśvasāra-Tantras, cited in Prāṇa-toṣiṇī, p. 24. She is ineffable and inconceivable: with form (Vikṛti), yet Herself (Mūla-prakṛti) formless. Mahānirvāṇa-Tantra, IV. 33-35. Thus Sāyāṇa (Rig-Veda. X, 129, 2) says that, whilst Māyā is Anirvācyā (indefinable), since it is neither Sat nor Asat, Cit is definable as Sat.

of the world from which it arises,[1] ultimately, as it is in itself (Svarūpa), Prakṛti-Śakti, like all else, is Consciousness, for Consciousness as Power and static Consciousness are one.[2] Consciousness, however, assumes the rôle of Prakṛti—that is, creative power—when evolving the universe. So substance consists of the Guṇas or modes of this natural principle which are called Sattva, Rajas, Tamas.[3] The general action of Śakti is to veil or contract consciousness. Prakṛti, in fact, is a *finitising* principle. To all seeming, it finitises and makes form in the infinite formless Consciousness.[4] So do all the Guṇas. But one does it less and another more. The first is Sattva-guṇa the function of which, relative to the other Guṇas, is to *reveal* consciousness. The greater the presence or power of Sattva-guṇa, the greater the approach to the condition of Pure Consciousness. Similarly, the function of Tamas Guṇa is to suppress or *veil* consciousness. The function of Rajas Guṇa is to *make active*—that is, it works on Tamas to suppress Sattva, or on Sattva to suppress Tamas.[5] The

---

[1] Kṛteh prārambho yasyāh. That is, by which creation (Sṛṣṭi,) maintenance (Sthiti), and dissolution (Laya) are done (Prakriyate kāryādikaṁ anayā).

[2] See Satyānanda's Comm. on 4th Mantra of Īśa Up. " The changeless Brahman which is consciousness appears in creation as Māyā which is Brahman (Brahmamayī) consciousness (Cidrūpiṇī), holding in Herself unbeginning (Anādi) Kārmik tendencies (Karma-saṁskāra) in the form of the three Guṇas. Hence She is Guṇamayī despite being Cinmayī. And as there is no second principle these Guṇas are Cit-Śakti."

[3] The three Guṇas *are* Prakṛti. The Devī, as in the form of Prakṛti, is called Triguṇātmikā (who is composed of the three Guṇas). All nature which issues from Her, the Great Cause (Mahā-kāraṇa-svarūpā), is also composed of the same Guṇās in different states of relation.

[4] See an article of mine in the *Indian Philosophical Review*, " Śakti and Māyā," reproduced in " Śakti and Śākta ".

[5] In the words of Professor P. Mukhyopadhyaya, dealing with the matter monistically, these are the three elements of the Life Stress on the surface of pure Consciousness—namely, presentation (Sattva), movement (Rajas), and veiling (Tamas), which are the three elements of creative evolution (" The Patent Wonder," p. 19).

object and the effect of evolution, as it is of all Sādhana, is to develop Sattva-guṇa. The Guṇas always co-exist in everything, but variously predominate. The lower the descent is made in the scale of nature the more Tamas Guṇa prevails, as in so-called "brute substance," which has been supposed to be altogether inert. The higher the ascent is made the more Sattva prevails. The truly Sāttvik man is a divine man, his temperament being called in the Tantras Divyabhāva.[1] Through Sattva-guṇa passage is made to Sat, which is Cit or pure Consciousness, by the Siddha-yogī, who is identified with Pure Spirit.

Prakṛti exists in two states, in one of which (so far as any effect is concerned)[2] She is quiescent. The Guṇas are then in stable equilibrium, and not affecting one another. There is no manifestation. This is the unmanifest (Avyakta), the potentiality of natural power (*naturą naturans*).[3] When, however, owing to the ripening of Karma, the time for creation takes place, there is a stirring of the Guṇas (Guṇakṣoba) and an initial vibration (Spandana), known in the Mantra-Śāstra as Cosmic Sound (Śabda-brahman). The Guṇas affect one another, and the universe made of these three Guṇas is created. The products of Prakṛti thus evolved are called Vikāra or Vikṛti.[4] Vikṛti is manifest (Vyakta) Prakṛti (*natura*

---

[1] Those in whom Rajas Guṇa is predominant, and who work that Guṇa to suppress Tamas, are Vīra (hero), and the man in whom the Tamas Guṇa prevails is a Paśu (animal).

[2] The three Guṇas are essentially changeful. Nāpariṇamya kṣaṇamapyavatiṣṭhante guṇāh (the guṇās do not remain for a moment without movement). Vācaspati-Miśra: Sāṁkhya-Tattva-Kaumudī, 16th Kārikā. The movement is twofold: (*a*) Sarūpa-pariṇāma or Sadṛśa-pariṇāma is dissolution, and (*b*) Virūpapariṇāma is evolution.

[3] This is, in fact the definition of Prakṛti as opposed to Vikṛti, Sattvarajastamasāṁ sāṁyāvasthā prakṛtih. Sāṁkhya-Kaumudī-Kārikā, 3; Sāṁkhya-Pravacana, I. 61.

[4] Vikāra or Vikṛti is something which is really changed, as milk into curd. The latter is a Vikṛti of the former. Vivarta is apparent

naturata). In the infinite and formless Prakṛti there appears a strain or stress appearing as form. On the relaxation of this strain in dissolution forms disappear in formless Prakṛti, who as manifested power (Śakti) re-enters the Brahman-Consciousness. These Vikṛtis are the Tattvas issuing from Prakṛti,[1] the Avidyā-Śakti—namely, the different categories of Mind, Senses and Matter.

The bodies are threefold: causal (Kāraṇa-śarīra, or Paraśarīra, as the Śaivas call it), subtle (Sūkṣma-śarīra), and gross (Sthūla-śarīra). These bodies in which the Ātmā is enshrined are evolved from Prakṛti-Śakti, and are constituted of its various productions. They form the tabernacle of the Spirit (Ātmā), which as the Lord is "in all beings, and who from within all beings controls them".[2] The body of the Lord (Īśvara) is pure Sattva-guṇa (Śuddha-sattva-guṇa-pradhāna).[3] This is the aggregate Prakṛti

---

but unreal change, such as the appearance of what was and is a rope as a snake. The Vedānta-sāra thus musically defines the two terms:

Satattvato's nyathāprathā vikāra ityudīritah
Atattvato's nyathāprathā vivarta ityudīritah.

Under V. 40, on page 422 *post*, the commentator speaks of Vikṛti as a reflection (Prati-biṁbatā) of Prakṛti. It is Prakṛti modified.

[1] As already explained, there are Tattvas which precede the Puruṣa-Prakṛti-Tattvas. Etymologically Tattva is an abstract derivation from pronoun "Tat" (that), or Thatness, and may, it has been pointed out, be compared with the Hæcceitas of Duns Scotus. The Tattva in a general sense is Truth or Brahman. But in the Sāṁkhya it has a technical sense, being employed as a concrete term to denote the eight "producers," the sixteen "productions," and the twenty-fifth Tattva or Puruṣa.

[2] Yah sarveṣu bhūteṣū tiṣṭhan: yah sarvāṇi bhūtānī antaro yamayati (Brih. Up., iii. 7, 15). The Jīva is in Māyāvāda thus Caitanya-rūpa with the Upādhi ajñāna and its effects, mind and body, and which is Abhimānin, or attributor to itself, of the waking, dreaming and slumber states.

[3] Śaṁkāra's Bhāṣya, II. 3-45. The Jīva is Caitanya distinguished by Upādhi. The latter term means distinguishing property, attribute, body, etc., and here body (Deha), senses (Indriya), mind (Manas, Buddhi), etc. (*ib.*, I. 2-6).

or Māyā of Him or Her as the Creator-Creatrix of all things. Jīva, as the Kulārṇava-Tantra[1] says, is bound by the bonds (Pāśa); Sadāśiva is free of them.[2] The former is Paśu, and the latter Paśupati, or Lord of Paśus (Jīvas). That is, Īśvarī[3] is not affected by Her own Māyā. She is all-seeing, all-knowing, all-powerful. Īśvara thus rules Māyā. Jīva is ruled by it. From this standpoint the Mother and Her child the Jīva are not, thus, the same. For the latter is a limited consciousness subject to error, and governed by that Māyā-śakti of Hers which makes the world seem to be different from what it in its essence is. The body of Jīva is therefore known as the individual Prakṛti or Avidya, in which there is impure Sattva, and Rajas and Tamas (Malina-sattva-guṇa-pradhāna). But in the Mother are all creatures. And so in the Triśatī[4] the Devī is called "in the form of one and many letters" (Ekānekākṣarākṛti). As Ekā She is the Ajñāna which is pure Sattva and attribute (Upādhi) of Īśvara; as Anekā She is Upādhi or vehicle of Jīva. Whilst Īśvara is one, Jīvas are many,[5] according to the diversity in the nature of the individual Prakṛti caused by the appearance of Rajas and Tamas in it in differing proportions. The Ātmā appears as Jīva in the various forms of the vegetable, animal, and human worlds.

The first or *Causal Body* of any particular Jīva, therefore, is that Prakṛti (Avidya-Śakti) which is the cause of the subtle and gross bodies of this Jīva which are evolved from it. This body lasts until Liberation, when the Jīvātmā

---

[1] Kulārṇava-Tantra.

[2] Pāśa-baddho bhavej jīvah pāśa-muktah sadāśivah (Kulārṇava-Tantra, IX. 48), upon which the author of the Prāṇa-toṣiṇī, who cites this passage, says: "Thus the identity of Śiva and Jīva is shown" (iti śivajīvayor aikyaṁ uktāṁ).

[3] Feminine of Īśvara. Some worship Śiva, some Devī. Both are one.

[4] Comm. by Śaṁkạra on v. 23.

[5] According to another Vedāntic view there is only one Jīva.

ceases to be such and is the Paramātmā or bodiless Spirit (Videha-mukti). The Jīva exists in this body during *dreamless sleep* (Suṣupti).

The second and third bodies are the differentiations through evolution of the causal body, from which first proceeds the subtle body, and from the latter is produced the gross body.

The *Subtle Body*, which is also called Linga Śarīra or Puryaṣṭaka, is constituted of the first evolutes (Vikṛti) from the causal Prakṛtic body—namely, the Mind (Antah-karaṇa), the internal instrument, together with the external instruments (Bāhya-karaṇa), or the Senses (Indriya), and their supersensible objects (Tanmātra).

The third or *Gross Body* is the body of "matter" which is the gross particular object of the senses [1] derived from the supersensibles.

Shortly, the subtle body may be described as the Mental Body, as that which succeeds is called the gross body of Matter. Mind is abstractedly considered by itself, that is, as dissociated from Consciousness which is never the case, an unconscious force which breaks up into particulars the Experience-Whole which is Cit. It is called the "working within" or "internal instrument" (Antah-karaṇa), and is one only, but is given different names to denote the diversity of its functions.[2] The Sāṁkhya thus speaks of Buddhi, Ahaṁkāra, Manas, to which the Vedānta adds Citta, being different aspects or attributes (Dharma) of Mind as displayed in the psychical processes by which the Jīva knows, feels and wills.

These may be considered from the point of view of evolution—that is, according to the sequence in which the

[1] The definition of a Bhūta (sensible matter) is that which can be seen by the outer organ, such as the eye, ear, and so forth.

[2] Sāṁkhya-Pravacana-Sūtra, II. 16. See "Mind" in "The World As Power".

limited experience of the Jīva is evolved—or from that in which they are regarded after creation, when the experience of concrete sense objects has been had. According to the former aspect, Buddhi or Mahat-Tattva is the state of mere presentation; consciousness of being only, without thought of " I " (Ahaṃkāra), and unaffected by sensations of particular objects (Manas and Indriyas). It is thus the impersonal Jīva Consciousness. Ahaṁkāra, of which Buddhi is the basis, is the personal consciousness which realizes itself as a particular " I," the experiencer. The Jīva, in the order of creation, first experiences in a vague general way without consciousness of the self, like the experience which is had immediately on waking after sleep. It then refers this experience to the limited self, and has the consciousness " I am So-and-so ".

Manas is the desire which follows on such experience, and the Senses (Indriya) and their objects are the means whereby that enjoyment is had which is the end of all will to life. Whilst, however, in the order of evolution Buddhi is the first principle, in the actual working of the Antahkaraṇa after creation has taken place, it comes last.

It is more convenient, therefore, to commence with the sense-objects and the sensations they evoke. The experiencer is affected by Matter in five different ways, giving rise in him to the sensations of hearing, touch and feel,[1] colour and form [2] and sight, taste, and smell.[3] But sensible

---

[1] See *post*; also section on Matter, in " The World As Power ".

[2] Rūpa is primarily colour. By means of colour form is perceived, for a perfectly colourless thing is not perceivable by the gross senses.

[3] The other objects of the senses are the speakable, prehensible, approachable, excitable (that which is within the genitals), and excretable. " Each sense is suited to a particular class of influences—touch to solid pressure, hearing to aerial pressure, taste to liquid, light to luminous rays." (Bain: " Mind and body," p. 22, 1892.)

See Sāṁkhya-Pravacana-Sūtra, II. 26-28, 40: Sāṁkhya-Tattva-Kaumudī, 27 Kārikā.

perception exists only in respect of particular objects and is thus perceived in its variations only. But there exist also general elements of the particulars of sense-perception. That general ideas may be formed of particular sense-objects, indicates, it is said,[1] their existence in some parts of the Jīva's nature as facts of experience; otherwise the generals could not be formed from the particulars given by the senses as the physical facts of experience. This general is called a Tanmātra, which means the "mere thatness" or abstract quality, of an object. Thus, the Tanmātra of a sound (Śabda-tanmātra) is not any particular sensible form of it, but the "thatness" of that sound—that is, that sound apart from any of its particular variations stated. The Tanmātras have, therefore, aptly been called the "generals of the sense particulars"[2]—that is, the general elements of sense perception. These necessarily come into existence when the senses (Indriya) are produced; for a sense necessitates something which can be the object of sensation. These Sūkṣma (subtle) Bhūtas, as they are also called, are not ordinarily themselves perceived, for they are supersensible (Atīndriya). Their existence is only mediately perceived through the gross particular objects of which they are the generals, and which proceed from them. They can be the objects of immediate (Pratyakṣa) perception only to Yogīs.[3] They are, like the gross sense-objects derived from them, five in number, namely, sound (Śabda-tanmātra), touch and feel[4] (Sparśa-tanmātra), colour and form (Rūpa-tanmātra), flavour (Rasa-tanmātra), and odour (Gandha-tanmātra) as

[1] See for this in greater detail J. C. Chatterji's "Kashmir Śaivaism."

[2] *Ib.*, see *post.*

[3] So it is said: Tāni vastūni tanmātrādīni pratyakṣa-viṣayāṇi (that is, to Yogīs).

[4] Whereby the thermal quality of things is perceived.

universals. Each of these evolves from that which precedes it.[1]

Sensations aroused by sense-objects are experienced by means of the outer instruments (Bāhya-karaṇa) of the Lord of the body, or senses (Indriya), which are the gateways through which the Jīva receives worldly experience. These are ten in number, and are of two classes: *viz.*, the five organs of sensation or perception (Jñānendriya), or ear (hearing), skin (feeling by touch), eye (sight), tongue (taste), and nose (smell); and the five organs of action (Karmendriya), which are the reactive response which the self makes to sensation—namely, mouth, hands, legs, anus, and genitals, whereby speaking, grasping, walking, excretion, and procreation are performed, and through which effect is given to the Jīva's desires. These are afferent and efferent impulses respectively.

The Indriya, or sense, is not the physical organ, but the faculty of mind operating through that organ as its instrument. The outward sense-organs are the usual means whereby on the physical plane the functions of hearing and so forth are accomplished. But as they are mere instruments and their power is derived from the mind, a Yogī may accomplish by the mind only all that may be done by means of these physical organs without the use of the latter.

With reference to their physical manifestations, but not as they are in themselves, the classes into which the Indriyas are divided may be described as the sensory and motor nervous systems. As the Indriyas are not the physical organs, such as ear, eye, and so forth, but faculties of the Jīva desiring to know and act by their aid, the Yogī claims to accomplish

[1] In a general way the last four correspond with the Vaiśeṣika Paramāṇus. There are differences, however. Thus, the latter are eternal (Nitya) and do not proceed from one another.

without the use of the latter all that is ordinarily done by their means. So a hypnotized subject can perceive things, even when no use of the special physical organs ordinarily necessary for the purpose is made.[1] The fact of there being a variety of actions does not necessarily involve the same number of Indriyas. An act of "going" done by means of the hand (as by a cripple) is to be regarded really as an operation of the Indriya of feet (Pādendriya), even though the hand is the seat of the Indriya for handling.[2] By the instrumentality of these Indriyas things are perceived and action is taken with reference to them. The Indriyas are not, however, sufficient in themselves for this purpose. In the first place, unless attention (Ālocana) co-operates there is no sensation at all. To be "absent-minded" is not to know what is happening.[3] Attention must therefore co-operate with the senses before the latter can "give" the experiencer anything at all.[4] Nextly, at one and the same moment the experiencer is subject to receive a countless number of sensations which come to and press upon him from all sides. If any of these is to be brought into the field of consciousness, it must be selected to the exclusion of others. The process of experience is the selection of a special section from out of a general whole, and then being engaged on it, so as to make it one's own, either as a particular object of thought or a particular field of operation.[5] Lastly, as Western psychology holds, the senses give not a completed whole, but a manifold—the manifold of sense. These

[1] See "Kashmir Śaivaism," by J. C. Chatterji, p. 120. Thus Professor Lombroso records the case of a woman who, being blind, read with the tip of her ear, tasted with her knees, and smelt with her toes.

[2] Tantrasāra Āhnika, 8.

[3] See "Kashmir Śaivaism," p. 112.

[4] So in the Bṛhadāraṇayaka-Upaniṣad, I. 3-27, it is said: "My Manas (mind) was diverted elsewhere. Therefore I did not hear."

[5] So, in the Text here translated *post*, Manas is spoken of as a doorkeeper who lets some enter, and keeps others outside.

"points of sensation" must be gathered together and made into a whole. These three functions of attention, selection, and synthesizing the discrete manifold of the senses, are those belonging to that aspect of the mental body, the internal agent (Antah-karaṇa), called Manas.[1] Just as Manas is necessary to the senses (Indriya), the latter are necessary for Manas. For the latter is the seat of desire, and cannot exist by itself. It is the desire to perceive or act, and therefore exists in association with the Indriyas.

Manas is thus the leading Indriya, of which the senses are powers. For without the aid and attention of Manas the other Indriyas are incapable of performing their respective offices; and as these Indriyas are those of perception and action, Manas, which co-operates with both, is said to partake of the character of both cognition and action.

Manas, through association with the eye or other sense, becomes manifold, being particularized or differentiated by its co-operation with that particular instrument, which cannot fulfil its functions except in conjunction with Manas.

Its function is said to be Saṁkalpa-Vikalpa, that is, selection and rejection from the material provided by the Jñānendriya. When, after having been brought into contact with the sense-objects, it selects the sensation which is to be presented to the other faculties of the mind, there is Saṁkalpa. The activity of Manas, however, is itself neither intelligent result nor moving feelings of pleasure or pain. It has not an independent power to reveal itself to the experiencer. Before things can be so revealed and realized as objects of perception, they must be made subject to the operation of Ahaṁkāra and Buddhi, without whose intelligent light they would be dark

---

[1] See "Kashmir Śaivaism," pp. 94-114. This is the Sāṁkhyan and Vedāntic definition. According to the Vaiśeṣika, Manas is that which gives knowledge of pleasure, pain, and Jīvātmā (I am So-and-so).

forms unseen and unknown by the experiencer, and the efforts of Manas but blind gropings in the dark. Nor can the images built up by Manas affect of themselves the experiencer so as to move him in any way until and unless the experiencer identifies himself with them by Ahaṁkāra—that is, by making them his own in feeling and experience. Manas, being thus an experience of activity in the dark, unseen and unrevealed by the light of Buddhi and not moving the experiencer until he identifies himself with it in feeling, is one in which the dark veiling quality (Tamas-guṇa) of Śakti Prakṛti is the most manifest.[1] This Guṇa also prevails in the Indriyas and the subtle objects of their operation (Tanmātra).

Ahaṁkāra the "I-maker" is self-arrogation[2]—that is, the realization of oneself as the personal "I" or self-consciousness of worldly experience in which the Jīva thinks of himself as a particular person who is in relation with the objects of his experience. It is the power of self-arrogation whereby all that constitutes man is welded into one Ego, and the percept or concept is referred to that particular thinking subject and becomes part of its experience. When, therefore, a sensation is perceived by Manas and determined by Buddhi, Ahaṁkāra says: "It is I who perceive it."

This is the "I" of phenomenal consciousness as distinguished from "this" the known. Buddhi functions with its support.[3] Buddhi considered with relation to the other faculties of experience is that aspect of the Antah-karaṇa

---

[1] See "Kashmir Śaivaism," p. 116, where the author cites the dictum of Kant that perceptions (Anschauung) without conceptions are blind.

[2] Abhimāna. Abhimānoऽhaṁkārah. See Sāṁkhya-Tattva-Kaumudī, 24 Kārikā, and Bk. II, Sūtra 16, Sāṁkhya-Pravacana-Sūtra.

[3] Taṁ ahaṁkāraṁ upajīvya hi buddhir adhyavasyati (Sāṃkhya-Tattva-Kaumudī), *supra*.

which determines (Adhyavasāyātmikā buddhih).[1] "A man is said to determine (Adhyavasyati) who, having perceived (Manas), and thought, 'I am concerned in this matter (Ahaṁkāra)' and thus having self-arrogated, comes to the determination, 'This must be done by me' (Kartavyaṁ etat mayā)."[2] "Must be done" here does not refer to exterior action only, but to mental action (Mānasī-kriyā) also, such as any determination by way of the forming of concepts and percepts ("It is so") and resolutions ("It must be done"). Buddhi pervades all effects whatever other than itself. It is the principal Tattva because it pervades all the instruments (Indriya), is the receptacle of all the Saṁskāras or Kārmic tendencies, and is in Sāṁkhya the seat of memory.[3] It is the thinking principle which forms concepts or general ideas acting through the instrumentality of Ahaṁkāra, Manas and the Indriyas. In the operations of the senses Manas is the principal; in the operation of Manas Ahaṁkāra is the principal; and in the operation of Ahaṁkāra Buddhi is the principal. With the instrumentality of all of these Buddhi acts, modifications taking place in Buddhi through the instrumentality of the sense functions.[4] It is Buddhi which is the basis of all cognition, sensation, and resolves, and makes over objects to Puruṣa, that is, Consciousness. And so it is said that Buddhi, whose characteristic is determination, is the charioteer; Manas, whose characteristic is Saṁkalpa-vikalpa, is the reins; and the Senses are the horses. Jīva is the Enjoyer (Bhoktā), that is, Ātmā conjoined with body,

---

[1] Sāṁkhya-Pravacana, II. 13. The Sūtra has Adhyavasāyo buddhih; but the Commentator points out that Buddhi is not to be identified with its functions. Buddhi is thus called Niścayakāriṇī.

[2] Sāṁkhya-Tattva-Kaumudī 23rd Kārikā: Sarva vyavahartā ālocya mattvā ahaṁ atrādhikṛta ityabhimatya kartavyaṁ etat mayā iti adhyavasyati.

[3] Sāṁkhya-Pravacana, II. 40-44.

[4] *Ibid.*, 45, 39.

senses, Manas and Buddhi.[1] In Buddhi Sattva-guṇa predominates; in Ahaṁkāra, Rajas, in Manas and the Indriyas and their objects, Tamas.

Citta[2] in its special sense is that faculty (Vṛtti) by which the Mind first recalls to memory (Smaraṇaṁ) that of which there has been previously Anubhava or pratyakṣa Jñāna—that is, immediate cognition. This Smaraṇaṁ exists only to the extent of actual Anubhava. For remembrance is the equivalent of, and neither more nor less than, what has been previously known;[3] remembrance being the calling up of that. Cintā, again, is that faculty whereby the current of thought dwells, thinks and contemplates upon (Cintā)[4] the subject so recalled by Smaraṇaṁ, and previously known and determined by Buddhi. For such meditation (Dhyāna) is done through the recall and fixing the mind upon past percepts and concepts. According to Vedānta, Buddhi determines but once only, and the further recall and thought upon the mental object so determined is the faculty of the separate mental category called Citta. Sāṁkhya, on the principle of economy of categories, regards Smaraṇaṁ and Cintā to be functions of Buddhi.[5] In the works here translated and elsewhere Citta is, however, currently used as a general term for the working mind—that is, as a synonym for the Antahkaraṇa.[6]

---

[1] Śaṁkara's Commentary on Kaṭhopaniṣad, 3rd Valli, 4th Mantra: Ātmendriyamanoyuktaṁ bhokteyāhur manīṣiṇah; and see Sāṁkhya-Pravacana, II. 47.

[2] Cetati anena iti cittaṁ.

[3] So the Pātañjala-Sūtra says: Anubhūta-viṣayāsaṁpramoṣah smṛtih (Nothing is taken away from the object perceived).

[4] Anusaṁdhānātmikā antahkaraṇa-vṛttir iti vedāntah. (It is the faculty of the Antahkaraṇa which investigates in the Vedānta.)

[5] Sāṁkhya-śāstre ca cintāvṛttikasya cittasya buddhāvevāntarbhāvah. (In the Sāṁkhya-Śāstra, Citta, the function of which is Cintā, is included in Buddhi, I. 64.)

[6] Cittaṁ antahkaraṇa-sāmānyaṁ (Citta is the Antahkaraṇa in general): Sāṁkhya-Pravacana-Bhāṣya.

To sum up the functions of the subtle body: the sense-objects (Bhūta, derived from Tanmātra) affect the senses (Indriya) and are perceived by Manas, are referred to the self by Ahaṁkāra, and are determined by Buddhi. The latter in its turn is illumined by the light of Consciousness (Cit), which is the Puruṣa; all the principles (Tattva) up to and including Buddhi being modifications of apparently unconscious Prakṛti. Thus all the Tattvas work for the enjoyment of the Self or Puruṣa. They are not to be regarded as things existing independently by themselves, but as endowments of the Spirit (Ātmā). They do not work arbitrarily as they will, but represent an organized co-operative effort in the service of the Enjoyer, the Experiencer or Puruṣa.

The subtle body is thus composed of what are called the "17," *viz.*, Buddhi (in which Ahaṁkāra is included), Manas, the ten senses (Indriya), and the five Tanmātras. No special mention is made of Prāṇa or Vital Principle by the Sāṁkhya, by which it is regarded as a modification of the Antahkaraṇa, and as such is implicity included. The Māyāvādins insert the Prāṇa pentad instead of the Tanmātra.[1]

The Jīva lives in his subtle or mental body alone when in the *dreaming* (Svapna) state. For the outside world of objects (Mahā-bhūta) is then shut out and the consciousness wanders in the world of ideas. The subtle body or soul is imperishable until Liberation is attained, when the Jīvātmā or seemingly conditioned consciousness ceases to be such and is the Supreme Consciousness or Paramātmā, Nirguṇa-Śiva. The subtle body thus survives the dissolution of the gross body of matter, from which it goes

---

[1] Sāṁkhya-Pravacana-Sūtra, III. 9. See Chapter on 'Power As Life' in "The World As Power".

forth (Utkramaṇa), and "reincarnates"[1] (to use an English term) until Liberation (Mukti). The Linga-śarīra is not all-pervading (Vibhu), for in that case it would be eternal (Nitya) and could not act (Kriyā). But it moves and goes (Gati). Since it is not Vibhu, it must be limited (Paricchinna) and of atomic dimension (Aṇu-parimāṇa). It is indirectly dependent on food. For though the material body is the food-body (Annamaya), Mind is dependent on it when associated with the gross body. Mind in the subtle body bears the Saṁskāras which are the result of past actions. This subtle body is the cause of the third or gross body.

The whole process of evolution is due to the presence of the will to life and enjoyment, which is a result of Vāsanā, or world-desire, carried from life to life in the Saṁskāras, or impressions made on the subtle body by Karma, which is guided by Īśvara. In its reaching forth to the world, the Self is not only endowed with the faculties of the subtle body, but with the gross objects of enjoyment on which those faculties feed. There, therefore, comes into being, as a projection of the Power (Śakti) of Consciousness, the *gross body* of matter called Sthūla-Śarīra.

The word Śarīra comes from the root "*Śṛ*" to decay; for the gross body is at every moment undergoing molecular birth and death until Prāṇa, or vitality, leaves the organism, which, as such, is dissolved. The Soul (Jīvātmā) is, when it leaves the body, no longer concerned therewith. There is no such thing as the resurrection of the same body. It turns to dust and the Jīva when it reincarnates does so in a new

[1] This is transmigration or pretyabhāva, which means "the arising again and again"—punarutpattih pretya bhāvah, as Gautama says. Pretya=having died, and Bhāva="the becoming (born into the world) again". "Again" implies habitualness: birth, then death, then birth, and so on, until final emancipation which is Mokṣa, or Apavarga (release), as the Nyāya calls it.

body, which is nevertheless, like the last, suited to give effect to its Karma.

The Sthūla-Śarīra, with its three Doṣas, six Kośas, seven Dhātus, ten Fires, and so forth,[1] is the perishable body composed of compounds of five forms of gross sensible matter (Mahā-bhūta), which is ever decaying, and is at the end dissolved into its constituents at death.[2] This is the Vedāntik body of food (Annamaya-Kośa), so called because it is maintained by food which is converted into chyle (Rasa), blood, flesh, fat, bone, marrow and seed-components of the gross organism. The Jīva lives in this body when in the *waking* (Jāgrat) state.

The human, physical, or gross body is, according to Western science, composed of certain compounds of which the chief are water, gelatine, fat, phosphate of lime, albumen, and fibrin, and of these water constitutes some two-thirds of the total weight. These substances are composed of simpler non-metallic and metallic elements, of which the chief are oxygen (to the extent of about two-thirds), hydrogen, carbon, nitrogen, calcium, and phosphorus. Again, to go one step farther back, though the alleged indestructibility of the elements and their atoms is still said by some to present the character of a "practical truth", well-known recent experiments go to re-establish the ancient hypothesis of a single Primordial Substance to which these various forms of matter may be reduced, with the resultant of the possible and hitherto derided transmutation of one element into another; since each is but one of the plural manifestations of the same underlying unity.

---

[1] See Introduction to my edition of Prapañcasāra-Tantra, Vol. III, "Tāntrik Texts".

[2] Decay and death are two of the six Ūrmis which, with hunger and thirst, grief and ignorance, are characteristics of the body (Deha-dharma): Prapañcasāra-Tantra, II.

Recent scientific research has shown that this original substance cannot be scientific " matter "—that is, that which has mass, weight and inertia. Matter has been dematerialized and reduced, according to current hypotheses, to something which differs profoundly from " matter " as known by the senses. This ultimate substance is stated to be Ether in a state of motion. The present scientific hypothesis would appear to be as follows: The ultimate and simplest physical factor from which the universe has arisen is motion of and in a substance called " Ether," which is not scientific " matter ". The motions of this substance give rise from the realistic point of view to the notion of " matter ". Matter is thus at base one, notwithstanding the diversity of its forms. Its ultimate element is on the final analysis of one kind, and the differences in the various kinds of matter depend on the various movements of the ultimate particle and its succeeding combinations. Given such unity of base, it is possible that one form of matter may pass into another. The Indian theory here described agrees with the Western speculations to which we have referred, that what the latter calls scientific or ponderable matter does not permanently exist, but says that there are certain motions or forces (five in number) which produce solid matter, and which are ultimately reducible to ether (Ākāśa). Ākāśa, however, and scientific " Ether " are not in all respects the same. The latter is an ultimate substance, not " matter," having vibratory movements and affording the medium for the transmission of light. Ākāśa is one of the gross forces into which the Primordial Power (Prakṛti-Śakti) differentiates itself. Objectively considered it is a vibration [1] in and of the

---

[1] It is Spanda-naśīla (vibratory), according to Sāṁkhya; for the products share the character of the original vibrating Prakṛti, and these products are not, like Prakṛti itself, all-pervading (Vibhu). The Vaiśeṣika-Sūtrakāra regards it as a motionless, colourless (Nīrūpa)

substance of Prakṛti of which it is a transformation in which the other forces are observed to be operating. Lastly, Ākāśa is not an ultimate, but is itself derived from the supersensible Tanmātra, with its quality (Guṇa) whereby Ākāśa affects the senses; and this Tanmātra is itself derived from the mental I-making principle (Ahaṁkāra), or personal consciousness produced from the superpersonal Jīva-consciousness as such (Buddhi), emanating from the root-energy, or Prakṛti-Śakti, the cause and basis of all forms of " material " force or substance. At the back of both " matter " and mind, there is the creative energy (Śakti) of the Supreme who is the cause of the universe and Consciousness itself.

Matter affects the Jīva in five different ways, giving rise in him to the sensations of smell, taste, sight, touch and feel, and hearing.

As already explained, the Tanmātras are supersensible, being abstract qualities, whilst the senses perceive their variations in particular objects only. These sense particulars are produced from the generals or Universals.

From the Śabda-Tanmātra and from the combinations of the latter with the other Tanmātras are produced the gross Bhūtas (Mahā-bhūta), which as things of physical magnitude perceivable by the senses approach the Western definition of discrete sensible " matter ". These five Mahā-bhūtas are Ākāśa (Ether), Vāyu (Air), Tejas (Fire), Āpas (Water) and Pṛthivī (Earth). Their development takes place from the Tanmātra, from one unit of that which is known in sensible matter as mass (Tamas), charged with energy (Rajas) by the gradual accretion of mass and redistribution of energy. The result of this is that each Bhūta is more gross than that which

continuum (Sarva-vyāpī). It is not an effect and is Vibhu, therefore it cannot vibrate (Gatikriyā). The Commentators argue that, as it is a Dravya or thing, it must possess the general quality (Dharma) of Dravya or Kṛyā—that is, action. See Chapter on ' Power As Matter ' in " The World As Power ".

precedes it until "Earth" is reached. These five Bhūtas have no connection with the English "elements" so called, nor, indeed, are they elements at all, being derived from the Tanmātras. Dynamically and objectively considered they are (proceeding from Ākāśa) said to be five forms of motion, into which Prakṛti differentiates itself: *viz.*, non-obstructive, all-directed motion radiating lines of force in all directions, symbolized as the "Hairs of Śiva"[1] affording the space (Ākāśa) in which the other forces operate; transverse motion[2] and locomotion in space (Vāyu); upward motion giving rise to expansion (Tejas); downward motion giving rise to contraction (Āpas); and that motion which produces cohesion, its characteristic of obstruction being the opposite of the non-obstructive ether in which it exists and from which it and the other Tattvas spring. The first is sensed by hearing through its quality (Guṇa) of sound (Śabda);[3] the second by touch through resistance and feeling;[4] the third by sight as colour;[5] the fourth by taste through flavour; and the fifth by the sense of smell through its odour, which is produced by matter only in so far as it partakes of the solid state.[6]

---

[1] "Kashmir Śaivaism," p. 132, where it is suggested that the lines of the magnetic field are connected with the lines of Dik (direction) as the lines of ethereal energy.

[2] Vāyu, as the Prapañcasāra-Tantra says, is characterized by motion (Calanapara). The Saṁskrit root Vā=to move. See Suśruta, Vol. II, p. 2, ed. Kavirāj Kuñjalala Bhiṣagratna.

[3] According to Western notions, it is the air which is the cause of sound. According to Indian notions, Ether is the substratum (Āśraya) of sound, and Air (Vāyu) is a helper (Sahakārī) in its manifestation.

[4] Touch is not here used in the sense of all forms of contact, for form and solidity are not yet developed, but such particular contact as that by which is realized the thermal quality of things.

[5] Fire is the name or that action which builds and destroys shapes.

[6] All matter in the solid state (Pārthiva) giving rise to smell is in the state of earth—*e.g.*, metals, flowers, etc.

The hard and stable obstructive " earth " is that which is smelt, tasted, seen, and touched, and which exists in space which is known by hearing—that is, the sounds in it. The smooth " water " is that which is tasted, seen, and touched in space. " Fire " is what is seen and touched —that is, felt as temperature—in space. " Air " is what is so felt in space. And sound which is heard is that by which the existence of the " Ether " is known. These Bhūtas when compounded make up the material universe. Each thing therein being thus made of all the Bhūtas, we find in the Tantras that form, colour and sound, are related, a truth which is of deep ritual significance. Thus, each of the sounds of speech or music has a corresponding form, which have now been made visible to the eye by the Phonoscope.[1] Thus the deaf may perceive sounds by the eye, just as by the Optophone and blind may read by means of the ear.

In the same Śāstra various colours and figures (Maṇḍalas) are assigned to the Tattvas to denote them. Ākāśa is represented by a transparent white circular diagram in which, according to some accounts, there are dots (Cidra = hole), thus displaying the interstices which Ākāśa produces; for Ākāśa, which is all-pervading, intervenes between each of the Tattvas which are evolved from it.

Vāyu is denoted by a smoky grey, six-cornered diagram;[2] Tejas, red, triangular diagram; Āpas, white, crescent-shaped diagram; and Pṛthivī, yellow, quadrangular diagram

---

[1] When words are spoken or sung into a small trumpet attached to the instrument, a revolving disk appears to break up into a number of patterns, which vary with the variations in sound.

[2] See as to this and other diagrams the coloured plates of the Cakras.

which, as the superficial presentation of the cube, well denotes the notion of solidity.

Similarly, to each Devatā also there is assigned a Yantra, or diagram, which is a suggestion of the form assumed by the evolving Prakṛti or body of that particular Consciousness.

The gross body is, then, a combination of the compounds of those Mahā-bhūtas, derivable from the Ākāśa (" Ether ") Tattva.

The Bhūtas and the Tanmātras, as parts of these compounds, pervade the body, but particular Bhūtas are said to have centres of force in particular regions. Thus the centres (Cakra) of " Earth " and " Water " are the two lower ones in the trunk of the body. " Fire " predominates in the central abdominal region, and " Air " and " Ether " in the two higher centres in the heart and throat. These five Tanmātras, five Bhūtas, and the ten senses (Indriyas) which perceive them, are known as the twenty gross Tattvas which are absorbed in Yoga in the centres of the bodily trunk. The remaining four subtle mental Tattvas (Buddhi, Ahaṁkāra, Manas and Prakṛti) have their special centres of activity in the head. Again, the Bhūtas may be specially displayed in other portions of the bodily organism. Thus, Pṛthivī displays itself as bone or muscles; Āpas as urine and saliva; Tejas as hunger and thirst; Vāyu in grasping and walking. Fire is manifold, its great mystery being saluted by many names. So Tejas manifests both as light and heat, for, as Helmholtz says, the same object may affect the senses in different ways. The same ray of Sunshine, which is called light when it falls on the eyes, is called heat when it falls on the skin. Agni manifests in the household and umbilical fires; as Kāmāgni in the Mūlādhāra centre; in Badabā or submarine fire and in the " Lightning " of the Suṣumṇā in the spinal column.

Matter, thus exists in the five states etheric,[1] aerial,[2] fiery,[3] fluid,[4] and solid.[5] Pṛthivī does not denote merely what is popularly called "Earth". All solid (Pārthiva) odorous substance is in the Pṛthivī state. All substance in the fluid (Āpya) state is in the Āpas state, as everything which has cohesive resistance is in that of Pṛthivī. This latter, therefore, is the cohesive vibration, the cause of solidity, of which the common earth is a gross compounded form. All matter in the aerial (Vāyava) condition is in the Vāyu state. These are all primary differentiations of cosmic matter into a universe of subtly fine motion. The Tattvas regarded objectively evoke in the Indriyas smell, taste, sight, touch and hearing.

The gross body is thus a combination of the compounds of these Mahā-Bhūtas, derivable ultimately from Ether (Ākāśa), itself evolved in the manner described.

The gross and subtle bodies above described are vitalized and held together as an organism by Prāṇa, which is evolved from the active energy (Kriyā-Śakti) of the Liṅga Śarīra. Prāṇa, or the vital principle, is the special relation of the Ātmā with a certain form of matter which by this relation the Ātmā organizes and builds up as a means of having experience.[6] This special relation constitutes the

---

[1] All-pervading (Sarva-vyāpī), though relatively so in Sāṁkhya, and colourless (Nīrūpa). As to vibration, *v. ante*.

[2] With movements which are not straight (Tiryag-gamana-śīla).

[3] Illuminating (Prakāśa) and heating (Tāpa).

[4] Liquid (Tarala), moving (Calanaśīla). It has the quality of Sneha, whereby things can be rolled up into a lump (Piṇda), as moistened flour or earth. Some solids things become liquid for a time through heat; and others become solids, the Jāti (species) of which is still water (Jalatva).

[5] Without hollow, dense (Ghana), firm (Dṛḍha), combined (Saṁghata) and hard (Kaṭina).

[6] "Hindu Realism," p. 84. See Chapter on 'Power As Life' in "The World As Power".

individual Prāṇa in the individual body. The cosmic all-pervading Prāṇa is not Prāṇa in this gross sense, but is a name for the Brahman as the author of the individual Prāṇa. The individual Prāṇa is limited to the particular body which it vitalizes, and is a manifestation in all breathing creatures (Prāṇī) of the creative and sustaining activity of the Brahman, who is represented in individual bodies by the Devī Kuṇḍalinī.

All beings, whether Devatas, men, or animals, exist only so long as the Prāṇa is within the body. It is the life-duration of all.[1] What life is has been the subject of dispute in India as elsewhere.[2] The materialists of the Lokāyata school considered life to be the result of the chemical combinations of the elements, in the same manner as the intoxicating property of spirituous liquors results from the fermentation of unintoxicating rice and molasses, or as spontaneous generation was supposed to occur under the influence of gentle warmth. This is denied by the Sāṁkhya. Though Prāṇa and its fivefold functions are called Vāyu, Life, according to this school, is not a Vāyu in the sense of a mere biomechanical force, nor any mere mechanical motion resulting from the impulsion of such Vāyu.

According to the view of this school, Prāṇa, or vitality, is the common function of the mind and all the senses, both sensory (Jñānendriya) and motor (Karmendriya), which result in the bodily motion. Just as several birds when confined in one cage cause that cage to move by themselves moving, so the mind and senses cause the body to move while they are engaged in their respective activities. Life is, then, a resultant of the various concurrent activities of other principles or forces in the organism.

1 Kauśītakī Upaniṣad, 3-2.

2 See Chapter on ' Power As Life ' in " The World As Power ".

The Vedāntists agree in the view that the Prāṇa is neither Vāyu nor its operation, but deny that it is the mere resultant of the concomitant activities of the organism, and hold that it is a separate independent principle and "material" form assumed by the universal Consciousness. Life is therefore a subtle principle pervading the whole organism which is not gross Vāyu, but is all the same a subtle kind of apparently unconscious force, since everything which is not the Ātmā or Puruṣa is, according to Māyāvāda-Vedānta and Sāṁkhya, unconscious or, in Western parlance "material" (Jada).[1] The gross outer body is heterogeneous (Paricchinna) or made up of distinct or well-defined parts. On the other hand, the Prāṇamaya self which lies within the Annamaya self is a homogeneous undivided whole (Sādhāraṇa) permeating the whole physical body (Sarva-piṇḍa-vyāpin). It is not cut off into distinct regions (Asādhāraṇa) (as is the Piṇda, or microcosmic physical body. Unlike the latter, it has no specialized organs each discharging a specific function. It is a homogeneous unity (Sādhāraṇa) present in every part of the body, which it ensouls as its inner self. Vāyu[2] which courses through the body is the manifestation, self-begotten, the subtle, invisible, all-pervading, divine energy of eternal life. It is so called from the fact of its coursing throughout the universe. Invisible in itself, yet its operations are manifest. For it determines the birth, growth and decay of all animated organisms, and as such it receives the

[1] See Commentary on Taittirīya Upaniṣad, edited by Mahādeva-Śāstri and Appendix C, by Dr. Brojendra Nath Seal, to Professor B. K. Sarkar's "The Positive Background of Hindu Sociology," where some further authorities are given. By unconscious in Vedānta is meant that thing is an object of consciousness, not that it is unconscious in itself for all is essentially consciousness.

[2] In the sense of Prāṇa. The Sanskrit root vā=to move. See Suśruta, Vol. II, p. 2, ed. by Kavirāj Kuñjalāla Bhiṣagratna.

homage of all created beings. As vital Vāyu it is instantaneous in action, radiating as nerve force through the organism in constant currents. In its normal condition it maintains a state of equilibrium between the different Doṣas[1] and Dhātus,[1] or root principles of the body. The bodily Vāyu is divided, as are the principles called Pitta[1] and Kapha,[1] into five chief divisions according to the differences in location and function. Vāyu, known in its bodily aspect as Prāṇa, the universal force of vital activity, on entry into each individual is divided into tenfold functions (Vṛtti) of which five are chief. The first or breathing, bears the same name (Prāṇa) as that given to the force considered in its totality—the function whereby atmospheric air with its pervading vitality, which has been first drawn from without into the bodily system, is expired.[2]

On the physical plane Prāṇa manifests in the animal body as breath through inspiration (Sa), or Śakti, and expiration (Ha), or Śiva. Breathing is itself a Mantra, known as the Mantra which is not recited (Ajapā-mantra), for it is said without volition.[3]

The divine current is the motion of Ha and Sa. This motion, which exists on all the planes of life, is for the earth plane (Bhūrloka) created and sustained by the Sun, the

---

[1] See Introduction to third volume of "Tāntrik Texts," where these terms are explained. The Devatās of these Dhātus are Ḍākinī and the other Śaktis in the Cakras. See "The World As Power".

[2] The Vāyus have other functions than those mentioned. The matter is here stated only in a general way. See Suśruta-Saṁhitā, cited *ante*. Prāṇa is not the physical breath, which is a gross thing, but that function of vital force which exhibits itself in respiration.

[3] Thus the Niruttara-Tantra (Chapter IV) says:

> Haṁ-kāreṇa bahir yāti sah-kāreṇa viśet punah,
> Haṁseti paramaṁ mantraṁ jīvo japati sarvadā.

By Haṁkāra it goes out, and by Sahkāra it comes in again. A jīva always recites the Supreme Mantra Hamsah. See also Dhyāna-bindu Up.

solar breath of which is the cause of human breath with its centrifugal and centripetal movements, the counterpart in man of the cosmic movement of the Haṁsah or Śiva-Śakti-Tattvas, which are the soul of the Universe. The Sun is not only the centre and upholder of the solar system,[1] but the source of all available energy and of all physical life on earth. Accompanying the sunshine there proceeds from the orb a vast invisible radiation, the pre-requisite of all vegetable and animal life. It is these invisible rays which, according to science, sustain the mystery of all physical life. The Sun as the great luminary is the body of the Solar God, a great manifestation of the Inner Spiritual Sun.[2]

Apāna, the downward "breath" which pulls against Prāṇa, governs the excretory functions; Samāna kindles the bodily fire and governs the processes of digestion and assimilation; Vyāna, or diffused "breathing," is present throughout the body, effecting division and diffusion, resisting disintegration, and holding the body together in all its parts; and Udāna, the ascending Vāyu, is the so-called "upward breathing". Prāṇa is in the heart; Apāna in the anus; Samāna in the navel; Udāna in the throat; and Vyāna pervades the whole body.[3] By the words "navel" and so forth it is not meant that the vāyu is in the navel itself but in that region of the body so designated—the abdominal region and its

---

[1] The Sun is said to hold the vast bulk of the total matter of the solar system, while it only carries about 2 per cent of its movement of momentum.

[2] The Yoga works speak of the Moon-Cit (Ciccandra). It is this spiritual moon which is shown on the cover of this book, embraced by the Serpent Kuṇḍalinī.

[3] Amṛtanāda-Upaniṣad, vv. 34, 35—Ānandāśrama Edition. Vol. XXIX, p. 43; Śāṇḍilya Up., Ch. I. See also, as to Prāṇa, Ch. II, Prapañcasāra-Tantra. It is also said that Prāṇa is at the tip of the nostrils (Nāsāgra-varttī), and others are also said to be elsewhere. These localities denote special seats of function. See "The World As Power".

centre the Maṇipūra-Cakra. The five minor Vāyus are Nāga, Kūrma, Kṛkara, Devadatta, and Dhanaṁjaya, which manifest in hiccup, closing and opening the eyes, digestion,[1] yawning, and in that Vāyu "which leaves not even the corpse". The functions of Prāṇa may be scientifically defined as follows: Appropriation (Prāṇa), Rejection (Apāna), Assimilation (Samāna), Distribution (Vyāna), and Utterance (Udāna). The Prāṇa represents the involuntary reflex action of the organism and the Indriyas one aspect of its voluntary activity.

In the case of the individualised Prāṇa, or principle which vitalizes the animal organism during its earth life, it may be said, when regarded as an independent principle, to be a force more subtle than that which manifests as terrestrial matter which it vitalises. In other words, according to this theory, the Ātmā gives life to the earth organisms through the medium of terrestrial Prāṇa, which is one of the manifestations of that Energy which issues from and is at base the all-pervading Ātmā, as Śakti.

Ātmā as such has no states, but in worldly parlance we speak of such. So the Māṇdukya-Upaniṣad[2] speaks of the four aspects (Pāda) of the Brahman.

Caitanya, or Consciousness in bodies, is immanent in the individual and collective gross, subtle, and causal bodies, and transcends them. One and the same Cit pervades and transcends all things, but is given different names to mark its different aspects in the Jīva. Cit, being immutable, has itself no states; for states can only exist in the products of the changing Prakṛti-Śakti. From, however, the aspect of Jīva several states exist, which, though informed by the

[1] Kṣudhākara; lit., "appetite-maker".

[2] This Upaniṣad gives an analysis of the states of Consciousness on all planes, and should be studied in connection with Gaudapāda's Kārikā on the same subject with Śaṁkarācārya's Commentary on the latter.

same Cit, may from this aspect be called states of consciousness.[1]

In the manifested world, Consciousness appears in three states (Avasthā), *viz.*[2]: waking (Jāgrat), dreaming (Svapna), and dreamless slumber (Suṣupti). In the waking state the Jīva is conscious of external objects (Bahih-prajña), and is the gross enjoyer of these objects through the senses (Sthūla-bhuk).[3] The Jīva in this state is called Jāgarī—that is, he who takes upon himself the gross body called Viśva. Here the Jīva consciousness is in the *gross body.*

In dreaming (Svapna) the Jīva is conscious of inner objects (Antah-prajña), and the enjoyer of what is subtle (Pra-vivikta-bhuk)—that is, impressions left on the mind by objects sensed in the waking state. The objects of dreams have only an external reality for the dreamer, whereas the objects perceived when awake have such reality for all who are in that state. The mind ceases to record fresh impressions, and works on that which has been registered in the waking state.

The first (Jāgrat) state is that of sense perception. Here the ego lives in a mental world of ideas, and the Jīva consciousness is in the *subtle body.* Both these states are states of duality in which multiplicity is experienced.[4]

---

[1] Described in detail *post.*

[2] See Māṇdukya-Upaniṣad (where these are analysed) with Gauḍapāda's Kārikā and Śaṁkarācārya's Commentary on the same.

[3] Māṇdukya Up., Mantra 3. Prapañcasāra-Tantra; Svairindriyair yadātmā bhuṅgte bhogān sa jāgaro bhavati (Ch. XIX, Tāntrik Texts, Vol. III). See Īśvara-pratyabhijñā: Sarvākṣa-gocaratvena yā tu bāhyatayā sthitā (cited by Bhāskararāya in Comm. to v. 62 of Lalitā).

[4] See Māṇdukya Up., Mantra 4. Īśvara-pratyabhijñā,

> ManomātrapatheSdhyakṣaviṣayatvena vibhramāt
> Spaṣṭāvabāsabhāvānāṁ sṛṣṭih svapnapadaṁ mataṁ
> (Cited in Lalitā, under v. 113.)

Prapañcasāra-Tantra: Saṁjñārahitair api tair asyānubhavo bhavet punah svapnah.

The third state, or that of dreamless sleep (Suṣupti), is defined as that which is neither waking nor dreaming, and in which the varied experiences of the two former states are merged into a simple experience (Ekībhūta), as the variety of the day is lost in the night without extinction of such variety. Consciousness is not objective (Bahih prajña) nor subjective (Antaḥ-prajña), but a simple undifferenced consciousness without an object other than itself (Prajñāna-ghana). In waking the Jīva consciousness is associated with mind and senses; in dreaming the senses are withdrawn; in dreamless slumber mind also is withdrawn. The Jīva, called Prajña, is for the time being merged in his *causal body*—that is, Prakṛti inseparably associated with Consciousness—that is, with that state of Consciousness which is the seed from which the subtle and gross bodies grow. The state is one of bliss. The Jīva is not conscious of anything,[1] but on awakening preserves only the notion, "Happily I slept; I was not conscious of anything."[2] This state is accordingly that which has as its object the sense of nothingness.[3] Whilst the two former states enjoy the gross and subtle objects respectively, this is the enjoyer of bliss only (Ānanda-bhuk)—that is, simple bliss without an object. The Lord is always the enjoyer of bliss, but in the first two states He enjoys bliss through objects. Here He enjoys bliss itself free from both subject and object. In this way the Suṣupti state approaches the Brahman Consciousness. But it is not that in its purity, because it, as the other two states are both associated with ignorance (Avidyā) the

---

[1] This state, when nothing is dreamt, is rarer than is generally supposed.

[2] See Pātañjala-Yoga-Sūtra: Sukhaṁ ahaṁ asvāpsaṁ na kincid avediṣaṁ iti smaraṇāt.

[3] Abhāva-pratyayālaṁhanāvṛttir nidra. See also Prapañcasāra-Tantra: Ātmanirudyuktatayā nairākulyaṁ bhavet suṣuptir api (Ch. XIX, Vol. III, of Tāntrik Texts).

first two with Vikṛti, and the last with Prakṛti. Beyond, therefore, the state there is the "fourth" (Turīya). Here the pure experience called Śuddha-vidyā is acquired through Samādhi-yoga, Jīva in the Suṣupti state is said to be in the causal (Kāraṇa) body, and Jīva in the Turīya state is said to be in the great causal (Mahā-kāraṇa) body.[1]

Beyond this there is, some say, a fifth state, "beyond the fourth" (Turīyātīta), which is attained through firmness in the fourth. Here the Īśvara-Tattva is attained. This is the Unmeṣa [2] state of consciousness, of which the Sadākhya-Tattva is the Nimeṣa.[2] Passing beyond "the spotless one attains the highest equality," and is merged in the Supreme Śiva.

The above divisions—Viśva, Taijasa, and Prājña—are those of the individual Jīva. But there is also the collective or cosmic Jīva, which is the aggregate of the individual Jīvas of each particular state.[3] In the macrocosm these collective[4] Jīvas are called Vaiśvānara (corresponding to the

---

[1] Bhāskararāya in his Comm. on Lalitā says: Ata eva suṣupti-dāśapanna-jīvopadheh kāraṇaśarīratvena turīyadaśāpanna-jīvopādheh mahākāraṇaśarīratvena vyavahārah.

Inasmuch as the Jīva in the Suṣupti state is possessed of the Kāraṇa-śarīra (causal body) the same Jīva in the Turīya state is understood to be possessed of the Great Causal Body (Mahākāraṇa-śarīratvena vyavahārah).

[2] Opening and closing of the eyes (of consciousness). The latter is the last stage before the perfect Śivā-consciousness is gained.

[3] Accounts vary in detail according as a greater or less number of stages of ascent are enumerated. Thus Nirvāṇa-Tantra, cited in Comm. to v. 43 *post*, says the Paramātmā is the Devatā in the Turīya state; and Prapañcasāra (Ch. XIX) says Jāgrat is Bīja, Svapna is Bindu, Suṣupti is Nāda, Turīya is Śakti, and the Laya beyond is Śānta.

[4] The nature of the collectivity is not merely a summation of units, but a collectivity the units of which are related to one another as parts of an organized whole. Thus Hiraṇyagarbha is he who has the consciousness of being all the Jīvas. Samaṣtyabhimānī Hiraṇyagarbhātmakah (Bhāskararāya, *op. cit.* v. 61). He is the aggregate of these Jīvas.

individual Viśva body), Hiraṇyagarbha, and Sūtrātmā[1] (corresponding to the individual Taijasa-body); and Īśvara is the name of the collective form of the Jīvas described as Prājña. Cosmically, these are the conscious Lords of the objective, subjective, and causal worlds, beyond which there is the Supreme Consciousness.

Supreme Yoga-experience and Liberation is attained by passing beyond the first three states of ordinary experience.

The Yoga-process is a return-movement to the Source which is the reverse of the creative movement therefrom. The order of production is as follows: Buddhi, then Ahaṁkāra, from the latter the Manas, Indriya and Tanmātra and from the last the Bhūta. As the seat of the Source is in the human body the cerebrum in which there is the greatest display of Consciousness, the seat of Mind is between the eyebrows and the seats of Matter in the five centres from the throat to the base of the spine. Commencement of the return movement is made here and the various kinds of Matter are dissolved into one another, and then into Mind and Mind into Consciousness as described later in Chapter V. To the question whether man can *here and now* attain the supreme state of Bliss, the answer in Yoga is " yes ".

---

[1] There is said to be this distinction between the two, that the Paramātmā manifested as the collective Antahkaraṇa is Hiraṇyagarbha, as the collective Prāṇa it is called Sūtrātma. When manifest through these two vehicles without differentiation it is Antaryāmin. See Bhāskararāya, *loc. cit.*

IV

MANTRA

Reference is made in the Text and in this Introduction to Śabda, Varṇa, Mantra. It is said that the letters (Varṇa) of the alphabet are distributed throughout the bodily centres on the petals of the lotuses, as is shown on Plates II-VII. In each of the lotuses there is also a Seed-Mantra (Bīja) of the Tattva of the centre. Kuṇḍalinī is both Light (Jyotirmayī) and Mantra (Mantramayī),[1] and Mantra is used in the process of rousing Her.

There is perhaps no subject in the Indian Śāstra which is less understood than Mantra. The subject is so important a part of the Tantra-Śāstra that its other title is Mantra-Śāstra. Commonly Orientalists and others describe Mantra as "prayer," "formulæ of worship," "mystic syllables," and so forth. Mantra science may be well-founded or not, but even in the latter case it is not the absurdity which some suppose it to be. Those who think so might except Mantras which are prayers, and the meaning of which they understand, for with prayer they are familiar. But such appreciation itself shows a lack of understanding. There is nothing necessarily holy or prayerful about a Mantra. Mantra is a power (Mantra-śakti) which lends itself impartially to any use. A man may be injured or killed by Mantra;[2] by Mantra a kind of union with the physical

[1] The first is the subtle, the second the gross form. See as regards the subject-matter of this Chapter the Author's "Garland of Letters".

[2] As in Māraṇaṁ and other of the Ṣat-karma. To quote an example which I have read in an account of an author nowise "suspect" as an

Śakti is by some said to be effected;[1] by Mantra in the initiation called Vedhadīkṣā there is such a transference of power from the Guru to the disciple that the latter swoons under the impulse of it;[2] by Mantra the Homa fire may and, according to ideal conditions, should be lighted;[3] by Mantra man is saved, and so forth. Mantra, in short, is a power (Śakti); power in the form of Sound. The root "*man*" means "to think".

The creative power of thought is now receiving increasing acceptance in the West. Thought-reading, thought-transference, hypnotic suggestion, magical projections (Mokṣaṇa), and shields (Grahaṇa),[4] are becoming known and practised, not always with good results. The doctrine is ancient in India, and underlies the practices to be found in the Tantras, some of which are kept in general concealed to

---

Occultist, Theosophist, etc.—General J. T. Harris noticed a scorpion close to the foot of a Sādhu. "Don't move," he said: "there is a scorpion by your foot." The Sādhu leaned over, and when he saw the scorpion he pointed at it with his fingers, on which the animal immediately and in the presence of the General shrivelled up and died. "You seem to have some powers already," the General said; but the Sādhu simply waived the matter aside as being of no importance ("China Jim": "Incidents in the Life of a Mutiny Veteran," by Major-General J. T. Harris, p. 74. Heinemann).

[1] An extraordinary use to which it is put, I am informed by some worshippers of the Bhairava-Mantra. The man projects the Mantra on to the woman, who then experiences the sensation of a physical union. The Viṣṇu-Purāṇa speaks of generation by will power.

[2] As the Kulārṇava-Tantra says, and as may be readily understood, such a Guru is hard to get. The disciple who receives this initiation gets all the powers of his initiator. It is said that there are Gurus who can at once make their disciples fit for the highest aims.

[3] As is stated to have actually happened lately in the house of a friend of a collaborator of mine. A man is alleged to have lit the fuel in Kuṣandikā-Homa simply by Mantra and the Bīja of fire ("Ram") without recourse to light or match.

[4] This Sanskrit term expresses not so much a "fence" to which use a Kavaca is put, but the knowledge of how a man may "catch" a Mantra projected at him.

prevent misuse.[1] What, however, is not understood in the West is the particular form of Thought-science which is Mantra-vidyā. Those familiar with Western presentment of similar subjects will more readily understand[2] when I say that, according to the Indian doctrine here described, thought (like mind, of which it is the operation) is a Power or Śakti. It is, therefore, as real, as outer material objects. Both are projections of the creative thought of the World-thinker. The root "*man*," which means 'to think', is also the root of the Sanskrit word for "Man," who alone of all creation is properly a thinker. Mantra is the manifested Śabda-brahman.

But what is Śabda or "sound"? Here the Śākta-Tantra-Śāstra follows the Mīmāmsā doctrine of śabda, with such modifications as are necessary to adapt it to its doctrine of Śakti. Sound (Śabda), which is a quality (Guṇa) of ether (Ākāśa), and is sensed by hearing, is two-fold—namely, lettered (Varnātmaka-śabda) and unlettered, or Dhvani (Dhvanyātmaka-śabda).[3] The latter is caused by the striking of two things together, and is meaningless. Śabda, on the contrary, which is Anāhata (a term applied to the Heart Lotus), is that Brahman sound which is not caused by the striking of two things together. Lettered sound is composed of sentences (Vākya), words (Pada), and letters

[1] In the Samhitā called Kulārṇava (not the Tantra of that name) Śiva, after referring to some terrible rites with the flesh of black cats, bats, and other animals, the soiled linen of a Candāla woman, the shroud of a corpse, and so forth, says; "Oh, Pārvati, my head and limbs tremble, my mouth is dried" (Hṛdayaṁ kampate mama, gātrāṇi mama kaṁpante, mukhaṁ śuṣyate Pārvatī), adding: "One must not speak of it, one must not speak, one must not speak, again and again I say it must not be spoken of" (Na vaktavyaṁ na vaktavyaṁ na vaktavyaṁ punah punah).

[2] It is because the Orientalist and missionary know nothing of occultism, and regard it as superstition, that their presentment of Indian teaching is so often ignorant and absurd.

[3] This Dhvani is the gross body of the Mantra. See the Author's "Garland of Letters".

(Varṇa). Such sound has a meaning.[1] Śabda manifesting as speech is said to be eternal.[2] This the Naiyāyikas deny, saying that it is transitory. A word is uttered, and it is gone. This opinion the Mīmāmsā denies, saying that the perception of lettered sound must be distinguished from lettered sound itself.[3] Perception is due to Dhvani caused by the striking of the air in contact with the vocal organs—namely, the throat, palate and tongue. Before there is Dhvani there must be the striking of one thing against another. It is not the mere striking which is the lettered Śabda. This manifests it. The lettered sound is produced by the formation of the vocal organs in contact with air, which formation is in response to the mental movement or idea, which by the will thus seeks outward expression in audible sound.[4] It is this perception which is transitory, for the Dhvani which manifests ideas in language is such. But lettered sound, as it is in itself—is eternal. It was not produced at the moment it was perceived. It was only manifested by the Dhvani. It existed before, as it exists after, such manifestation, just as a jar in a dark room which is revealed by a flash of lightning is not then produced, nor does it cease to exist on its ceasing to be perceived through the disappearance of its manifester, the lightning. The air in contact with the voice organs reveals sound in the form of the letters of the alphabet, and

---

[1] When the word "Ghata" is uttered, then there arises in the mind the idea of a jar. When the Mantra of a Divinity is uttered there arises the idea of the Deity whose name it is.

[2] Not as audible sounds (Dhvani), but as that which finds auditory expression in audible sounds. The sensible expressions are transient. Behind them is the eternal Logos (Śabda-brahman), whose manifestation they are.

[3] Samaṁ tu tatra darśanaṁ ("But alike is the perception thereof").

[4] This is only one form in which letters find sensible expression. Thus writing gives visual expression, and to the blind perforated dots give tactual expression.

their combinations in words and sentences. The letters are produced for hearing by the effort of the person desiring to speak, and become audible to the ear of others through the operation of unlettered sound or Dhvani. The latter being a manifester only, lettered Śabda is something other than its manifester.

Before describing the nature of Śabda in its different forms of development it is necessary to understand the Indian psychology of perception. At each moment the Jīva is subject to innumerable influences which from all quarters of the universe pour upon him. Only those reach his Consciousness which attract his attention, and are thus selected by his Manas. The latter attends to one or other of these sense impressions, and conveys it to the Buddhi. When an object (Artha) is presented to the mind and perceived, the latter is formed into the shape of the object perceived. This is called a mental Vṛtti (modification), which it is the object of Yoga to suppress. The mind as a Vṛtti is thus a representation of the outer object. But in so far as it is such represention it is as much an object as the outer one. The latter—that is, the physical object—is called the gross object (Sthūla-artha), and the former or mental impression is called the subtle object (Sūkṣma-artha). But besides the object there is the mind which perceives it. It follows that the mind has two aspects, in one of which it is the perceiver and in the other the perceived in the form of the mental formation (Vṛtti) which in creation precedes its outer projection, and after the creation follows as the impression produced in the mind by the sensing of a gross physical object. The mental impression and the physical object exactly correspond, for the physical object is, in fact, but a projection of the cosmic imagination, though it has the same reality as the mind has; no more and no less. The mind is thus both cognizer (Grāhaka) and cognized (Grāhya), revealer (Prakāśaka) and revealed

(Prakāśya), denoter (Vācaka) and denoted (Vāchya). When the mind perceives an object it is transformed into the shape of that object. So the mind which thinks of the Divinity which it worships (Iṣta-devatā) is at length, through continued devotion, transformed into the likeness of that Devatā. By allowing the Devatā thus to occupy the mind for long it becomes as pure as the Devatā. This is a fundamental principle of Tāntrik Sādhana or religious practice. The object perceived is called Artha, a term which comes from the root "Ri" which means to get, to know, to enjoy. Artha is that which is known, and which therefore is an object of enjoyment. The mind as Artha—that is, in the form of the mental impression—is a reflection of the outer object or gross Artha. As the outer object is Artha, so is the interior subtle mental form which corresponds to it. That aspect of the mind which cognizes is called Śabda or Nāma (name), and that aspect in which it is its own object or cognized is called Artha or Rūpa (form). The outer physical object of which the latter is, in the individual, an impression is also Artha or Rūpa, and spoken speech is the outer Śabda. Subject and object are thus from the Mantra aspect Śabda and Artha—terms corresponding to the Vedāntic Nāma and Rūpa, or concepts and concepts objectified. As the Vedānta says, the whole creation is Nāma and Rūpa. Mind is the power (Śakti), the function of which is to distinguish and identify (Bheda-samsarga-vṛtti Śakti).

Just as the body is causal, subtle and gross, so is Śabda, of which there are four states (Bhāva), called Parā, Paśyantī, Madhyamā and Vaikharī—terms further explained in Section V of this Introduction. Parā sound is that which exists of the differentiation of the Mahābindu before actual manifestation. This is motionless causal Śabda in Kuṇḍalinī in the Mūlādhāra centre of the body. That aspect of it in which it commences to move with a general—that is, non-particularized—motion (Sāmānya-spanda) is Paśyantī, whose place is from the Mūlādhāra to the Maṇipūra-Cakra, the next centre. It is here associated with Manas. These represent the motionless and first moving Īśvara aspect of Śabda. Madhyamā sound is associated with Buddhi. It is Hiraṇyagarbha Śabda (Hiraṇyagarbha-rūpa) extending from Paśyantī to the heart. Both Madhyamā sound, which is the inner "naming" by the cognitive aspect of mental movement, as also its Artha or subtle (Sūkṣma) object (Artha), belong to the mental or subtle body (Śūkṣma or Linga-śarīra). Perception is dependent on distinguishing and identification. In the perception of an object that part of the mind which identifies and distinguishes, or the cognizing part, is subtle Śabda, and that part of it which takes the shape of the object (a shape which corresponds with the outer thing) is subtle Artha. The perception of an object is thus consequent on the stimultaneous functioning of the mind in its twofold aspect as Śabda and Artha, which are in indissoluble relation with one another as cognizer (Grāhaka) and cognized (Grāhya). Both belong to the subtle body. In creation Madhyamā-Śabda first appeared. At that moment there was no outer Artha. Then the cosmic mind projected this inner Madhyamā Artha into the world of sensual experience, and named it in spoken speech (Vaikharī-Śabda). The last or Vaikharī-Śabda is uttered speech developed in the throat issuing from the mouth. This is Virāt-Śabda. Vaikharī-Śabda is therefore language or gross lettered sound. Its corresponding Artha is the physical or gross object which language denotes. This belongs to the gross body (Sthūla-śarīra). Madhyamā-Śabda is mental movement or ideation in its cognitive aspect, and Madhyamā Artha is the mental impression of the gross object. The inner thought-movement in its aspect as Śabdārtha, and considered both in its knowing aspect (Śabda) and as the subtle known object (Artha), belong to the subtle body (Sūkṣma-śarīra). The cause of these two is the first general movement towards particular ideation (Paśyantī) from the motionless cause, Para-śabda, or Supreme Speech. Two forms of inner or hidden speech, causal and subtle, accompanying mind movement, thus precede and lead up to spoken language. The inner forms of ideating movement constitute the subtle, and the uttered sound the gross, aspect of Mantra, which is the manifested Śabda-brahman.

The gross Śabda, called Vaikharī or uttered speech, and the gross Artha, or the physical object denoted by that speech, are the projection of the subtle śabda and Artha through the initial activity of the Śabda-brahman into the world of gross sensual perception. Therefore in the gross physical world Śabda means language—that is, sentences, words and letters, which are the expression of ideas and are Mantra. In the subtle or mental world Madhyamā Śabda is the mind which "names" in its aspect as cognizer, and Artha is the same mind in its aspect as the mental object of its cognition. It is defined to be the outer in the form of the mind. It is thus similar to the state of dreams (Svapna): as Para-śabda is the causal dreamless (Suṣupti) and Vaikharī the waking (Jāgrat) state. Mental Artha is a Saṁskāra, an impression left on the subtle body by previous experience, which is recalled when the Jīva re-awakes to world experience and recollects the experience temporarily lost in the cosmic dreamless state (Suṣupti) which is dissolution (Mahā-pralaya). What is it which arouses this Saṁskāra? As an effect (Kārya) it must have a cause (Kāraṇa). This Kāraṇa is the Śabda or name (Nāma), subtle or gross, corresponding to that particular Artha. When the word "Ghata" is uttered this evokes in the mind the image of an object—a jar—just as the presentation of that object does. In the Hiraṇyagarbha state Śabda as Saṁskāra worked to evoke mental images. The whole is thus Śabda and Artha—that is, name and form (Nāma-Rūpa). These two are inseparably associated. There is no Śabda without Artha or Artha without Śabda. The Greek word Logos also means thought and word combined. There is thus a double line of creation, Śabda and Artha, ideas and language together with their objects. Speech, as that which is heard, or the outer manifestation of Śabda, stands for the Śabda creation. The Artha creation are the inner and outer objects seen by the mental or physical vision. From the cosmic creative standpoint the mind comes first, and from it is evolved the physical world according to the ripened Saṁskāras, which led to the existence of the particular existing universe. Therefore the mental Artha precedes the physical Artha, which is an evolution in gross matter of the former. This mental state corresponds to that of dreams (Svapna) when man lives in the mental world only. After creation, which is the waking (Jāgrat) state, there is for the individual an already existing parallelism of names and objects.

Uttered speech is a manifestation of the inner naming or thought. This thought-movement is similar in men of all races. When an Englishman or an Indian thinks of an object, the image is to both the same, whether evoked by the object itself or by the utterance of its name. Perhaps for this reason a thought-reader whose cerebral centre is *en rapport* with that of another may read the hidden "speech"—that is, the thought of one whose spoken speech he cannot understand. Thus, whilst the thought-movement is similar in all men, the expression of it as Vaikharī-Śabda differs. According to tradition, there was once a universal language. According to the Biblical account, this was so before the confusion of tongues at the Tower of Babel. Nor is this unlikely when we consider that difference in gross speech is due to difference of races evolved in the course of time. If the instruments by, and conditions under, which thought is revealed in speech were the same for all men, then there would be but one language. But now this is not so. Racial characteristics and physical conditions, such as the nature of the vocal organs, climate, inherited impressions, and so forth, differ. Therefore, so also does language. But for each particular man speaking any particular language the uttered name of any object is the gross expression of his inner thought-movement. It evokes that movement and again expresses it. It evokes the idea and the idea is Consciousness as mental operation. That operation can be so intensified as to be itself creative. This is Mantra-caitanya.

From the above account it will be understood that, when it is said that the "letters" are in the six bodily Cakras, it is not to be supposed that it is intended to absurdly affirm that the letters as written shapes, or as the uttered sounds which are heard by the ear, are there. The letters in this sense—that is, as gross things—are manifested only in speech and writing. This much is clear. But the precise significance of this statement is a matter of great difficulty. There is, in fact, no subject which presents more difficulties than Mantra-vidyā, whether considered generally or in relation to the particular matter in hand. In the first place, one must be constantly on guard against falling into a possible trap—namely, the taking of prescribed methods of realization for actualities in the common sense of that term. The former are conventional, the latter are real. Doubts on this matter are increased by some variations in the descriptive accounts. Thus in some Ganeśa is the Devatā of the Mūlādhāra. In the Text here translated it is Brahmā. Similarly this Text gives Ḍākinī in the Mūlādhāra as the Devatā of the Asthi-Dhātu (bony substance). When sitting in the prescribed Āsana (posture), the bones are gathered up around this Cakra, and, moreover, from it as the centre of the body the bones run up and downwards. Another account, however, given to me places Devī Śākinī here.[1] Mistakes have also to be reckoned with, and can only be ascertained and rectified by a comparison of several MSS.[2] Again, four letters are said to be on the petals of the Mūlādhāra Lotus—namely, Va, Śa, Ṣa, and Sa. Why are these said to be there? Various statements have been made to me. As there are certain letters which are ascribed to each form of sensible matter (Bhūta), it seems obvious to suggest that the Earth letters (Pārthiva-varṇa) are in the Earth centre. But an examination on this basis does not bear the suggestion out. Next, it is said that the letters have colours, and the letters of a particular colour are allocated to the lotuses of the same colour. The Text does not support this theory. It has been said that certain letters derive from certain Devatās. But the letters produce the Devatā, for these are the Artha of Mantra as Śabda. I have been also told that the letters are placed according to their seat of pronunciation (Uccāraṇa). But it is replied that the Mūlādhāra is the common source of this (Uccāraṇa-sthāna) for all.[3] Again, it is said that the

---

[1] This account, which may be compared with that of the Text, is as follows:

Bone (Asthi-dhātu): Mūladhāra-cakra; Devī Śākinī.
Fat (Meda-dhātu): Svādhiṣṭhāna-cakra; Devī Kākinī.
Flesh (Māmsa-dhātu): Maṇipūra-cakra; Devī Lākinī.
Blood (Rakta-dhātu): Anāhata-cakra; Devī Rākinī.
Skin (Tvak-dhātu): Viśuddha-cakra; Devī Ḍākinī.
Marrow (Majjā-dhātu): Ājñā-cakra; Devī Hākinī.

In the Sahasrāra-Padma are all Dhātus beginning with Śukra (semen).

[2] Thus in the text given me, from which I quote, the four letters of the Mūlādhāra are given as Va, Śa, Ṣa and La. The latter should, according to other accounts, be Sa.

[3] This is true, but nevertheles there may be special seats of pronunciation for each letter or class of letters. As apparently supporting this suggestion it may be noted that the vowel sounds are placed in the throat centre, and Ha and Kṣa above.

letters on the petals are Bījas or seed-Mantras of all activities (Kriyā) connected with the Tattva of the centre, each letter undergoing variations according to the vowels.[1] All beings in Pṛthivī (Earth) Tattva, should be meditated upon in the Mūlādhāra. Here are therefore (as we might expect), the organs of feet (Pādendriya), the action of walking (Gamana-kriyā), smell (Gandha), the quality of Pṛthivī, the sense of smell (Ghrāṇa), Nivṛtti-Kalā,[2] and Brahmā (Lord of the Tattva). But we are also told that the letters Va, Śa, Ṣa and Sa are the Ātmā and Bījas of the four Vedas,[3] of the four Yugas,[4] of the four oceans,[5] which are therefore called Catur-varṇātmaka, or in the self of the four letters. It is true that the four Vedas are in, and issue from, Para-śabda, the seat of which is the Mūlādhāra. For Veda in its primary sense is the world as idea in the mind of the creative Brahman, portions of which have been revealed to the Ṛṣis (seers) and embodied in the four Vedas. But why should Va be the seed of the Ṛgveda, Śa of the Yajurveda, and so forth? The ritual explanation, as given in the Rudra-yāmala (xiv. 73, xv. 2, xvi. 1, 2) is that the petal Va is Brahmā (Rajo-guṇa), and is the Bīja of Ṛk; Śa is Viṣṇu (Sattva-guṇa), and Śa, being Puṇḍarīkātmā, is the Bīja of Yajus; Ṣa is Rudra (Tamo-guṇa), and is the Bīja of Sāma, Sa is the Bīja of Atharva, as it is the Bīja of Śakti.[6] These four are in Para-śabda in Mūlādhāra. It seems to me (so far as my studies in

[1] I am informed that the subject is dealt with in detail in the Kuṇḍalinī-kalpataru, and in particular in the Adhyātma-sāgara, neither of which MSS. have I yet seen.

[2] See Author's "Garland of Letters" (Kalās of the Śaktis). Samāna-Vāyu is also located here.

[3] Va of Ṛk, Śa of Yajus, Ṣa of Sāma and Sa of Atharva-Veda.

[4] The four ages—Satya, Treta, Dvāpara and Kali.

[5] Of sugarcane juice, wine, ghee (Ghṛta), milk.

[6] See Rudra-yāmala XVII, where priority is given to Atharva as dealing with Ācāra of Śakti. From Atharva arose Sāma, from Sāma, Yajus, and from the latter Ṛk.

the Śāstra have yet carried me) that the details of the descriptions of the centres are of two kinds. There are, firstly, certain facts of objective and universal reality. Thus, for example, there are certain centres (Cakra) in the spinal column. The principle of solidity (Pṛthivī-Tattva) is in the lowest of such centres, which as the centre of the body contains the static or potential energy called Kuṇḍalinī-Śakti. The centre as a lotus is said to have four petals, because of the formation and distribution of the Yoga-nerves[1] (Nāḍī) at that particular point. Solidity is denoted aptly by a cube, which is the diagram (Yantra) of that centre. The consciousness of that centre as Devatā is also aptly borne on an elephant, the massive solidity of which is emblematical of the solid earth principle (Pṛthivī). The forces which go to the making of solid matter may, by the Yogī, be seen as yellow. It may be that particular substances (Dhātu) of the body and particular Vṛtti (qualities) are connected with particular Cakras, and so forth.

There are, however, another class of details which have possibly only symbolical reality, and which are placed before the Sādhaka for the purposes of instruction and meditation only.[2] The letters as we know them—that is, as outer speech—are manifested only after passing through the throat. They cannot therefore exist as such in the Cakras. But they are said to be there. They are there, not in their gross, but in their subtle and causal forms. It is these subtle forms which are called Mātṛkā. But as such forms they are Śabda of and as ideating movements, or are the cause thereof. Consciousness, which is itself (Svarūpa) soundless (Nih-śabda), in its supreme form (Para-śabda)

[1] The term "nerve" is used for default of another equivalent. These Nāḍīs, called Yogā-Nāḍīs, are not, like the Nāḍīs of physiology, gross things, but subtle channels along which the life-force works in bodies.

[2] See the Demchog Tantra, Published as the seventh volume of "Tāntrik-Texts".

assumes a general undifferentiated movement (Sāmānya-spanda), then a differentiated movement (Viśeṣa-spanda), issuing in clearly articulate speech (Spaṣta-tara-spanda). The inner movement has outer correspondence with that issuing from the lips by the aid of Dhvani. This is but the Mantra way of saying that Consciousness moves as Śakti, and appears as subject (Śabda) and object (Artha) at first in the subtle form of Mind and its contents generated by the Saṁskāras, and then in the gross form of language as the expression of ideas and of physical objects (Artha), which the creative or Cosmic Mind projects into the world of sensual experience to be the source of impressions to the individual experiencer therein. It is true that in this sense the letters, as hidden speech or the seed of outer speech, are in the Cakras, but the allocation of particular letters to particular Cakras is a matter which, if it has a real and not merely symbolical significance, must receive the explanation given in my "Śakti and Sākta".

In each of the Cakras there is also a Bīja (seed) Mantra of each of the Tattvas therein. They are the seed of the Tattva, for the latter springs from and re-enters the former. The Natural Name of anything is the sound which is produced by the action of the moving forces which constitute it. He therefore, it is said, who mentally and vocally utters with creative force the natural name of anything, brings into being the thing which bears that name. Thus "Ram" is the Bīja of fire in the Maṇipūra-Cakra. This Mantra "Ram" is said to be the expression in gross sound (Vaikharī-Śabda) of the subtle sound produced by the forces constituting fire. The same explanation is given as regards "Lam" in the Mūlādhāra, and the other Bījas in the other Cakras. The mere utterance,[1] however, of "Ram" or any other Mantra

[1] The mind must in worship with form (Sākāra) be centred on the Deity of Worship (Iṣta-devatā), and in Yoga on the light form (Jyotirmaya-rūpa). It is said, however, that mere repetition of a Mantra

is nothing but a movement of the lips. When, however, the Mantra is "awakened"[1] (Prabuddha)—that is, when there is Mantra-caitanya (Mantra-consciousness)—then the Sādhaka can make the Mantra work. Thus in the case cited the Vaikharī-Śabda, through its vehicle Dhvani, is the body of a power of Consciousness which enables the Mantrin to become the Lord of Fire.[2] However this may be, in all cases it is the creative thought which ensouls the uttered sound which works now in man's small "magic," just as it first worked in the "grand magical display" of the World Creator. His thought was the aggregate, with creative power, of all thought. Each man is Śiva, and can attain His power to the degree of his ability to consciously realize himself as such. For various purposes the Devatās are invoked. Mantra and Devatā are one and the same. A Mantra-Devatā is Śabda and Artha, the former being the name, and the latter the Devatā whose name it is. By practice (Japa) with the Mantra the presence of the Devatā is invoked. Japa or repetition of Mantra is compared to the action of a man shaking a sleeper to wake him up. The two lips are Śiva and Śakti. Their movement is the coition (Maithuna) of the two. Śabda which issues therefrom is in the nature of Seed or Bindu. The Devatā thus produced is, as it were, the "son" of the Sādhaka. It is not the Supreme Devatā (for it is actionless) who appears, but in all cases an emanation

without knowing its meaning will produce *some* benefit or that which arises from devotion. The subject of natural Name is dealt with in the author's "Garland of Letters".

[1] Thought is not then only in the outer husk, but is vitalized through its conscious centre.

[2] Some attain these powers through worship (Upāsanā) of Agni Vetāla, a Devayoni; some of Agni Himself. The former process, which requires 12,000 Japa, is given in Śābara-tantra. In the same way objects are said to be moved, though at a distance from the operator, by the worship of Madhumatī-Devī. A higher state of development dispenses with all outer agents.

produced by the Sādhaka for his benefit only.[1] In the case of worshippers of Śiva a Boy-Śiva (Bāla Śiva) appears, who is then made strong by the nurture which the Sādhaka gives to his creation. The occultist will understand all such symbolism to mean that the Devatā is a form of the consciousness of Sādhaka which the latter arouses and strengthens, and gains good thereby. It is his consciousness which becomes the boy Śiva, and when strengthened the full-grown Divine power itself. All Mantras are in the body as forms of consciousness (Vijñāna-rūpa). When the Mantra is fully practised it enlivens the Saṁskāra, and the Artha appears to the mind. Mantras are thus a form of the Saṁskāra of Jīvas, the Artha of which becomes manifest to the consciousness which is fit to perceive it. The essence of all this is—concentrate and vitalize thought and will power. But for such a purpose a method is necessary—namely, language and determined varieties of practice according to the end sought. These, Mantra-vidyā (which explains what Mantra is) also enjoins.

The causal state of Śabda is called Śabda-brahman—that is, the Brahman as the cause of Śabda and Artha. The unmanifest (Avyakta) power or Śabda, which is the cause of manifested Śabda and Artha, uprises on the differentiation of the Supreme Bindu from Prakṛti in the form of Bindu through the prevalence of Kriyā[2] Śakti. Avyakta Rava or Śabda (unmanifested sound) is the principle of sound as such (Nāda-mātra), that is undifferentiated sound, not specialized in the form of letters, but which is, through

[1] If Sūrya (Sun-God) be invoked, it is an emanation which comes and then goes back to the sun.

[2] See, v. 12: Śāradā.

> Kriyā-śakti-pradhānāyāh śabda-śabdārtha-kāraṇam,
> Prakṛtir bindu-rūpiṇyāh-śabda-brahmābhavat param.

In plain English this means, in effect, that increasing activity in the Consciousness about to create (Bindu) produces that state in which it is the cause of subject and object, as mind and matter.

creative activity, the cause of manifested Śabda and Artha.[1] It is the Brahman considered as all-pervading Śabda, undivided, unmanifested, whose substance is Nāda and Bindu, the proximate creative impulse in Para-śiva and proximate cause of manifested Śabda and Artha.[2] It is the eternal partless Sphota[3] which is not distinguished into Śabda and Artha, but is the Power by which both exist and are known. Śabda-brahman is thus the kinetic ideating aspect of the undifferentiated Supreme Consciousness of philosophy, and the Saguṇa-Brahman of religion. It is Cit-śakti vehicled by undifferentiated Prakṛti-śakti—that is, the creative aspect of the one Brahman who is both transcendent and formless (Nirguṇa), and immanent and with form (Saguṇa).[4] As the Haṭha-yoga-pradīpikā says:[5] "Whatever is heard in the form of sound is Śakti. The absorbed state (Laya) of the Tattvas (evolutes of Prakṛti) is that in which no form exists.[6] So long as there is the notion of Ether, so long is sound heard. The soundless is called

[1] Tena śabdārtharūpa-viśiṣṭasya śabda-brahmatvaṁ avadhāritam (Prāṇa-toṣiṇī, 13).

[2] See Prāṇa-toṣiṇi, p. 10; Rāghava-Bhatta, Comm. v. 12, Ch. I, Sāradā.

Sṛṣṭyunmukha-paramaśiva-prathamollāsamātraṁ akhaṇdo vyakto nādabindumaya eva vyāpako brahmātmakah śabdah.

[3] Sphota, which is derived from *Sphut*, to open (as a bud does), is that by which the particular meaning of words is revealed. The letters singly, and therefore also in combination, are non-significant. A word is not the thing, but that through which, when uttered, there is cognition of the thing thereby denoted. That which denotes the thing denoted is a disclosure (Sphota) other than these letters. This Sphota is eternal Śabda.

[4] It is to be noted that of five Bhutas, Ākāśa and Vāyu belonging to the formless division (Amūrtta), and the remaining three to the form division (Mūrtta). The first is sensed by hearing. Śabda is vibration for the ear as name. Agni, the head of the second division, is sensed as form (Rūpa). Artha is vibration to the eye (mental or physical) or form.

[5] Ch. IV, vv. 101, 102.

[6] Yatkiṁcin nādarūpeṇa Śrūyate śaktir eva sā,
Yas tattvānto nirākārah sa eva parameśvarah.

Para-brahman or Paramātmā."[1] Śabda-brahman thus projects itself for the purpose of creation into two sets of movement—namely, firstly the Śabda (with mental vibrations of cognition) which, passing through the vocal organs, becomes articulate sound; and, secondly, Artha movements denoted by Śabda in the form of all things constituting the content of mind and the objective world. These two are emanations from the same Conscious Activity (Śakti) which is the Word (Vāk or "Logos"), and are in consequence essentially the same. Hence the connection between the two is permanent. It is in the above sense that the universe is said to be composed of the letters. It is the fifty[2] letters of the Sanskrit alphabet which are denoted by the garland of severed human heads which the naked[3] Mother, Kālī, dark like a threatening raincloud, wears as She stands amidst bones and carrion beasts and birds in the burning-ground on the white corpse-like (Śava-rūpa) body of Śiva. For it is She who "slaughters"—that is, withdraws all speech and its objects into Herself at the time of the dissolution of all things (Mahā-pralaya).[4] Śabda-brahman is the Consciousness (Caitanya) in all creatures. It assumes the form of Kuṇḍalī, and abides in the body of all breathing creatures (Prāṇī), manifesting itself by letters in the form of prose and verse.[5] In the sexual

[1] Tāvad ākāśasaṁkalpo yāvacchabdah pravartate,
Nihśabdaṁ tatparaṁ brahma paramātmeti gīyate.

[2] Sometimes given as fifty-one.

[3] She is so pictured because She is beyond Māyā (Māyātītā). She is the "Bewilderer of all" by Her Māyā, but is Herself unaffected thereby. This Kālī symbolism is explained in the Svarūpa-vyākhyā of the "Hymn to Kālī" (Karpūrādi-Stotra).

[4] The same symbolism is given in the description of the Heruka in the Buddhist Demchog Tantra.

[5] Caitanyaṁ sarvabhūtāṇāṁ śabda-brahmeti me matih,
Tat prāpya kuṇḍalīrūpaṁ prāṇināṁ dehamadhyagaṁ,
Varṇātmanāvirbhavati gadyapadyādi-bhedatah. (Śāradā-Tilaka, Ch. I.)

symbolism of the Śākta-Tantras, seed (Bindu)[1] issued upon the reversed union[2] of Mahākāla and Mahākālī, which seed, ripening in the womb of Prakṛti, issued as Kuṇḍalī in the form of the letters (Akṣara). Kuṇḍalī as Mahāmātṛkā-sundarī has fifty-one coils, which are the Mātṛkās or subtle forms of the gross letters or Varṇa which is the Vaikharī form of the Śabda at the centres. Kuṇḍalī when with one coil is Bindu; with two, Prakṛti-Puruṣa; with three, the three Śaktis (Iccha, Jñāna, Kriyā) and three Guṇas (Sattva, Rajas, Tamas); with the three and a half She is then actually creative with Vikṛti; with four She is the Devī Ekajatā, and so on to Śrīmātṛkotpattisundarī with fifty-one coils.[3] In the body, unmanifested Para-śabda is in Kuṇḍalī-Śakti. That which first issues from it is in the lowest Cakra, and extends upwards though the rest as Paśyantī, Madhyamā and Vaikharī-Śabda. When Śakti first "sees"[4] She is Paramā-Kalā[5] in the mother-form (Ambikārūpā), which is supreme speech (Parā-vāk) and supreme peace (Paramā śāntā). She "sees" the manifested Śabda from Paśyantī to Vaikharī. The Paśyantī[6] state of Śabda is that in which Icchā-Śakti (Will) in the form of a goad[7] (Aṁkuśākāra) is about to display the universe, then

---

[1] The term Bindu also means a drop as of semen.

[2] Viparīta-maithuna. Śakti is above Śiva, and moving on and in coition with Him because She is the active and He the inert Consciousness.

[3] Śaktisaṁgama-Tantra, first Ullāsa Utpattikhāṇḍa. When with the ten coils She is the well-known Daśamahāvidyā.

[4] The first movement in creation, called Īkṣaṇa ("seeing") in Veda. To see is to ideate.

[5] Paramā=supreme or first. Kalā=Vimarśa-Śakti of Ātmā. She is, as such, the first cause of all the letters.

[6] Paśyantī=She who "sees" (Īkṣaṇa).

[7] Here the crooked line (Vakra-rekhā) comes first, and the straight second. Possibly this may be the line rising to form the triangular pyramid.

in seed (Bīja) form. This is the Śakti Vāmā.[1] Madhyamā-Vāk, which is Jñāna (knowledge), and in the form of a straight line (Ṛjurekhā), is Jyeṣṭhā-Śakti. Here there is the first assumption of form as the Mātṛkā (Mātṛkātvam upapannā), for here is a particular motion (Viśeṣa-spanda). The Vaikharī state is that of Kriyā Śakti, who is the Devī Raudri, whose form is triangular [2] and that of the universe. As the former Śakti produces the subtle letters of Mātṛkā which are the Vāsanā,[3] so this last is the Śakti of the gross letters of words and their objects.[4] These letters are the Garland of the Mother issuing from Her in Her form as Kuṇḍalinī-Śakti, and absorbed by Her in the Kuṇḍalinī-yoga here described.

---

[1] So called because she "vomits forth" the universe (Vamanāt vāmā iti).

[2] Śṛṅgātaka—that is, a triangular pyramidal figure of three dimensions.

[3] That is, Sāṁskāra or revived impression, which is the seed of the ideating Cosmic Consciousness.

[4] Yoginīhṛdaya-Tantra, Saṁketa I.

V

THE CENTRES OR LOTUSES (CAKRA, PADMA)

At this stage we are in a position to pass to a consideration of the Cakras, which may shortly be described as subtle centres of operation in the body of the Śaktis or Powers of the various Tattvas or Principles which constitute the bodily sheaths. Thus the five lower Cakras from Mūlādhāra to Viśuddha are centres of the Bhūtas, or five forms of sensible matter. The Ājñā and other Cakras in the region between it and the Sahasrāra are centres of the Tattvas constituting the mental sheaths, whilst, the Sahasrāra or thousand-petalled lotus at the top of the brain, is the blissful abode of Parama Śiva-Śakti which is the state of pure Consciousness.

A description of the Cakras involves, in the first place, an account of the Western anatomy and physiology of the central and sympathetic nervous systems; secondly, an account of the Tāntrik nervous system and Cakras; and, lastly, the correlation, so far as that is possible, of the two systems on the anatomical and physiological side, for the rest is in general peculiar to Tāntrik occultism.

The Tāntrik theory regarding the Cakras and Sahasrāra is concerned on the *Physiological* side, or Bhogāyatna aspect, with the central spinal system, comprising the brain or encephalon, contained within the skull, and the spinal cord, contained within the vertebral column (Merudaṇḍa). It is to be noted that, just as there are five centres (Cakras) hereinafter described, the vertebral column itself is divided into five regions, which, commencing from the lowest, are the coccygeal, consisting of four imperfect vertebræ, often united together into one bone called the coccyx; the sacral region, consisting of five vertebræ united together to form a single bone, the sacrum; the lumbar region, or region of the loins, consisting of five vertebræ; the dorsal region, or region of the back, consisting of twelve vertebræ; and the cervical region, or region of the neck, consisting of seven vertebræ. As exhibited by segments, the cord shows different characteristics in different regions. Roughly speaking, these correspond to the regions which are assigned to the governing control of the Mūlādhāra, Svādhiṣṭhāna, Maṇipūra, Anāhata and Viśuddha centres, or Cakras or Lotuses (Padma). The central system has relation with the periphery through the thirty-one spinal and twelve cranial nerves, which are both afferent and efferent or sensory and motor, arousing sensation or stimulating action. Of the cranial nerves, the last six arise from the spinal bulb (medulla), and the other six, except the olfactory and optic nerves, from the parts of the brain just in front of the bulb. Writers of the Yoga and Tantra schools use the term Nāḍī, by preference, for nerves. They also, it has been said, mean cranial nerves when they speak of Sirās, never using the latter for arteries, as is done in the medical literature.[1] It must, however, be noted that the Yoga Nāḍīs are not the ordinary material nerves, but subtler lines of direction along which the vital forces go. The spinal nerves, after their exit from the intervertebral foramina, enter into communication with the gangliated cords of the sympathetic nervous system, which lie on each side of the vertebral column. The spinal cord extends in

[1] Dr. Brojendranath Seal, p. 337, Appendix to Professor Benoy Kumar Sarkar's "Positive Background of Hindu Sociology". The word Dhaminī is also used for nerve. It is to be noted, however, that the present work uses Sirās for other than cranial nerves, for in v. I, it calls Iḍā and Piñgalā-Nāḍīs or Sirās.

the case of man from the upper border of the atlas, below the cerebellum, passing into the medulla, and finally opening into the fourth ventricle of the brain, and descends to the second lumbar vertebra, where it tapers to a point, called the *filum terminale.* I am told that microscopic investigations by Dr. Cunningham have disclosed the existence of highly sensitive grey matter in the *filum terminale*, which was hitherto thought to be mere fibrous cord. This is of importance, having regard to the position assigned to the Mūlādhāra and the Serpent Power. It is continued in this for a variable distance, and then ends blindly. Within the bony covering is the cord, which is a compound of grey and white brain matter, the grey being the inner of the two, the reverse of the position on the encephalon. The cord is divided into two symmetrical halves, which are connected together by a commissure in the centre of which there is a minute canal called the central spinal canal (wherein is the Brahmanāḍī), which is said to be the remnant of the hollow tube from which the cord and brain were developed.[1] This canal contains cerebro-spinal fluid. The grey matter viewed longitudinally forms a column extending through the whole length of the cord, but the width is not uniform. There are special enlargements in the lumbar and cervical regions which are due mainly to the greater amount of grey matter in these situations. But throughout the whole cord the grey matter is specially abundant at the junctions of the spinal nerves, so that a necklace arrangement is visible, which is more apparent in the lower vertebrates, corresponding to the ventral ganglionic chain of the invertebrates.[2] The white matter consists of tracts or columns of nerve fibres. At the upper border of the atlas, or first cervical vertebra, the spinal cord passes into the medulla oblongata below the cerebellum. The centre canal

[1] See Ferrier's "Functions of the Brain".

[2] *Ibid.*, 7.

opens into the fourth ventricle of the brain. The cerebellum is a development of the posterior wall of the hindermost of the three primary dilatations of the embryonic cerebro-spinal tube, the fourth ventricle constituting the remnant of the original cavity. Above this is the cerebrum, which with the parts below it is an enlarged and greatly modified upper part of the cerebro-spinal nervous axis. The spinal cord is not merely a conductor between the periphery and the centres of sensation and volition, but is also an independent centre or group of centres. There are various centres in the spinal cord which, though to a considerable extent autonomous, is connected together with the higher centres by the associating and longitudinal tracts of the spinal cord.[1] All the functions which are ascribed primarily to the spinal centres belong also in an ultimate sense to the cerebral centres. Similarly, all the "Letters" which exist distributed on the petals of the lotuses exist in the Sahasrāra. The centres influence not only the muscular combinations concerned in volitional movements, but also the functions of vascular innervation, secretion, and the like, which have their proximate centres in the spinal cord. The cerebral centres are said, however, to control these functions only in relation with the manifestations of volition, feeling, and emotion; whereas the spinal centres with the subordinate sympathetic system are said to constitute the mechanism of unconscious adaptation, in accordance with the varying conditions of stimuli which are essential to the continued existence of the organism. The medulla, again, is also both a path of communication between the higher centres and the periphery and an independent centre regulating functions of the greatest importance in the system. It is to be noted that the nerve fibres which carry motor impulses descending from the brain to the spinal cord cross

[1] See Ferrier's "Functions of the Brain," p. 80.

over rather suddenly from one side to the other on their way through the spinal bulb (medulla), a fact which has been noted in the Tantras in the description of the Mukta Triveṇī. The latter is connected by numerous afferent and efferent tracts with the cerebellum and cerebral ganglia. Above the cerebellum is the cerebrum, the activity of which is ordinarily associated with conscious volition and ideation and the origination of voluntary movements. The notion of Consciousness, which is the introspective subject-matter of psychology, must not, however, be confused with that of physiological function. There is therefore no organ of consciousness, simply because " Consciousness " is not an organic conception, and has nothing to do with the physiological conception of energy, whose inner introspective side it presents.[1] Consciousness in itself is the Ātmā. Both mind and body, of which latter the brain is a part, are veiled expressions of Consciousness, which in the case of matter is so veiled that it has the appearance of unconsciousness. The living brain is constituted of gross sensible matter (Mahābhūta) infused by Prāṇa or the life-principle. Its material has been worked up so as to constitute a suitable vehicle for the expression of Consciousness in the form of Mind (Antah-karaṇa). As Consciousness is not a property of the body, neither is it a mere function of the brain. The fact that mental consciousness is affected or disappears with disorder of the brain proves the necessity of the latter for the expression of *such* consciousness, and not that consciousness is inherent alone in brain or that it is the property of the same. On each side of the vertebral column there is a chain of ganglia connected with nerve fibre, called the sympathetic cord (Iḍā and Piṅgalā), extending all the way from the base of the skull to the coccyx. This is in

---

[1] Auguste Forel's " Hygiene of Nerves and Mind," p. 95.

communication with the spinal cord. It is noteworthy that there is in the thoracic and lumbar regions a ganglion of each chain corresponding with great regularity to each spinal nerve, though in the cervical region many of them appear to be missing; and that extra large clusters of nervous structure are to be found in the region of the heart, stomach and lungs, the regions governed by the Anāhata, Maṇipūra, and Viśuddha, respectively, the three upper of the five Cakras hereinafter described. From the sympathetic chain on each side nerve fibres pass to the viscera of the abdomen and thorax. From these, nerves are also given off which pass back into the spinal nerves, and others which pass into some of the cranial nerves; these are thus distributed to the blood-vessels of the limbs, trunk, and other parts to which the spinal or cranial nerves go. The sympathetic nerves chiefly carry impulses which govern the muscular tissue of the viscera and the muscular coat of the small arteries of the various tissues. It is through the sympathetic that the tone of the blood vessels is kept up by the action of the vaso-motor centre in the spinal bulb. The sympathetic, however, derives the impulses which it distributes from the central nervous system; these do not arise in the sympathetic itself. The impulses issue from the spinal cord by the anterior roots of the spinal nerves, and pass through short branches into the sympathetic chains. The work of the sympathetic systems controls and influences the circulation, digestion and respiration.[1]

The anatomical arrangement of the central nervous system is excessively intricate, and the events which take place in that tangle of fibre, cell and fibril, are, on the other hand, even now almost unknown.[2] And so it has been admitted that in the description of the physiology of the

[1] See Foster and Shore's "Physiology," pp. 206, 207.

[2] "Manual of Physiology," by G. N. Stewart, 5th edition, p. 657 (1906).

central nervous system we can as yet do little more than trace the paths by which impulses *may* pass between one portion of the system and another, and from the anatomical connections deduce, with more or less probability, the nature of the physiological nexus which its parts form with each other and the rest of the body.[1] In a general way, however, there may (it is said) be reasons to suppose that there are nervous centres in the central system related in a special way to special mechanisms, sensory, secretory, or motor, and that centres, such as the alleged genito-spinal centre, for a given physiological action exist in a definite portion of the spinal cord. It is the subtle aspect of such centres as expressions of Consciousness (Caitanya) embodied in various forms of Māyā-Śakti which is here called Cakra. These are related through intermediate conductors with the gross organs of generation, micturition, digestion, cardiac action, and respiration in ultimate relation with the Muladhāra, Svādhiṣṭhāna, Maṇipūra, Anāhata, and Viśuddha Cakras respectively, just as tracts have been assigned in the higher centres as being in special, even if not exclusive, relation with various perceptive, volitional, and ideative processes.

With this short preliminary in terms of modern Western physiology and anatomy, I pass to a description of the Cakras and Nāḍīs (nerves), and will then endeavour to correlate the two systems.

The conduits of Prānik or vital force are the nerves called Nāḍī, which are reckoned to exist in thousands in the body. "As in the leaf of the Aśvattha tree (*Ficus religiosa*), there are minute fibres, so is the body permeated by Nāḍīs."[2] Nāḍī is said in v. 2 to be derived from the root *nad*, or motion.

---

[1] *Ibid.*

[2] Shāṇḍilya Up., Ch. I, where the Nāḍīs are given and their purification spoken of; Dhyāna-bindu Up., and as to Suṣuṁnā see Maṇḍala-brāhmaṇa Up., First Brāhmaṇa.

For here the Prāṇa or Life Principle moves. The Bhūta-śuddhi Tantra speaks of 72,000, the Prapañcasāra-Tantra of 300,000, and the Śiva-Saṁhitā of 350,000; but of these, whatever be their total extent, only a limited number are of importance. Some are gross Nāḍīs, such as the physical nerves, veins and arteries, known to medical science. But they are not all of this gross or physical and visible character. They exist, like all else, in subtle forms, and are known as Yoga-Nāḍīs. The latter may be described as subtle channels (Vivara) of Prānik or vital energy. The Nāḍīs are, as stated, the conduits of Prāṇa. Through them its solar and lunar currents run. Could we see them, the body would present the appearance of those maps which delineate the various ocean currents. They are the paths along which Prāṇa-śakti goes. They therefore belong to the vital science as life-element, and not to the medical Śāstra (Vaidya-śāstra). Hence the importance of the Sādhana, which consists of the physical purification of the body and its Nāḍīs. Purity of body is necessary if purity of mind is to be gained in its extended Hindu sense. Purification of the Nāḍīs is perhaps the chief factor in the preliminary stages of this Yoga; for just as their impurity impedes the ascent of Kuṇḍalī-śakti, their purity facilitates it. This is the work of Prānāyāma (v. *post*).

Of these Nāḍīs, the principal are fourteen, and of these fourteen Iḍā, Piṅgalā, and Śuṣumṇā are the chief. Of these three, again, Suṣumṇā is the greatest, and to it all others are subordinate; for by the power of Yoga (Yogabala) Prāṇa is made to go through it, and, passing the Cakras, leave the body through the Brahma-randhra. It is situate in the interior of the cerebro-spinal axis, the Merudaṇḍa, or spinal column, in the position assigned to its interior canal, and extends from the basic plexus, the Tāttvik centre called the Mūlādhāra, to the twelve-petalled lotus in the pericarp of the Sahasrāra-Padma, or thousand-petalled lotus. Within the fiery red Tāmasik Suṣuṁnā is the lustrous Rājasik Vajrā or Vajriṇī-Nāḍī, and within the latter the pale nectar-dropping Sāttvik Citrā or Citriṇī. The interior of the latter is called the Brahma-Nāḍī. The first is said to be fire-like (Vahni-svarūpa), the second sun-like (Sūrya-svarūpa), and the third moon-like (Candra-svarūpa).[1] These are the threefold aspect of the Śabda-brahman. The opening at the end of the Citriṇī-Nāḍī is called the door of Brahman (Brahma-dvāra), for through it the Devī Kuṇḍalī enters to ascend.[2] It is along this last-mentioned Nāḍī, known as the Kula-Mārga and the "Royal Road," that the Śakti Kuṇḍalinī is led in the process hereafter described.

Outside this nerve are the two Nāḍīs, the pale Iḍā or Śaśī (Moon) and the red Piṅgalā or Mihira (Sun), which are connected with the alternate breathing from the right to the left nostril and *vice versa*.[3] The first, which is "feminine" (Śakti-rūpā) and the embodiment of nectar (Amṛta-vigrahā), is on the left; and the second, which is "masculine" as being in the nature of Rudra (Raudrāmikā), is on the right. They both indicate Time or Kāla, and Suṣuṁna devours Kāla. For on that path entry is made into timelessness. The three are also known as Gangā (Iḍā), Yamunā (Piṅgalā) and Sarasvatī (Suṣuṁnā), after the names of the three sacred rivers of India. The Mūlādhāra is the meeting-place of the

---

[1] Hence She is called in the Lalitā-Sahasranāma (v. 106) Mūlādhārāṁbujārūḍhā. Fire, Sun and Moon are aspects of the differentiated Parabindu or Kāmakalā (v. *ante*). See the Chapter on Sun, Moon and Fire in "Garland of Letters"

[2] The Sun generally represents poison, and the moon nectar (Shāṇḍilya Up., Ch. I). Both were obtained at the churning of the ocean, and represent the upbuilding and destructive forces of Nature.

[3] The Hindus have long known that breathing is done through one nostril for a period of time and then through the other. In Prāṇāyāma to make the breathing change one nostril is closed. But the skilled Yogī can shift the breathing at his will without closing a nostril with his fingers. At the moment of death breathing is through both nostrils at one and the same time.

three "rivers," and hence is called Yukta-triveṇī. Proceeding from the Ādhāra lotus, they alternate from right to left and left to right, thus going round the lotuses. According to another account, their position is that of two bows on either side of the spinal cord. An Indian medical friend tells me that these are not discrepant accounts, but represent different positions according as Iḍā and Piṅgalā exist inside or outside the spinal cord. When they reach the space between the eyebrows known as the Ājñā-Cakra, they enter the Suṣuṁnā, making a plaited knot of three called Mukta-triveṇī. The three "Rivers," which are again united at this point, flow separately therefrom, and for this reason the Ājñā-Cakra is called Mukta-triveṇī. After separation, the Nāḍī which proceeded from the right testicle goes to the left nostril, and that from the left testicle to the right nostril. It has been said that the distinction made between the heating "Sun" and cooling "Moon" is that which exists between the positive and negative phases of the same subject-matter, positive and negative forces being present in every form of activity. Piṅgalā is thus, according to this view, the conduit of the positive solar current, and Iḍā of the negative lunar current. There are also, as we have seen, interior solar and lunar Nāḍīs in the fiery Suṣuṁnā where the two currents meet.[1] These are all but microcosmic instances of the vaster system of cosmic matter, every portion of which is composed of three Guṇas (Triguṇātmaka) and the threefold Bindus, which are Sun, Moon, and Fire.

As regards nerve cords and fibres, cranial and spinal nerves, and the connected sympathetic nerves, Dr. Brojendranath Seal says: "With the writers on the Yoga, all the Śirās, and such of the Dhamanīs as are not vehicles of vital

[1] Similarly, there are three Nāḍīs which in Latāsādhanā are worshipped in the Madanāgāra—*viz.*, Cāndri, Saurī, Āgneyī, representing the sun, moon and fire.

current, metabolic fluid, lymph, chyle, or blood, are cranial nerves, and proceed from the heart through the spinal cord to the cranium. These cranial nerves include pairs for the larynx and the tongue, for the understanding and use of speech, for the raising and lowering of the eyelids, for weeping, for the sensations of the special senses etc., a confused and unintelligent reproduction of Suśruta's classification. But the enumeration of the spinal nerves with the connected sympathetic chain and ganglia is a distinct improvement on the old anatomists."[1]

He then continues: "The Suṣumnā is the central cord in the vertebral column (Brahma-daṇḍa or Meru). The two chains of sympathetic ganglia on the left and right are named Iḍā and Piṅgalā respectively. The sympathetic nerves have their main connection with Suṣumnā at the solar plexus (Nābhi-cakra). Of the seven hundred nerve cords of the sympathetic spinal system (see Saṅgītaratnākara), the fourteen most important are:[2]

"1. Suṣumnā, in the central channel of the spinal cord. 2. Iḍā, the left sympathetic chain, stretching from under the left nostril to below the left kidney in the form of a bent bow. 3. Piṅgalā, the corresponding chain on the right. 4. Kuhū, the pudic nerve of the sacral plexus, to the left of the spinal cord. 5. Gāndhārī, to the back of the left sympathetic chain, supposed to stretch from below the corner of the left eye to the left leg. It was evidently supposed that some nerves of the cervical plexus came down through the spinal cord and joined on to the great sciatic

[1] P. 340, Appendix to Professor Sarkar's "Positive Background of Hindu Sociology", subsequently published in his "Positive Sciences of the Hindus". The author annexes a plan which attempts to give a rough idea of the relative positions of the principal nerves of the sympathetic spinal system.

[2] Some of these are referred to in the present work: see v. 1.

nerve of the sacral plexus. 6. Hasti-jihvā, to the front of the left sympathetic chain, stretching from below the corner of the left eye to the great toe of the left foot, on the same supposition as before. Pathological facts were believed to point to a special nerve connection between the eyes and the toes. 7. Sarasvatī, to the right of Suṣumnā, stretching up to the tongue (the hypoglossol nerves of the cervical plexus). 8. Pūṣā, to the back of the right sympathetic chain, stretching from below the corner of the right eye to the abdomen (a connected chain of cervical and lumbar nerves). 9. Payasvinī, between Pūṣā and Sarasvatī, auricular branch of the cervical plexus on the left. 10. Śaṅkhinī, between Gāndhārī and Sarasvatī, auricular branch of the cervical plexus on the left. 11. Yaśasvinī, to the front of the right sympathetic chain, stretching from the right thumb to the left leg (the radial nerve of the brachial plexus continued on to certain branches of the great sciatic). 12. Vāruṇā, the nerves of the sacral plexus, between Kuhū and Yaśasvinī, ramifying over the lower trunk and limbs. 13. Viśvodarā, the nerves of the lumbar plexus, between Kuhū and Hasti-jihvā ramifying over the lower trunk and limbs. 14. Alambuṣā, the coccygeal nerves, proceeding from the sacral vertebræ to the urinogenitary organs."[1]

The Tattvas in the body pervaded by Prāṇa have certain special centres of predominance and influence therein, which are the Cakras (centres or circles or regions) or Padmas (lotuses) of which this work is a description.

Inside the Meru, or spinal column, are the six main centres of Tattvik operation, called Cakras or Padmas, which are the seats of Śakti, as the Sahasrāra above is the abode of

---

[1] Citing Saṅgītaratnākara, Ślokas 144-156; also the Yogārṇava-Tantra. This account has in parts been criticized by an Indian medical friend, who tells me that it is in those parts influenced too much by Western physiology.

Śiva.[1] These are the Mūlādhāra, Svādhiṣṭhāna, Maṇipūra, Anāhata, Viśuddha and Ājñā, which *in the physical body* are said to have their correspondences in the principal nerve plexuses and organs, commencing from what is possibly the sacro-coccygeal plexus to the "space between the eyebrows," which some identify with the pineal gland, the centre of the third or spiritual eye, and others with the cerebellum. The Cakras[2] themselves are, however, as explained later, centres of Consciousness (Caitanya) as extremely subtle force (Śakti); but the gross regions which are built up by their coarsened vibrations, which are subject to their influence, and with which loosely and inaccurately they are sometimes identified, have been said to be various plexuses in the trunk of the body and the lower cerebral centres mentioned. In the portion of the body below the Mūlādhāra are the seven lower worlds, Pātāla and others, together with the Śaktis which support all in the universe.

The first centre, or Mūlādhāra-Cakra, which is so called from its being the root of Suṣumnā where Kuṇḍalī rests,[3] is at the place of meeting of the Kaṇḍa (root of all the Nāḍīs) and the Suṣumnā-Nāḍī, and is in the region midway between the genitals and the anus. It is thus the centre of the body for men.[4] By this and similar statements made as regards the other lotuses, it is not meant that the Cakra proper is in the region of the gross body described, but that it is *the subtle centre* of that gross region, such centre existing in the spinal column which forms its axis. The reader must bear this

---

[1] Varāha Up., Ch. V.

[2] See Ch. V, Varāha Up. and Dhyānabindu Up. and Ch. III, Yogakuṇḍalī Up.

[3] Derived from Mūla (root) and Ādhāra (support).

[4] Śāṇḍilya Up., Ch. I, where also the centres for birds and other animals are given. In some diagrams (Kashmir "Nāḍī-cakra") Kuṇḍalī is represented above the position given in the Text.

observation in mind in the descriptions of the Cakras, or an erroneous notion will be formed of them. This crimson Mūlādhāra lotus [1] is described as one of four petals, the Vṛttis of which are the four forms of bliss known as Paramānanda, Sahajānanda, Yogānanda and Vīrānanda.[2] On these four petals are the golden letters Vaṁ (वं), Śaṁ (शं), Ṣaṁ (षं), and Saṁ (सं).[3] Each letter in its Vaikharī form is a gross manifestation of inner or subtle Śabda. On the petals are figured the letters, which are each a Mantra, and as such a Devatā. The petals are configurations made by the position of the Nāḍīs at any particular centre, and are in themselves Prāṇa-śakti manifested by Prāṇa-vāyu in the living body. When that Vāyu departs they cease to be manifest. Each letter is thus a particular Śabda or Śakti and a surrounding (Āvaraṇa) Devatā of the Principal Devatā and its Śakti of the particular Cakra. As Śakti they are manifestations of Kuṇḍalī and in their totality constitute Her Mantra body, for Kuṇḍalī is both light (Jyotirmayī) and Mantra (Mantramayī). The latter is the gross or Sthūla aspect of which Japa is done. The former is the Sūkṣma or subtile aspect which is led up to in Yoga. Their specific enumeration and allocation denote the differentiation in the body of the total Śabda. This Lotus is the centre of the yellow Pṛthivī, or "Earth" Tattva, with its quadrangular Maṇḍala, the Bīja or Mantra of which Tattva is Laṁ (लं).[4]

---

[1] This and other lotuses hang head downwards except when Kuṇḍalī passes through them, when they turn upwards.

[2] These Vṛttis or qualities (see *post*) denoting four forms of bliss are not given in the text here translated, but in Tarkālankāra's Commentary to the Mahānirvāṇa-Tantra.

[3] In this and other cases meditation is done from the right (Dakṣiṇāvartena). See v. 4, Ṣat-cakra-nirupaṇa cited as S.N.

[4] The Dhyānabindu Up. associates the Bījas with the five Prāṇas. Thus "Laṁ" is associated with Vyāna.

At this centre is the Pṛthivī-Tattva, the Bīja of which is "La", with Bindu or the Brahmā-consciousness presiding over this centre or "Laṁ" which is said to be the expression in gross (Vaikharī) sound of the subtle sound made by the vibration of the forces of this centre. So, again, the subtle Tejas Tattva and its Bīja Raṁ is in the Maṇipūra-Cakra, and the gross fire known as Vaiśvānara is in the physical belly, which the subtle centre governs. This Bīja represents in terms of Mantra the Tattva regnant at this centre, and its essential activity. With the symbolism used throughout this work, Bīja is said to be seated on the elephant Airāvata, which is here located. This and the other animals figured in the Cakras are intended to denote the qualities of the Tattvas there regnant. Thus, the elephant is emblematic of the strength, firmness, and solidity, of this Tattva of "Earth". They are, further, the vehicles (Vāhana) of the Devatās there. Thus in this Cakra there is the seed-mantra (Bīja) of Indra, whose vehicle is the elephant Airāvata. The Devatā of the centre is, according to the Text, the creative Brahmā, whose Śakti is Sāvitrī.[1] There also is the Śakti known as Dākinī,[2] who, as also the other Śaktis, Lākinī and the rest, which follow, are the Śaktis of the Dhātus or bodily substances[3] assigned to this and the other centres. Here is the "female" triangle or Yoni known as Traipura, which is the Śaktipīṭha, in which is set the "male" Śiva-linga, known as Svayaṁbhu, of the shape and colour of a young leaf, representing, as do all Devīs and Devas, the Māyā-Śakti and Cit-Śakti aspects of the Brahman as manifested in the particular centres (vv. 4-14). The lingas are four—

---

[1] The Creator is called Savitā because He creates.

[2] Who, according to Sammohana-Tantra, Ch. II, acts as keeper of the door.

[3] *Viz.*, chyle, blood, flesh, fat, bone, marrow, seed.

Svayaṁbhu, Bāṇa, Itara, Para. According to the Yoginīhṛdaya-Tantra[1] (Ch. I), they are so called because they lead to Cit. They are the Pīṭhas, Kāmarūpa and the rest because they reflect Cit (Citsphurattādhāratvāt). They are Vṛttis of Manas, Ahaṁkāra, Buddhi, Citta. To the first three are assigned certain forms and colours—namely, yellow, red, white, triangular, circular; as also certain letters—namely, the sixteen vowels, the consonants Ka to Ta (soft), and Tha to Sa. Para is formless, colourless and letterless, being the collectivity (Samaṣṭi) of all letters in the form of bliss. The Traipura is the counterpart in the Jīva of the Kāmakalā of the Sahasrāra. The Devī Kuṇḍalinī, luminous as lightning, shining in the hollow of this lotus like a chain of brilliant lights, the World-bewilderer who maintains all breathing creatures,[2] lies asleep coiled three and a half times[3] round the Linga, covering with Her head the Brahma-dvāra.[4]

The Svādhiṣṭhāna-Cakra is the second lotus proceeding upwards, and is, according to the commentary, so called after Sva or the Paraṁ Lingaṁ.[5] It is a vermilion lotus of six petals placed in the spinal centre of the region at the root of the genitals. On these petals are the letters like lightning: Baṁ (बं), Bhaṁ (भं), Maṁ (मं), Yaṁ (यं), Raṁ (रं), Laṁ (लं). "Water" (Ap) is the Tattva of this Cakra, which is known as the white region of Varuṇa. The Tāttvik Maṇḍala is in the shape of a crescent moon[6] (Ardhendurūpa-

[1] Yoginīhṛdaya Tantra, Ch. I.

[2] See v. 49, S. N.

[3] These correspond with the three and a half Bindus of which the Kubjikā Tantra speaks. See *ante*.

[4] Entrance to the Suṣumnā.

[5] For another definition see Dhyānabindu Up., where all the Cakras are named. Another derivation is "own abode" (of Śakti).

[6] The diagrams or maṇḍalas symbolic of the elementals are also given, as here stated, in the first chapter of the Śāradā-Tilaka and in the

lasitam). The Bīja of water (Varuṇa) is "Vaṁ". This, the Varuṇa-Bīja, is seated on a white Makara[1] with a noose in his hand. Hari (Viṣṇu) and Rākinī Śakti of furious aspect, showing Her teeth fiercely, are here (vv. 14—18).

Above it, at the centre of the region of the navel, is the lotus Maṇipūra (Nābhi-padma), so called, according to the Gautamīya-Tantra, because, owing to the presence of the fiery Tejas, it is lustrous as a gem (Maṇi).[2] It is a lotus of ten petals on which are the letters Ḍaṁ (डं), Ḍhaṁ (ढं), Ṇaṁ (णं), Taṁ (तं), Thaṁ (थं), Daṁ (दं), Dhaṁ (धं), Nam (नं), Paṁ (पं), Phaṁ (फं). This is the triangular region of the Tejas-Tattva. The triangle has three Svastikas. The red Bīja of fire, "Raṁ" is seated on a ram, the carrier of Agni, the Lord of Fire. Here is the old red Rudra smeared with white ashes, and the Śakti Lākinī who as the Devatā of this digestive centre is said to be "fond of animal food, and whose breasts are ruddy with the blood and fat which drop from Her mouth". Lākinī and the other special Śaktis of the centres here named are the Śaktis of the Yogī himself—that is, Śaktis of the Dhātus assigned to each of his bodily centres, and concentration on this centre may involve the satisfaction of the appetites of this Devatā. The Śaktis of the higher centres are not meat-eaters. From these three centres the gross Virāt, waking body, is evolved (vv. 19—31).

Next above the navel lotus (Nābhi-padma) is the Anāhata, in the region of the heart, which is red like a Bandhūka flower, and is so called because it is in this place that Munis

---

Viśvasāra-Tantra, cited at p. 25 of the Prāṇa-toṣiṇī, with the exception that, according to the Viśvasāra Tantra, the Maṇḍala of water is not a crescent, but eight-cornered (Aṣṭāśra). Different Tantras give different descriptions. See Śāradā, Ch. I.

[1] An animal like an alligator. See Plate III.

[2] For another derivation, derived from Samaya worship, see Commentry on the Lalitā-Sahasranāma, vv. 88, 99.

or Sages hear that "sound (Anāhata-śabda) which comes without the striking of any two things together", or the "sound" of the Śabda-brahman, which is here the Pulse of Life. For it is here that the Puruṣa (Jīvātmā) dwells. This lotus is to be distinguished from the Heart Lotus of eight petals, which is represented in the place below it, where in mental worship the Patron Deity (Iṣta-devatā) is meditated upon. (See Plate V.) Here is the Tree which grants all desires (Kalpataru) and the jewelled Altar (Maṇi-piṭha) beneath it. As the Viśvasāra-Tantra cited in the Prāṇa-toṣini says: "Śabda-brahman is said to be Deva Sadāśiva. That Śabda is said to be in the Anāhata-cakra. Anāhata is the great Cakra in the heart of all beings. Oṁkāra is said to be there in association with the three Guṇas." [1] The Mahā-svacchandra-Tantra says: [2] "The great ones declare that Thy blissful form, O Queen, manifests in Anāhata, and is experienced by the mind inward-turned of the Blessed Ones, whose hairs stand on end and whose eyes weep with joy." This is a lotus of twelve petals with the vermilion letters Kaṁ (कं), Khaṁ (खं), Gaṁ (गं), Ghaṁ (घं), Ṅaṁ (ङं), Caṁ (चं), Chaṁ (छं), Jaṁ (जं), Jhaṁ (झं), Jñaṁ (ञं), Ṭaṁ (टं), Ṭhaṁ (ठं). This is the centre of the Vāyu-Tattva. According to v. 22, the region of Vāyu is six-cornered (that is formed by two triangles, of which one is inverted) and its colour that of smoke by reason of its being surrounded by masses of vapour.[3] Its Bīja "Yaṁ"

---

[1] P. 10.

Śabda-brahmeti taṁ prāha sākṣād devah sadāśivah,
Anāhateṣu cakreṣu sa śabdah parikīrttnate.
Anāhataṁ mahācakraṁ hṛdaye sarvajantuṣu,
Tatra omkāra ityukto guṇatraya-samanvitah.

[2] Cited by Bhāskararāya's Comm. on Lalitā, v. 121, on the title of the Devī as Nāda-rūpā; and in v. 218, where she is described as Nādarūpiṇī, referring also to Yoginīhṛdaya-Tantra.

[3] According to the Śāradā, Ch. I (and to the same effect Prapañcasāra-Tantra) the colours of the Bhūtas are as follows: Ākāśa (ether) is transparent (Svaccha); Vāyu (air) is black (Kṛṣṇa); Agni (fire) is

is seated on a black antelope which is noted for its fleetness, and is the Vāhana of "Air" (Vāyu), with its property of motion. Here are Īśa, the Overlord of the first three Cakras; the Śakti Kākinī garlanded with human bones, whose "heart is softened by the drinking of nectar"; and the Śakti in the form of an inverted triangle (Trikoṇa), wherein is the golden Bāṇa-Linga, joyous with a rush of desire" (Kāmodgamollasita), and the Haṁsa as Jīvātmā, like "the steady flame of a lamp in a windless place" (vv. 22—27). The Ātmā is so described because, just as the flame is undisturbed by the mind, so the Ātmā is in itself unaffected by the motions of the world.[1]

The seventeenth verse of the Ānanda-Laharī mentions that the Devatās Vaśinī and others are to be worshipped in the two last-mentioned Cakras. Vaśinī and others are eight in number.[2]

(1) Vaśinī, (2) Kāmeśvarī, (3) Modinī, (4) Vimalā, (5) Aruṇā, (6) Jayinī, (7) Sarveśvarī, and (8) Kālī or Kaulinī. These are respectively the Presiding Deities of the following eight groups of letters: (1) अ to अः, 16 letters; (2) क to ङ, 5 letters; (3) च to ञ, 5 letters; (4) ट to ण, 5 letters; (5) त to न, 5 letters; (6) प to म, 5 letters; (7) य to व, 4 letters; (8) श to क्ष or ळ, 5 letters.

The other beings in v. 17 of Ānanda-Laharī refer to the twelve Yoginīs, who are: (1) Vīdyā-yoginī, (2) Recikā, (3) Mocikā, (4) Amṛtā, (5) Dīpikā, (6) Jñānā, (7) Āpyāyanī, (8) Vyapinī, (9) Medhā, (10) Vyoma-rūpā, (11) Siddhi-rūpā, and (12) Lakṣmi-yoginī.

---

red (Rakta); Ap water is white (Śveta); and Pṛthivī (earth) is yellow (Pīta).

[1] This steady, still, state is that of the Ātmā as such. See Maṇḍala-brāhmaṇa Up., Brāhmaṇas II, III.

[2] "Saundarya Lahari", Ganesh & Co. (Madras) Private Ltd., pp. 40-41.

These twenty Deities (eight Vaśinīs and twelve Yoginīs) are to be worshipped in Maṇipūra and Anāhata centres. In respect of this, the Commentator quotes a verse from the Tāittirīyāraṇyaka, and gives a description of these Deities, their respective colours, place, and so forth.

At the spinal centre of the region at the base of the throat (Kaṇṭha-mūla) is the Viśuddha-Cakra or Bhāratī-sthāṇa,[1] with sixteen petals of a smoky purple hue, on which are the sixteen vowels with Bindu thereon—that is, Aṁ (अं), Āṁ (आं), Iṁ (इं), Īṁ (ईं), Uṁ (उं), Ūṁ (ऊं), Ṛṁ (ऋं), Ṝṁ (ॠं), Lriṁ (ऌं), Lrīṁ (ॡं), Eṁ (एं) Aim (ऐं), Om (ओं), Auṁ (औं), and the two breathings Aṁ (अं), Ah, (अः). According to the Devī-Bhāgavata (VII. 35), the Cakra is so called because the Jīva is made pure (Viśuddha) by seeing the Haṁsa. Here is the centre of the white circular Ākāśa or Ether Tattva, the Bīja of which is "Haṁ". Ākāśa is dressed in white and mounted on a white elephant. Its Maṇḍala is in the form of a circle.[2] Here is Sadāśiva in his androgyne or Ardhanārīśvara Mūrti, in which half the body is white and the other half gold. Here also is the white Śakti Śākinī, whose form is light (Jyoti-svarūpa). Here, too, is the lunar region, "the gateway of the Great Liberation". It is at this place that the Jñānī "sees the three forms of time" (Trikāladarśī). As all things are in the Ātmā, the Jñānī who has realized the Ātmā has seen them (vv. 28—31). Above the Viśuddha, at the root of the palate, is a minor Cakra called Lalanā, or in some Tantras Kalā-Cakra, which is not mentioned in the works here translated. It is a red lotus with twelve petals bearing

[1] That is, abode of the Devī of speech.

[2] This is sometimes represented as a circle with a number of dots in it, for as the Prapañcasāra-Tantra says, Ākāśa has innumerable Suṣira —that is, Chidra, or spaces between its substance. It is because of its interstitial character that things exist in space.

the following Vṛtti or qualities: Śraddhā (faith), Saṁtoṣa (contentment), Aparādha (sense of error), Dama (self-command), Māna (anger),[1] Sneha (affection),[2] Śuddhatā (purity), Arati (detachment), Saṁbhrama (agitation),[3] Ūrmi (appetite).[4] (*V. post.*)

Before summarising the previous description, it is to be here observed that the Commentator Kālīcaraṇa states the principle of this Yoga to be that that which is grosser is merged into that which is more subtle (Sthulānāṁ sūkṣme layah). The grosser are lower in the body than the more subtle. The gross which are in and below the Mūlādhāra or connected with it are: (1) the Pṛthivī-Tanmātra; (2) the Pṛthivī Maha-bhūtā; (3) the nostrils with their sense of smell, which is the grossest of the senses of knowledge (Jñānendriya), and which is the quality (Guṇa) of the Pṛthivī Tanmātra; and (4) the feet, which are the grossest of the senses of action (Karmendriya), and "which have Pṛthivī (earth) for their support". Here the nostrils are classified as the grossest of the Jñānendriyas, because therein is the sense which perceives the quality (Guṇa) of smell of the grossest Tanmātra (Gandha), from which is derived the Pṛithivī Sthūla-Bhūta. Thus the Jñānendriyas have a relation with the Tanmātras through their Guṇas (qualities), for the perception of which these senses exist. In the case, however, of the senses of action (Karmendriya), no such relation appears to exist between them and the Tanmātras. In the order of successive merging or Laya, the feet occur in the

---

[1] This term is generally applied to cases arising between two persons who are attached to one another, as man and wife.

[2] Usually understood as affection towards those younger or lower than oneself.

[3] Through reverence or respect.

[4] Or it may refer to the six which are technically called ūrmi—that is, hunger, thirst, sorrow, ignorance (moha), decay, and death.

same grade as earth, hands in the same grade as water, anus in the same grade as fire, penis in the same grade as air, and mouth in the same grade as ether; not, apparently, because there is any direct relation between earth and feet, water and hands, fire and anus, and so forth, but because these organs are in the same order of comparative subtlety as earth, water, and fire, and so forth. Hands are supposed to be subtler agents than feet; the anus[1] a subtler agent than the hands; the penis a subtler agent than the anus; and the mouth a subtler agent than the penis. This is also the order in which these agents are situated in the body, the hands coming second because they find their place between the feet and the anus when the arms are given their natural vertical positions. It is to be remembered in this connection that the Tantras here follow the Sāṁkhya, and state the scheme of creation as it occurs also in the Purāṇas, according to which the Jñānendriyas and Karmendriyas and the Tanmātras issue from different aspects of the threefold Ahaṁkāra. There is a relation between the senses and the Tanmātras in the created Jīva, according to the Vedānta, for the senses are related to the Tanmātras, but the order, in that case, in which the senses occur is different from that given in this work. For, according to the Vedāntik scheme, earth is related to the sense of smell and penis; water to the sense of taste and anus; fire to the sense of sight and feet; air to the sense of touch and hands; and ether to the sense of hearing and mouth. Another explanation, seemingly artificial, however, which has been given, is as follows: The feet are associated with "Earth" because the latter alone has the

[1] At first sight this might appear not to be so, but the importance of the anus is well known to medical experts, its sensitivity having even given rise to what has been called a "psychology of the anus".

power of support, and the feet rest on it. "Water" is associated with the hands because in drinking water the hand is used. The word Pāṇi, which means hands, is derived from the root Pā, to drink (Pīyate anena iti pāṇi). "Fire" is associated with the anus because what is eaten is consumed by fire in the stomach, and the residue is passed out through the anus, whereby the body becomes pure. "Air" is associated with the penis because in procreation the Jīvātmā as Prāṇa-Vāyu throws itself out through the penis. And so the Śruti says: "Ātmā itself is reborn in the son" (Ātmāvai jāyate putrah). "Ether" is associated with the mouth because by the mouth sound is uttered, which is the Guṇa (quality) of ether (Ākāśa).

Hitherto we have dealt with the comparatively gross Tattvas. According to this work, the twenty grosser Tattvas are associated (4 × 5) as in the following table:

Centre in which dissolved	*Grosser Tattvas*
1. Mūlādhāra	... Gandha (smell) Tanmātra; Pṛthivī-Tattva (earth); the Jñānendriya of smell;[1] the Karmendriya of feet.
2. Svādhiṣṭhāna	... Rasa (taste) Tanmātra; Ap-Tattva (water); the Jñānendriya of taste; the Karmendriya of hands.
3. Maṇipūra	... Rūpa (sight) Tanmātra; Tejas-Tattva (fire); the Jñānendriya of sight; the Karmendriya of anus.
4. Anāhata	... Sparśa (touch) Tanmātra; Vāyu-Tattva (air); the Jñānendriya of touch; the Karmendriya of penis.
5. Viśuddha	... Śabda (sound) Tanmātra; Ākāśa-Tattva (ether); the Jñānendriya of hearing; the Karmendriya of mouth.

[1] The nose is a centre at which sexual excitement may be aroused or subdued. Though the reproductive organ is higher up than the Mūlādhāra the sexual force ultimately proceeds from the latter.

It will be observed that with each of the elements is associated an organ of sensation (Jñānendriya) and action (Karmendriya). In Chapter II of the Prapañcasāra-Tantra it is said: "Ether is in the ears, air in the skin, fire in the eyes, water in the tongue, and earth in the nostrils." The Karmendriyas are possibly so arranged because the Tattvas of the respective centres in which they are placed are, as above stated, of similar grades of subtlety and grossness. As explained below, each class of Tattvas is dissolved in the next higher class, commencing from the lowest and grossest centre, the Mūlādhāra. So far the Tattvas have been those of the "matter" side of creation.

Progress is next made to the last or Ājñā-Cakra, in which are the subtle Tattvas of Mind and Prakṛti. The Cakra is so called because it is here that the command (Ājñā) of the Guru is received from above. It is a lotus of two white petals between the eyebrows, on which are the white letters Haṁ (हं) and Kṣaṁ (क्षं). This exhausts the fifty letters. It will have been observed that there are fifty petals and fifty letters in the six Cakras. In the pericarp is the great Mantra "Oṁ". Each Lotus has either two or four more petals than the one immediately below it, and the number of the petals in the Viśuddha-Cakra is the sum of the preceeding differences. Here are Paramaśiva in the form of Haṁsa (Haṁsa-rūpa), Siddha-kālī, the white Hākinī-Śakti "elated by draughts of ambrosia", the inverted triangle or Yonī (Trikoṇa), and the Itara Linga, shining like lightning, which is set in it. The three Lingas are thus in the Mūlādhāra, Anāhata, and Ājñā-Cakras respectively; for here at these three 'Knots' or Brahma-granthis the force of Māyā Śakti is in great strength. And this is the point at which each of the three groups of Tattvas associated with Fire, Sun, and Moon, converge.[1] The

[1] *V. post.*

phrase "opening the doors" refers to passage through these Granthis. Here in the Ājñā is the seat of the subtle Tattvas, Mahat and Prakṛti. The former is the Antahkaraṇa with Guṇas—namely, Buddhi, Citta, Ahaṁkāra and its product Manas (Sasaṁkalpa-vikalpaka). Commonly and shortly it is said that Manas is the Tattva of the Ājñā Cakra. As, however, it is the mental centre, it includes all the aspects of mind above stated, and the Prakṛti whence they derive, as also the Ātmā in the form of the Praṇava (Oṁ) its Bīja. Here the Ātmā (Antarātmā) shines lustrous like a flame. The light of this region makes visible all which is between the Mūla and the Brahma-randhra. The Yogī by contemplation of this lotus gains further powers (Siddhi), and becomes Advaitācāra-vādī (Monist). In cọnnection with this Padma, the text (S. N., v. 36) explains how detachment is gained through the Yonī-Mudrā. It is here that the Yogī at the time of death places his Prāṇa, and then enters the supreme primordial Deva, the Purāṇa (ancient) Puruṣa, "who was before the three worlds, and is known by the Vedānta". The same verse describes the method (Prāṇāropaṇa-prakāra). From the last centre and the causal Prakṛti is evolved the subtle body which individually is known as Taijas, and collectively (that is, the Īśvara aspect) as Hiraṇya-garbha. The latter term is applied to the manifestation of the Paramātmā in the Antah-karaṇa; as displayed in Prāṇa it is Sūtrātmā; and when manifested through these two vehicles without differentiation it is known as the Antar-yāmin. The Cakras are the bodily centres of the world of differentiated manifestation, with its gross and subtle bodies arising from their causal body, and its threefold planes of consciousness in waking, sleeping, and dreamless slumber.

Above the Ājñā-cakra (vv. 32—39) there are the minor Cakras called Manas and Soma, not mentioned in the texts here translated. The Manas Cakra is a lotus of six petals, on the petals of which are (that is, which is the seat of) the sensations of hearing, touch, sight, smell, taste, and centrally initiated sensations in dream and hallucination. Above this, again, is the Soma-Cakra, a lotus of sixteen petals, with certain Vṛttis which are detailed latter.[1] In this region are " the house without support " (Nirālaṁbapurī), " where Yogīs see the radiant Īśvara," the seven causal bodies (v. 39) which are intermediate aspects of Ādyā Śakti, the white twelve-petalled lotus by the pericarp of the Sahasrāra (vv. 32—39), in which twelve-petalled lotus is the A-ka-ṭha triangle, which surrounds the jewelled altar (Maṇipīṭha) on the isle of gems (Maṇidvīpa), set in the Ocean of Nectar,[2] with Bindu above and Nāda below, and the Kāmakalā triangle and the Guru of all, or Parama-śiva. Above this, again, in the pericarp, are the Sūrya and Candra-Maṇḍalas, the Para-bindu surrounded by the sixteenth and seventeenth digits of the moon circle. In the Candra-Maṇḍala there is a triangle. Above the Moon is Mahā-vayu, and then the Brahma-randhra with Mahā-śaṃkhinī.

The twelve-petalled lotus and that which is connected with it is the special subject of the short book Pādukā-pañcaka-Stotra here translated, which is a hymn by Śiva in praise of the " Fivefold Footstool ", with a commentary by Śrī-Kālīcaraṇa. The footstools are variously classified as follows: According to the first classification they are—(1) the white twelve-petalled lotus in the pericarp of the Sahasrāra lotus. Here there is (2) the inverted Triangle the abode of Śakti called " A-ka-ṭha ". (3) The region of the Altar (Maṇipītha), on each side of which are Nāda and

---

[1] *V. post.*

[2] In mental worship the jewelled altar of the Iṣṭadevatā is in the eight-petalled lotus below Anāhata (see Plate V). The Isle of Gems is a supreme state of Consciousness, and the Ocean of Nectar is the infinite Consciousness Itself. As to the causal bodies, see " Garland of Letters ".

Bindu. The eternal Guru, " white like a mountain of silver," should be meditated upon, as on the Jewelled Altar (Maṇipītha). (4) The fourth Pādukā is the Haṁsa below the Antarātmā; and (5) the Triangle on the Pīthā. The differences between this and the second classification are explained in the notes to v. 7 of the Pādukā. According to this latter classification they are counted as follows: (1) The twelve-petalled lotus; (2) the triangle called A-ka-tha; (3) Nāda-Bindu; (4) the Maṇipītha-Maṇḍala; and (5) the Haṁsa, which makes the triangular Kāmakalā. This Triangle, the Supreme Tattva, is formed by the three Bindus which the text calls Candra (Moon), Sūrya (Sun), and Vahni (Fire) Bindus, which are also known as Prakāśa, Vimarśa,[1] and Miśra-Bindu. This is the Haṁsa known as the triangular Kāmakalā, the embodiment of Puruṣa-Prakṛti, The former is the Bindu Haṁkāra at the apex of the triangle, and the two other Bindus called Visarga or Sa are Prakṛti. This Kāmakalā is the Mūla (root) of Mantra.

The Śabdabrahman with its threefold aspect and energies is represented in the Tantras by this Kāmakalā, which is the abode of Śakti (Abalālayam). This is the Supreme Triangle, which, like all Yonī-pīṭhas, is inverted. It may be here noted that Śakti is denoted by a triangle because of its threefold manifestation as Will, Action, and Knowledge (Icchā, Kriyā, Jñāna). So, on the material plane, if there are three forces, there is no other way in which they can be brought to interact except in the form of a triangle in which, while they are each separate and distinct from one another, they are yet related to each other and form part of one whole. At the corners of the Triangle there are two Bindus, and at the apex a single Bindu. These are the Bindus of Fire (Vahni-bindu), Moon

[1] As to this term see "Mahāmāyā" and "Kāmakalāvilāsa," by A. Avalon.

(Candra-bindu), and Sun (Sūrya-bindu).[1] Three Śaktis emanate from these Bindus, denoted by the lines joining the Bindus and thus forming a triangle. These lines are the line of the Śakti Vāmā, the line of the Śakti Jyeṣṭhā, and the line of the Śakti Raudrī. These Śaktis are Volition (Icchā), Action (Kriyā), and Cognition (Jñāna). With them are Brahmā, Viṣṇu, and Rudrā, associated with the Guṇas, Rajas, Sattva, and Tamas.

The lines of the triangle emanating from the three Bindus or Haṁsa are formed by forty-eight letters of the alphabet. The sixteen vowels beginning with A form one line; the sixteen consonants beginning with Ka form the second line; and the following sixteen letters beginning with Tha form the third line. Hence the triangle is known as the A-ka-tha triangle. In the inner three corners of the triangle are the remaining letters Ha, Lla, Kṣa. The Yāmala thus speaks of this abode, " I now speak of Kāmakalā," and, proceeding, says: " She is the eternal One who is the three Bindus, the three Śaktis, and the three Forms (Tri-Mūrti)." The Bṛhat-Śrī-krama, in dealing with Kāmakalā, says: " From the Bindu (that is, the Para-bindu) She has assumed the form of letters (Varṇāvayava-rūpiṇī)." The Kālī Urdhvāmnāya says: " The threefold Bindu (Tri-bindu) is the supreme Tattva, and embodies in itself Brahmā, Viṣṇu, and Śiva." [2] The triangle which is composed of the letters has emanated from the Bindu. These letters are known as the Mātṛkā-Varṇa. These form the

---

[1] The Kāmakalāvilāsa says: " Bindu-trayamayas tejas-tritayah " (three Bindus and three fires). " Tripurasundarī sits in the Cakra which is composed of Bindus (Bindumaye-cakre), Her abode being the lap of Kāmeśvara, whose forehead is adorned by the crescent moon. She has three eyes, which are Sun, Moon, and Fire."

[2] The Māhesvari-Saṁhitā says: " Sūrya, Candra, and Vahni, are the three Bindus; and Brahmā, Viṣṇu, and Saṁbhu are the three lines."

body of Kula-kuṇḍalinī[1] the Śabdabrahman, being in their Vaikharī state various manifestations of the primal unmanifested "sound" (Avyaktanāda).

They appear as manifested Śabda on the self-division of the Parā-bindu; for this self-division marks the appearance of the differentiated Prakṛti.

The commentary on the Pādukā-pañcaka (v. 3) says that the Bindu is Parā-Śakti itself, and its variations are called Bindu, Nāda, and Bīja, or Sun, Moon, and Fire; Bindu, the sun, being red, and Nāda, the moon, being white.[2] These form the Cinmaya or Ānandamaya-kośa or sheaths of consciousness and bliss (Pādukā-pañcaka, v. 3). The two Bindus making the base of the triangle are the Visarga (*ib.*, v. 4). In the Āgama-kalpadruma it is said: "Haṁkāra is Bindu or Puruṣa, and Visarga is Sah or Prakṛti. Haṁsah is the union of the male and female, and the universe is Haṁsah." The triangular Kāmakalā is thus formed by Haṁsah (*ib.*). The Haṁsa-pītha is composed of Mantras (*ib.*, v. 6).

As this subject is of great importance, some further authorities than those referred to in the work here translated are given. In his commentary to v. 124 of the Lalitā, in which the Devī is addressed as being in the form of Kāmakalā (Kāmakalārūpā), Bhāskararāya says: "There are three Bindus and the Hārdha-kalā.[3] Of these Bindus the first is called Kāma, and the Hakārārdha is named Kalā."[4] He adds that the nature of Kāmakalā is set forth in the

---

[1] The Kāmakalāvilāsa says: "Ekapañcāṣadakṣarātma" (She is in the form of the 51 letters). See A. Avalon's edition and translation of "Kāmakalāvilāsa".

[2] This appears to be in conflict with the previous statement of Rāghava-Bhatta, that Bindu is Moon and Nāda the Sun.

[3] Also called Hakārārdha—that is, half the letter Ha (ह).

[4] Bindu-trayaṁ hārdha-kalā ca ityatra prathamo binduh kāmākhyā Caramā-kalā ca iti pratyāhāra-nyāyena kāmakaletyuch-yate.

Kāmakalā-vilāsa in the verses commencing "Supreme Śakti (Parā-Śakti) is the manifested union of Śiva and Śakti in the form of seed and sprout," and ending with the lines "Kāma (means) desire, and Kalā the same. The two Bindus are said to be the Fire and Moon."[1] Kāma, or creative Will, is both Śiva and Devī, and Kalā is their manifestation. Hence it is called Kāmakalā. This is explained in the Tripurā-siddhānta: "O, Pārvati, Kalā is the manifestation of Kāmeśvara and Kāmeśvarī. Hence She is known as Kāmakalā."[2] Or she is the manifestation (Kalā) of desire (Kāma)[3] that is, of Icchā. The Kālikā-Purāṇa says: "Devī is called Kāma because She came to the secret place on the blue peak of the great mountain Kailāsa along with Me for the sake of desire (Kāma): thus Devī is called Kāma. As She is also the giver or fulfiller of desire, desiring, desirable, beautiful, restoring the body of Kāma (Manmatha) and destroying the body of Kāma, hence She is called Kāma."[4] After Śiva (with whom She is one) had destroyed Kāma, when he sought by the instilment of passion to destroy His Yoga; so She (with whom He is one) afterwards gave a new body to the "Bodiless One" (Anaṅga). They destroy the worlds and take them to themselves through the cosmic Yoga path,

---

[1] Tasyāh svarūpaṁ sphuṭa-śiva-śaktī-samāgama-bījāṁkurarūpiṇī parā śaktirityārabhya kāmah kamanīyatayā kalā ca dahanendu-vigrahau bindū ityantena nirṇītaṁ kāmakalāvilāse tadrūpetyarthaha (*ib.*).

[2] Kāmayoh kaleti vā, taduktaṁ, tripurā-siddhānte:

Tasya kāmeśvarākhyasya kāmeśvaryāś ca parvati.
Kalākhyā salīlā sā ca khyātā kāmakaleti sā.

[3] Kāmaś cāsau kalārūpā ceti vā.

[4] Kāmapadamatra-vācyatāyāh Kālīpurāṇe pratipādanāt.

Kāmārtham āgatā yasmān mayā sārdhaṁ mahā-girau.
Kāmākhyā procyate devī nīlakūtarahogatā.
Kāmadā kāminī kāṁyā kāntā kāmāṅgadāyinī.
Kāmāṅganāśinī yasmāt kāmākhyā tena kathyate.
Iti ṣadakṣaramidaṁ nāma (*ib.*).

and again by Their desire and will (Icchā) recreate them. These Bindus and Kalā are referred to in the celebrated Hymn, "Wave of Bliss" (Ānandalaharī).[1]

This Devī is the great Tripura-sundarī. Bhāskararāya's Guru Nṛsiṃhānandanātha wrote the following verse, on which the disciple commentates: "I hymn Tripurā, the treasure of Kula,[2] who is red of beauty; Her limbs like unto those of Kāmarāja, who is adored by the three Devatas[3] of the three Guṇas; who is the desire (or will) of Śiva;[4] who dwells in the Bindu and who manifests the universe." She is called (says the commentator cited)[5] Tripurā, as She has three (Tri) Puras (*lit.*, cities), but, here meaning Bindus, angles, lines, syllables, etc. The Kālikā-Purāṇa says: "She has three angles (in the triangular Yonī) as well as three circles (the three Bindus), and her Bhūpura[6] has three lines. Her Mantra

---

[1] Mukhaṁ binduṃ kṛtvā kucayugaṁ adhas tasya tadadho
Hakārārdhaṁ dhyāyet haramahiṣi te manmathakalāṁ (v. 19).

(Let him contemplate on the first Bindu as the face of the Devī, and on the other two Bindus as Her two breasts, and below that on the half Ha.) Half Ha is the Yonī, the womb, and origin of all. See Lalitā, v. 206.

[2] Kulanidhi. In its literal ordinary sense Kula means race or family, but has a number of other meanings: Śakti (Akula is Śiva), the spiritual hierarchy of Gurus, the Mūlādhāra, the doctrine of the Kaula-Tāntriks, etc.

[3] Viśṇu, Brahmā and Rudra of the Sattva, Rajas and Tamas qualities respectively.

[4] This is the Commentator's meaning of Ekām tām. Ekā—a+i=e. According to the Viśva Dictionary, "A" has among other meanings that of Īśa or Śiva, and, according to the Anekārtha-dhvani-mañjarī Lexicon, I=Manmatha, that is, Kāma, or desire. Ekā is therefore the spouse of Śiva, or Śivakāma, the desire or will of Śiva.

[5] Introduction to Lalitā.

[6] The portion of the Yantra which is of common form and which encloses the particular design in its centre. Reference may, however, also be here made to the three outer lines of the Śrī-cakra.

is said to be of three syllables,[1] and She has three aspects. The Kuṇḍalinī energy is also threefold, in order that She may create the three Gods (Brahmā, Viṣṇu, Rudra). Thus, since She the supreme energy is everywhere triple, She is called Tripura-sundarī." [2] These syllables are said by the commentator last cited [3] to be the three Bījas of the three divisions (of the Pañcadaśī)—*viz.*, Vāgbhava, Kāmarāja, and Śakti, which according to the Vāmakeśvara-Tantra are the Jñāna-Śakti which confers salvation, and the Kriyā- and Icchā-Śaktis.

Three "Pāda" are also spoken of as Tripurā—white, red, and mixed.[4] Elsewhere, as in the Varāha-Purāṇa, the Devī is said to have assumed three forms—white, red, and black; that is, the Supreme energy endowed with the Sāttvik, Rājasik, and Tāmasik qualities.[5] The one Śakti becomes three to produce effects.

---

[1] *V. post.* The Kāma-Bīja is Klīṁ. Klīṁkārā is Śivakāma. Here Īm means the Kāmakalā in the Turīya state through which Mokṣa is gained, and hence the meaning of the saying (*ib.*, v. 176) that he who hears the Bīja without Ka and La does not reach the place of good actions—that is, he does not go to the region attained by good actions, but to that attainable by knowledge alone (see *ib.*, v. 189, citing Vāmakeśvara-Tantra).

[2] Other instances may be given, such as the Tripurārṇava, which says that the Devī is called Tripurā because She dwells in the three Nāḍīs (Suṣumnā, Piṅgalā, and Iḍā; *v. post*) and in Buddhi, Manas, Citta (*v. post*).

[3] V. 177.

[4] According to a note of R. Anantakṛṣna-Śāstri, translator of the Lalitā, p. 213, the three "feet" are explained in another work of Bhāskararāya as follows: White, the pure Saṁvit (Consciousness) untainted by any Upādhis; red, the Parāhaṁta (Supreme Individuality), the first Vṛtti (modification) from the Saṁvit; and the mixed—the above mentioned as one inseparable modification (the Vṛtti) of "I". These are known as the "three feet" (Caraṇa-trītaya), or Indu (white), Agni (red), Ravi (mixed).

[5] So also the Devī Bhāgavata Pr. says: "The Śāmbhavī is white; Śrī-vidyā red; and Śyāmā, black." The Yantra of Śrī-vidyā is the Śrī-cakra mentioned.

In the Kāmakalā meditation (Dhyāna) the three Bindus and Hārdha-kalā are thought of as being the body of the Devī Tripura-sundarī. The Commentator on the verse of the Ānandalaharī cited says:[1] "In the fifth sacrifice (Yajña) let the Sādhaka think of his Ātmā as in no wise different from, but as the one only Śiva; and of the subtle thread-like Kuṇḍalinī which is all Śaktis, extending from the Ādhāra lotus to Parama-Śiva. Let him think of the three Bindus as being in Her body (Tripura-sundarī), which Bindus indicate Icchā, Kriyā, Jñāna—Moon, Fire, and Sun; Rajas, Tamas, Sattva; Brahmā, Rudra, Viṣṇu; and then let him meditate on the Cit-kalā who is Śakti below it." [2]

The Bindu which is the "face" indicates Viriñci[3] (Brahmā) associated with the Rajas Guṇa. The two Bindus which are the "breasts," and upon which meditation should be done in the heart, indicate Hari[4] (Viṣṇu) and Hara[5] (Rudra) associated with the Sattva and Tamas Guṇas. Below them meditate in the Yoni upon the subtle Cit-kalā, which indicates all three Guṇas, and which is all these three Devatās.[6] The meditation given in the Yoginī-Tantra is as

---

[1] Saṁkarācārya-granthāvalī (Vol. II), ed. Śrī Prasanna-Kumāra Śāstrī. The editor's notes are based on the Commentary of Acyutānanda-Svāmī.

[2] Atha pañcamayāge abhedabuddhyā ātmānaṁ śiva-rūpaṁ ekātmānaṁ vibhāvya ādhārāt paramaśivāntaṁ sūtrarūpāṁ sūkṣmāṁ kuṇḍalinīṁ sarvaśakti-rūpāṁ vibhāvya sattva-rajas-tamoguṇa-sūcakaṁ brahmā-viṣṇu-śiva-śaktyātmakaṁ sūryāgnicandrarūpaṁ bindu-trayaṁ tasyā aṅge vibhāvya adhaś citkalāṁ dhyāyet (Comm. to v. 19).

[3] That is, He who creates, from *Vi+rich*.

[4] He who takes away or destroys (harati) all grief and sin.

[5] The same.

[6] Mukhaṁ binduṁ kṛtvā rajoguṇasūcakaṁ viriñcyātmakaṁ binduṁ mukhaṁ kṛtvā, tasyādho hṛdaya-sthāne sattva-tamo-guna-sūcakaṁ hariharātmakaṁ bindudvayaṁ kucayugaṁ kṛtvā, tasyādhah yoniṁ guṇa-traya-sūcikāṁ hari-hara-viriñcyātmikāṁ sūkṣmāṁ citkalāṁ hakārārdhaṁ kṛtvā yonyantargata-trikoṇākṛtiṁ kṛtvā dhyāyet (*ib.*).

follows: "Think of three Bindus above Kalā, and then that from these a young girl sixteen years old springs forth, shining with the light of millions of rising suns, illuminating every quarter of the firmament. Think of Her body from crown to throat as springing from the upper Bindu, and that her body from throat to middle, with its two breasts and three belly lines of beauty (Trivalī), arise from the two lower Bindus. Then imagine that the rest of Her body from genitals to feet is born from Kāma. Thus formed, She is adorned with all manner of ornaments and dress, and is adored by Brahmā, Īśa, and Viṣṇu. Then let the Sādhaka think of his own body as such Kāmakalā."[1] The Śrītattvārṇava says: "The glorious men who worship in that body in Sāmarasya[2] are freed from the waves of poison in the untraversable sea of the world (Saṁsāra)."

To the same effect are the Tāntrik works the Śrī-krama[3] and Bhāva-cūdāmaṇi[4] cited in the Commentary to the Ānandalaharī. The first says: "Of the three Bindus, O Mistress of the Devas, let him contemplate the first as the mouth and in the heart the two Bindus as the two breasts. Then let him meditate upon the subtle Kalā Hakārārdha in the Yoni." And the second says: "The face in the form of Bindu, and below twin breasts, and below them the

---

[1] See p. 199, *et seq.*, Nityapūjā-paddhati, by Jaganmohana-Tarkālaṁkāra.

[2] That is equal feeling; or being one with; union of Śiva and Śakti.

[3] Tathā ca Śrīkrame:

> Bindutrayasya deveśi prathamaṁ devi vaktrakaṁ,
> Bindudvayaṁ stanadvandvaṁ hṛdi sthāne niyojayet.
> Hakārādhaṁ kalāṁ sūkṣmāṁ yonimadhye vicintayet.

[4] Taduktaṁ Bhāva-cūdāmanau:

> Mukhaṁ binduvadākāraṁ Tadadhah kuca-yugmakaṁ
> Tadadhaśca hakārārdhaṁ Supariṣkṛtamaṇḍalaṁ.

The second line of this verse is also printed Tadadhah saparārdhaṁ cha. But this means the same thing. Sapara is Hakāra, as Ha follows Sa. For further Dhyānas and mode of meditation, see p. 199 of the Nityapūjā paddhati of Jaganmohana-Tarkālaṁkāra.

beauteous form of the Hakārārdha." The three Devatās Brahmā, Viṣṇu, and Rudra, with their Śaktis, are said to take birth from the letters A, U, M, of the Oṁkāra or Praṇava.[1] Ma, as the Prapañcasāra-Tantra [2] says, is the Sun or Ātmā among the letters, for it is Bindu. From each of these ten Kalās arise.

Verse 8 of the first work translated says that in the Mūlādhāra centre there is the Triangle (Trikoṇa) known as Traipura, which is an adjective of Tripura. It is so called because of the presence of the Devī Tripurā within the Ka inside the triangle. This Ka is the chief letter of the Kāma Bīja, and Kaṁ [3] is the Bīja of Kāminī, the aspect of Tripura-sundarī in the Mūlādhāra. Here also, as the same verse says, there are the three lines Vāmā, Jyeṣṭhā, and Raudrī and, as the Ṣaṭcakra-vivṛti adds, Icchā, Jñāna, and Kriyā.[4] Thus the Traipura-Trikoṇa is the gross or Sthūla aspect of that subtle (Sukṣma) Śakti which is below the Sahasrāra, and is called Kāmakalā. It is to this Kāminī that in worship the essence of Japa (Tejo-rūpajapa) is offered, the external Japa being offered to the Devata, worshipped in order that the Sādhaka may retain the fruits of his worship.[5] There are also two other Liṅgas and Trikoṇas at the Anāhata and Ājñā centres, which are two of the Knots or Granthis, and which are so called because Māyā is strong

---

[1] Pheṭkāriṇī-Tantra, Ch. I:

> Tebhya eva samutpannā varṇā ye viṣṇu-śūlinoh
> Mūrtayah śakti-saṁyuktā ucyante tāh krameṇa tu.

And so also Viśvasāra-Tantra (see Prānatoṣinī, 10):

> Śivo brahmā tathā viṣṇurokāre ca pratiṣṭhitāh,
> Akāraś ca bhaved brahmā Ukārah saccidātmakah,
> Makāro rudra ityukṭa iti tasyārthakalpanā.

[2] Ch. III.

[3] Nityapūjā-paddhati, p. 80, by Jaganmohana-Tarkālaṁkāra.

[4] See p. 117, *post.*

[5] Nityapūjā-paddhati, *loc. cit.*

at these points of obstruction, at which each of the three groups converge. The Traipura-Trikoṇa is that, however, in the Mūlādhāra which is the grosser correspondence of the Kāmakalā, which is the root (Mūlā) of all Mantras below the Sahasrāra, and which, again, is the correspondence in Jīva of the Tri-bindu of Īśvara.

Before, however, dealing in detail with the Sahasrāra, the reader will find it convenient to refer to the tables on pp. 141 and 142, which summarize some of the details above given upto and including the Sahasrāra.

In the description of the Cakras given in this work, no mention is made of the moral and other qualities and things (Vṛtti) which are associated with the Lotuses in other books, such as the Adhyātmaviveka,[1] commencing with the root-lotus and ending with the Soma-Cakra. Thus, the Vṛttis, Praśraya, Aviśvāsa, Avajñā, Mūrcchā, Garvanāśa, Krūratā,[2] are assigned

---

[1] Quoted in the Dīpikā to v. 7 of the Haṁsopaniṣad and see Śaṁgītaratnākara, Ch. I, Prakaraṇa ii.

(1) Mūlādhāra—Parama, Sahaja, Vīrānanda, Yogānanda.

(2) Svādhiṣṭhāna—Praśraya, Krūratā, Garvanāśa, Mūrcchā, Avajñā, Aviśvāsa.

(3) Maṇipūra—Suṣupti, Tṛṣṇā, Īrṣyā, Piśunatā, Lajjā, Bhaya, Ghṛṇā, Moha, Kaṣāya, Viṣāditā.

(4) Anāhata—Laulyapraṇāśa, Prakata, Vitarka, Anutāpitā, Āśā, Prakāśa, Cintā, Samūhā, Samatā, Daṁbha, Vaikalya, Viveka, Ahaṁkṛti.

(5) Viśuddhi—Prāṇava, Udgītha, Huṁphaṭ, Vaṣat, Svadhā, Svāhā, Namaḥ, Amṛta, Ṣadja, Ṛṣabha, Gāndhāra, Madhyama, Pañcama, Dhaivata, Niṣāda, Viṣa.

(6) Lalanā-Cakra—Mada, Māna, Sneha, Śoka, Khedla, Lubdhatā, Arati, Saṁbhrama, Ūrmi, Śraddhā, Toṣa, Uparodhitā.

(7) Ājña-Cakra—Sattva āvirbhāva, Raja āvirbhāva, Tama āvirbhāva.

(8) Manas-Cakra—Svapna, Rasopabhoga, Ghrāṇa, Rūpopalaṁbha, Sparśa, Śabdabodha.

(9) Sahasrāra or Soma-Cakra—Kṛpā, Kṣamā, Ārjava, Dhairya, Vairāgya, Dhṛti, Sammada, Hāsya, Romāñcanicaya, Dhyanāśru, Sthiratā, Gāṁbīrya, Udyama, Acchatva, Audārya, Ekāgratā.

[2] Credulity, suspicion, disdain, delusion (or disinclination), false knowledge (*lit.*, destruction of everything which false knowledge leads to), pitilessness.

to Svādhiṣṭhāna: Lajjā, Piśunatā, Īrśā, Tṛṣṇā, Suṣupti, Viṣāda, Kaṣāya, Moha, Ghṛṇā, Bhaya,[1] to the Maṇipūra; Āśa, Cintā, Ceṣṭā, Samatā, Daṁbha, Vikalatā, Ahaṁkāra, Viveka, Lolatā, Kapaṭatā, Vitarka, Ānutāpa to Anāhata[2]; Kṛpā, Mṛduta, Dhairya, Vairāgya, Dhṛti, Saṁpat, Hāsya, Romāñca, Vinaya, Dhyāna, Susthiratā, Gāṁbhīrya, Udyama, Akṣobha, Audārya, Ekāgratā,[3] to the secret Soma-cakra; and so forth. In the Mūlādhāra, which has been described as the "source of a massive pleasurable æthesia," there are the four forms of bliss already mentioned; in the Viśuddha the seven subtle "tones," Niṣāda, Ṛṣabha, Gāndhāra, Ṣadja, Madhyama, Dhaivata, Pañcama; certain Bījas, Huṁphat, Vauṣat, Vaṣat, Svadhā, Svāhā, Namah; in the eighth petal "venom," and in the sixteenth "nectar";[4] and in the petals and pericarp of the Ājñā the three Guṇas and in the former the Bījas, Haṁ and Kṣaṁ; and in the six-petalled Manas-Cakra above the Ājña are Śabda-jñāna, Sparśa-jnāna, Rūpa-jñāna, Āghrāṇopalabdhi, Rasopabhoga, and Svapna, with their opposites, denoting the sensations of the sensorium—hearing, touch, sight, smell, taste, and centrally initiated sensations in dream and hallucination. It is stated that particular Vṛttis are assigned to a particular lotus, because of a connection between such Vṛtti and the operation of the Śaktis of the Tattva at the centre to which it is assigned. That they exist at any particular Cakra is said to

---

[1] Shame, treachery, jealousy, desire, supineness, sadness, worldliness, ignorance, aversion (or disgust), fear.

[2] Hope, care or anxiety, endeavour, mineness (resulting in attachment), arrogance or hypocrisy, sense of languor, egoism or self-conceit, discrimination, covetousness, duplicity, indecision, regret.

[3] Mercy, gentleness, patience or composure, dispassion, constancy, prosperity (spiritual), cheerfulness, rapture or thrill, humility or sense of propriety, meditativeness, quietude or restfulness, gravity (of demeanour), enterprise or effort, emotionlessness (being undisturbed by emotion), magnanimity, concentration.

[4] Both were extracted at the churning of the ocean, and, as so spoken of, represent the destructive and upbuilding forces of the world.

be shown by their disappearance when Kuṇḍalī ascends through the Cakra. Thus the bad Vṛttis of the lower Cakras pass away in the Yogī who raises Kuṇḍali above them.

Moral qualities (Vṛtti) appear in some of the lower Cakras in the secret twelve-petalled lotus called the Lalanā (and in some Tantras Kalā) Cakra, situate above the Viśuddha, at the root of the palate (Tālumūla), as also in the sixteen-petalled lotus above the Manas-Cakra, and known as the Soma-Cakra. It is noteworthy that the Vṛtti of the two lower Cakras (Svādhiṣṭhāna and Maṇipūra) are all bad; those of the Anāhata centre are mixed,[1] those of the Lalanā-Cakra are predominantly good, and those of the Soma-Cakra wholly so; thus indicative of an advance as we proceed from the lower to the higher centres, and this must be so as the Jīva approaches or lives in his higher principles. In the twelve-petalled white lotus in the pericarp of the Sahasrāra is the abode of Śakti, called the Kāmakalā, already described.

Between Ājñā and Sahasrāra, at the seat of the Kāraṇa-Śarīra of Jīva, are the Varṇāvalī-rupā Viloma-Śaktis, descending from Unmanī to Bindu. Just as in the Īśvara or cosmic creation there are seven creative Śaktis from Sakala Parameśvara to Bindu; and in the microcosmic or Jīva creation seven creative Śaktis from Kuṇḍalinī, who is in the Mūlādhāra, to Bindu, both of which belong to what is called the Anuloma order:[2] so in the region between the Ājñā-Cakra and Sahasrāra, which is the seat of the causal body (Kāraṇa-Śarīra) of Jīva, there are seven Śaktis,[3] which,

[1] *E.g.*, with Dambha (arrogance) Lolatā (covetousness), Kapatatā (duplicity), we find Āśā (hope), Ceṣṭā (endeavour), Viveka (discrimination).

[2] That is, the ordinary as opposed to the reversed (viloma) order. Thus, to read the alphabet as A to Z is anuloma; to read it backwards, Z to A, is viloma. In the above matter, therefore anuloma is evolution (sṛṣṭi) or the forward movement, and viloma (nivṛtti) the path of return.

[3] See "Garland of Letters," Chapter on "Causal Śaktis of the Praṇava".

commencing with the lowest, are Bindu (which is in Īśvara-Tattva), Bodhinī, Nāda, Mahānāda or Nādānta (in Ṣadakhya-Tattva), Vyāpikā, Samanī (in Śakti-Tattva), and Unmanī (in Śiva-Tattva). Though these latter Śaktis have a cosmic creative aspect, they are not here co-extensive with and present a different aspect from the latter. They arc not co-extensive, because the last-mentioned Śaktis are,

Cakra	Situation	Number of Petals	Letters on Same	Regnant Tattva and its Qualities	Colour of Tattva
Mūlādhāra	Spinal centre of region below genitals	4	va, śa, ṣa, sa	Pṛthivī; cohesion, stimulating sense of smell	Yellow
Svādhiṣṭhāna	Spinal centre of region above the genitals	6	ba, bha, ma, ya, ra, la	Ap; contraction, stimulating sense of taste	White
Maṇipūra	Spinal centre of region of the navel	10	ḍa, ḍha ṇa, ta, tha, da, dha, na pa, pha	Tejas; expansion, producing heat and stimulating sight-sense of colour and form	Red
Anāhata	Spinal centre of region of the heart	12	ka, kha, ga, gha, ṅa, ca, ccha, ja, jha, jña, ṭa, ṭha	Vāyu; general movement, stimulating sense of touch	Smoky
Viśuddha	Spinal centre of region of the throat	16	the vowels a, ā, i, ī, u, ū, ṛ, ṝ, ḷ, ḹ, e, ai, o, au, aṃ, aḥ	Ākāśa; space-giving, stimulating sense of hearing	White
Ājñā	Centre of region between the eyebrows	2	ha and kṣa	Manas (mental faculties)	...

Above the Ájñā is the causal region and the Lotus of a thousand petals, with all the letters, wherein is the abode of the Supreme Bindu Paraśiva.

Shape of Mandala	Bija and its Vahana (Carrier)	Devata and its Vahana	Śakti of the Dhatu	Linga and Yoni	Other Tattvas here Dissolved
Square	Laṁ on the Airāvata elephant	Brahmā on Haṁsa	Ḍākini	Svayaṁbhu and Traipura-Trikoṇa	Gandha (smell) Tattva; smell (organ of sensation); feet (organ of action)
Cresent	Vaṁ on Makara	Viṣṇu on Garuda	Rākinī	...	Rasa (taste) Tattva; taste (organ of sensation); hand (organ of action)
Triangle	Raṁ on a ram	Rudra on a bull	Lākinī	...	Rūpa (form and colour; sight) Tattva; sight (organ of sensation); anus (organ of action)
Six-pointed hexagon	Yaṁ on an antelope	Īśā	Kākinī	Bāṇa and Trikoṇa	Sparśa (touch and feel) Tattva; touch (organ of sensation); penis (organ of action)
Circle	Haṁ on a white elephant	Sadāśiva	Sākinī	...	Śabda (sound) Tattva; hearing (organ of sensation; mouth (organ of action)
...	Oṁ	Śaṁbhu	Hākinī	Itara and Trikoṇa	Mahat, the Sūkṣma Prakṛti called Hiraṇyagarbha (v. 52)

as here mentioned, Śaktis of the Jīva. Haṁsa, Jīva or Kuṇḍalī is but an infinitesimal part of the Para-bindu. The latter is in the Sahasrāra, or thousand-petalled lotus, the abode of Īśvara, who is Śiva-Śakti and is the seat of the aggregate Kuṇḍalī or Jīva. And hence it is said that all the letters are here twentyfold ($50 \times 20 = 1,000$). In the Sahasrāra are Para-bindu, the supreme Nirvāṇa-Śakti, Nirvāṇa-Kalā, Amā-Kalā,[1] and the fire of Nibodhikā. In the Para-bindu is the empty void (Śūnya) which is the supreme Nirguṇa-Śiva.

Another difference is to be found in the aspect of the Śaktis. Whilst the cosmic creative Śaktis are looking outwards and forwards (Unmukhī), the Śaktis above the Ājñā are in Yoga, looking backwards towards dissolution. The Īśvara of the Sahasrāra is not then the creative aspect of Īśvara. There He is in the Nirvāṇa mood, and the Śaktis leading up to Nirvāṇa-Śakti are "upward moving," that is, liberating Śaktis of the Jīva.

These seven states or aspects of Bindumaya-paraśakti (see p. 424, *post*) leading up to Unmanī, which are described in this and other Tāntrik books, are called causal forms (Kāraṇa-rūpa). The commentary to the Lalitā[2] apparently enumerates eight, but this seems to be due to a mistake, Śakti and Vyāpikā being regarded as distinct Śaktis instead of differing names for the third of this series of Śaktis.

Below Visarga (which is the upper part of the Brahmarandhra, in the situation of the fontanelle) and the exit of Śaṅkhinī-Nāḍī is the Supreme White (or, as some call it, variegated) Lotus of a thousand petals (see vv. 41—49 *post*) known as the Sahasrāra, on which are all the letters of the Sanskrit alphabet, omitting according to some the cerebral Lakāra, and according to others Kṣa. These are repeated

[1] See "Garland of Letters," Chapter on "Kalās of the Śaktis".

[2] V. 121. Lalitā-Sahasranāma.

twenty times to make the 1,000, and are read from beginning to end (Anuloma), going round the Lotus from right to left. Here is Mahā-vāyu and the Candra-maṇḍala, in which is the Supreme Bindu (O), "which is served in secret by all the Devas". Bindu implies Guṇa, but it also means the void of space, and in its application to the Supreme Light, which is formless, is symbolical of its decaylessness. The subtle Śūnya (Void), which is the Ātmā of all being (Sarvātmā), is spoken of in vv. 42—49. Here in the region of the Supreme Lotus is the Guru, the Supreme Śiva Himself. Hence the Śaivas call it Śivasthāna, the abode of bliss where the Ātmā is realized. Here, too, is the Supreme Nirvāṇa-Śakti, the Śakti in the Para-bindu, and the Mother of all the three worlds. He who has truly and fully known the Sahasrāra is not reborn in the Samsāra, for he has by such knowledge broken all the bonds which held him to it. His earthly stay is limited to the working out of the Karma already commenced and not exhausted. He is the possessor of all Siddhi, is liberated though living (Jīvanmukta), and attains bodiless liberation (Mokṣa), or Videha-Kaivalya, on the dissolution of his physical body.

In the fourteenth verse and commentary thereon of the Ānandalaharī, the Deity in the Sahasrāra is described.[1]

"She is above all the Tattvas. Every one of the six centres represents a Tattva. Every Tattva has a definite number of rays. The six centres, or Cakras, are divided into three groups. Each of these groups has a knot or apex where converge the Cakras that constitute that group. The names of the groups are derived from those of the Presiding Deities. The following table clearly puts the above:

---

[1] See Paṇḍit R. Anantakṛṣṇa Śāstrī, "Saundarya Lahari," p. 36 (Ganesh & Co., (Madras) Private Ltd.) The passage within quotation marks is taken from that work.

See "Wave of Bliss," by A. Avalon.

No.	Name of Cakra	Name of Tattva	No. of Rays of Tattva	Name of Group	Name of Converging Point	Remarks
1 2	Mūlādhāra Svādhiṣṭhāna	Bhū Agni	56 } 62 }	Agni Khaṇḍa	Rudra- granthi	In Sahasrāra the rays are numberless, eternal and unlimited by space.
3 4	Maṇipūra Anāhata	Apas Vāyu	52 } 54 }	Sūrya	Viṣṇu granthi	There is another Candra here whose rays are countless and evershining.
5 6	Viśuddha Ājñā	Ākāśa Manas	72 } 64 }	Candra	Brahma granthi	
			360			

"Lakṣmīdhara quotes the Taittirīyāraṇyaka in support of his commentary, from which we have taken the notes above given. The extracts which he makes from 'Bhairava-Yāmala' are very valuable. In discoursing about Candrā, Śiva addresses (vv. 1—17, Candra-jñānavidyāprākaraṇa) Pārvati, his consort, thus:

"'Welcome, O Beauty of the three worlds, welcome is Thy question. This knowledge (which I am about to disclose) is the secret of secrets, and I have not imparted it to anyone till now. (But I shall now tell thee the grand secret. Listen, then, with attention:)'

"'Śrī-cakra (in the Sahasrāra) is the form of Parā-Śakti. In the middle of this Cakra is a place called Baindava, where She, who is above all Tattvas, rests united with Her Lord Sadāśiva. O Supreme One, the whole Cosmos is a Śrī-cakra formed of the twenty-five Tattvas—5 elements + 5 Tanmātras + 10 Indriyas + Mind + Māya, Śuddha-vidyā, Maheśa, and Sadāśiva.[1] Just as it is in Sahasrāra, so

[1] Māyā to Sadāśiva are the Śiva-Tattvas described in "Garland of Letters".

cosmically, also, Baindava is above all Tattvas. Devī, the cause of the creation, protection, and destruction, of the universe, rests there ever united with Sadāśiva, who as well is above all Tattvas and ever-shining. Uncountable are the rays that issue forth from Her body; O good one, they emanate in thousands, lakhs—nay, crores. But for this light there would be no light at all in the universe. . . 360 of these rays illumine the world in the form of Fire, Sun, and Moon. These 360 rays are made up as follows: Agni (Fire) 118, Sun 106, Moon 136. O Śaṁkari, these three luminaries enlighten the macrocosm as well as the microcosm, and give rise to the calculation of time—the Sun for the day, the Moon for the night, Agni (Fire) occupying a mean position between the two.' [1]

"Hence they constitute (or are called) Kāla (time), and the 360 days (rays) make a year. The Veda says: 'The year itself is a form of the Lord. The Lord of time, the Maker of the world, first created Marīci (rays), etc., the Munis, the protectors of the world. Everything has come to exist by the command of Parameśvarī.'

"Diṇḍima takes a quite different view of this verse. He interprets it as meaning that, having already described the Antaryāga (inner worship), the author recommends here the worship of the Āvaraṇa-Devatās, *i.e.*, Deities residing in each of the Cakras or centres without propitiating whom it is impossible for the practitioner to lead the Kuṇḍalinī through these Cakras. He enumerates all the 360 Deities and describes the mode of worshipping each of them.

"There are other commentators who understand the 360 rays esoterically, and connect the same with the 360 days of the year, and also with the human body. Every commentator quotes the Taittirīyāraṇyaka, first chapter, to

---

[1] See "Wave of Bliss," ed. A. Avalon.

support his views. Thus it seems that Taittirīyāraṇyaka contains much esoteric matter for the mystic to digest. The first chapter of the Āraṇyaka referred to is chanted in worshipping the Sun. It is called Āruṇam because it treats of Aruṇā (red-coloured Devī)." [1]

An Indian physician and Saṁskritist has expressed the opinion that better anatomy is given in the Tantras than in the purely medical works of the Hindus.[2] It is easier, however, to give a statement of the present and ancient physiology than to correlate them. Indeed, this is for the present a difficult matter. In the first place, the material as regards the latter is insufficiently available and known to us, and those Hindu scholars and Sādhakas (now-a-days, probably not numerous) who are acquainted with the subject are not conversant with Western physiology, with which it is to be compared. It is, further, possible to be practically acquainted with this Yoga without knowing its physiological relations. Working in what is an unexplored field, I can only here put forward, on the lines of the Text and such information as I have gathered, explanations and suggestions which must in some cases be of a tentative character, in the hope that they may be followed up and tested by others.

It is clear that the Meru-daṇḍa is the vertebral column, which as the axis of the body is supposed to bear the same relation to it as does Mount Meru to the earth. It extends from the Mūla (root) or Mūlādhāra to the neck. It and the connected upper tracts, spinal bulb, cerebellum, and the like, contain what has been described as the central system

[1] P. 38 of Paṇḍit Anantakṛṣṇa-Śāstrī's "Saundaryalahari", Ganesh & Co. (Madras) Private Ltd.

[2] Dr. B. D. Basu, of the Indian Medical Service, in his Prize Essay on the Hindu System of Medicine, published in the *Guy's Hospital Gazette* (1889), cited in Vol. XVI, "Sacred Books of the Hindus," by Professor Benoy Kumar Sarkar.

of spinal nerves (Nāḍī) and cranial nerves (Śiro-nāḍī). The Suṣuṁnā, which is undoubtedly a Nāḍī within the vertebral column, and as such is well described by the books as the principal of all the Nāḍīs, runs along the length of the Meru-daṇḍa, as does the spinal cord of Western physiology, if we include therewith the *filum terminale.* If we include the *filum,* and take the Kaṇḍa to be between the anus and penis, it starts from practically the same (sacro-coccygeal) region, the Mūlādhāra, and is spoken of as extending to the region of the Brahma-randhra,[1] or to a point below the twelve-petalled lotus (v. 1)—that is, at a spot below but close to the Sahasrāra, or cerebullum, where the nerve Citriṇī also ends. The position of the Kaṇḍa is that stated in this work (v. 1). It is to be noted, however, that according to the Haṭha-yoga-pradīpikā the Kaṇḍa is higher up, between the penis and the navel.[2] The place of the union of Suṣuṁnā and Kaṇḍa is known as the "Knot" (Granthi-ṣṭhāna), and the petals of the Mūla lotus are on four sides of this (v. 4). It is in this Suṣuṁnā (whatever for the moment we take it to be) that there are the centres of Prāṇa-Śakti or vital power which are called Cakras or Lotuses. The spinal cord ends blindly in the *filum terminale,* and is apparently closed there. The Suṣuṁnā is said to be closed at its base, called the "gate of Brahman" (Brahma-dvāra) until, by Yoga, Kuṇḍalī makes its way through it. The highest of the six centres called Cakra in the Suṣuṁnā is the Ājñā, a position which corresponds frontally with the space between the eyebrows (Bhrū-madhya), and at the back with the pineal gland, the pituitary body, and the top of the cerebellum. Close by it is the Cakra called Lalanā, and in some Tantras Kalā

---

[1] Sammohana-Tantra, II, 7, or according to the Tripurā-sāra-samuccaya, cited in v. 1, from the head to the Ādhāra.

[2] *V. post.*

Cakra which is situate at the root of—that is, just above—the palate (Tālumūla). Its position as well as the nature of the Ājñā would indicate that it is slightly below the latter.[1] The Suṣuṁnā passes into the ventricles of the brain, as does the spinal cord, which enters the fourth ventricle.

Above the Lalanā are the Ājñā-Cakra with its two lobes and the Manas-Cakra with its six lobes, which it has been suggested are represented in the physical body by the Cerebellum and Sensorium respectively. The Soma-Cakra above this, with its sixteen "petals," has been said to comprise the centres in the middle of the Cerebrum above the Sensorium. Lastly, the thousand-petalled lotus Sahasrāra corresponds to the upper Cerebrum of the physical body, with its cortical convolutions, which will be suggested to the reader on an examination of the Plate VIII, here given, of that centre. Just as all powers exist in the seat of voluntary action, so it is said that all the fifty "letters" which are distributed throughout the spinal centres of the Suṣuṁnā exist here in multiplied form—that is, 50×20. The nectar-rayed moon[2] is possibly the under-part of the brain, the convolutions or lobes of which, resembling half-moons, are called Candrakalā, and the mystic mount Kailāsa is undoubtedly the upper brain. The ventricle connected with the spinal cord is also semi-lunar in shape.

As above stated, there is no doubt that the Suṣuṁnā is situated in the spinal column, and it has been said that it represents the central canal. It is probable that its general position is that of the central canal. But a query may be raised if it is meant that the canal alone is the Suṣuṁnā. For the latter Nāḍī, according to this work, contains within it two

[1] Vide "Introduction to Tantra-Śāstra" pp. 49-51 for a brief description of the Cakras, including Lalanā and Kalā Cakras.

[2] See Śiva-Saṁhitā, II, 6.

others—namely, Vajriṇī and Citriṇī. There is thus a threefold division. It has been suggested that the Suṣumnā when not considered with its inner Nāḍīs as a collective unit, but as distinguished from them, is the white nervous matter of the spinal cord, Vajriṇī the grey matter, and Citriṇī the central canal, the inner Nāḍī of which is known as the Brahma-nāḍī, and, in the Śiva-saṁhitā, Brahma-randhra.[1] But as against such suggestion it is to be noted that v. 2 of this work describes Citriṇī as being as fine as a spider's thread (Lūtā-tantūpameya), and the grey matter cannot be so described, but is a gross thing. We must therefore discard this suggestion, and hold to the opinion either that the central canal is the Suṣumnā or that the latter is in the canal, and that within or part of it are two still more subtle and imperceptible channels of energy, called Vajriṇī and Citriṇī. I incline to the latter view. The true nature of the Citriṇī-Nāḍī is said in v. 3 to be pure intelligence (Śuddha-bodha-svabhāvā) as a force of Consciousness. As v. 1 says, the three form one, but considered separately they are distinct. They are threefold in the sense that Suṣumnā, who is tremulous like a woman in passion," is as a whole composed of "Sun," "Moon," and "Fire," and the three Guṇas. It is noteworthy in this connection that the Kṣurikā-Upaniṣad,[2] which speaks of the Suṣumnā, directs the Sādhaka "to get into the white and very subtle Nāḍī, and to drive Prāṇa-vāyu through it." These three, Suṣumnā, Vajriṇī, and Citriṇī, and the central canal, or Brahma-nāḍī, through which, in the Yoga here described, Kuṇḍalinī, passes, are all, in any case, part of the spinal cord. And, as the Śiva-saṁhitā and all other Yoga

[1] Ch. II, v. 18.

[2] Ed. Ānandāśrama Series XXIX, p. 145. Prāṇa does not here mean gross breath, but that which in the respiratory centres appears as such and which appears in other forms in other functions and parts of the body.

works say, the rest of the body is dependent on Suṣumnā, as being the chief spinal representative of the central nervous system. There seems also to be some ground to hold that the Nāḍīs, Iḍā and Piṅgalā, or "moon" and "sun," are the left and right sympathetic cords respectively on each side of the "fiery" Suṣumnā. It is to be noted that, according to one and a common notion reproduced in this work, these Nāḍīs, which are described as being pale and ruddy respectively (v. 1), do not lie merely on one side of the cord, but cross it alternating from one side to the other (see v. 1), thus forming with the Suṣumnā and the two petals of the Ājñā-Cakra the figure of the Caduceus of Mercury, which, according to some represents them. Elsewhere (v. 1), however it is said that they are shaped like bows. That is, one is united with Suṣumnā and connected with the left scrotum. It goes up to a position near the left shoulder, bending as it passes the heart, crosses over to the right shoulder, and then proceeds to the right nostril. Similarly, the other Nāḍī connected with the right scrotum passes to the left nostril. It has been suggested to me that Iḍā and Piṅgalā are blood-vessels representing the Inferior Vena Cava and Aorta. But the works and the Yoga process itself indicate not arteries, but nerves. Iḍā and Piṅgalā when they reach the space between the eyebrows make with the Suṣumnā a plaited threefold knot called Triveṇī and proceed to the nostrils. This, it has been said, is the spot in the medulla where the sympathetic cords join together or whence they take their origin.

There remains to be considered the position of the Cakras. Though this work speaks of six, there are, according to some, others. This is stated by Viśvanātha in his Ṣatcakra-Vivṛti. Thus we have mentioned Lalanā, Manas, and Soma Cakras. The six here given are the principal ones. Indeed, a very long list exists of Cakras or Ādhāras, as some call them. In a modern Sanskrit work called "Advaitamārtaṇḍa" the author[1] gives twenty, numbering them as follows: (1) *Ādhāra*, (2) Kuladīpa, (3) Vajra or Yajña, (4) *Svādhiṣṭhāna*, (5) Raudra, (6) Karāla, (7) Gahvara, (8) Vidyāprada, (9) Trimukha, (10) Tripada, (11) Kāla-daṇḍaka, (12) Ukāra, (13) Kāladvāra, (14) Karamgaka, (15) Dīpaka, (16) Ānanda-lalitā, (17) *Maṇipūraka*, (18) Nākula, (19) Kāla-bhedana, (20) Mahotsāha. Then for no apparent reason, many others are given without numbers, a circumstance, as well as defective printing, which makes it difficult in some cases to say whether the Sanskrit should be read as one word or two.[2] They are apparently Parama, Pādukaṁ, Padaṁ (or Pādakaṁ-padaṁ), Kalpa-jāla, Poṣaka, Lolama, Nādāvarta, Triputa, Kamkālaka, Putabhenana, Mahā-granthivirākā, Bandha-jvalana (printed as Bandhe-jvalana), *Anāhata*, Yantraputa (printed Yatro), Vyomacakra, Bodhana, Dhruva, Kalākandalaka, Krauñcabheruṇḍa-vibhava, Dāmara, Kula-phīṭhaka, Kula-kolāhala, Hālavarta, Mahad-bhaya, Ghorābhairava, *Viśuddhi*, Kanṭhaṁ, Uttamaṁ (*quære* Viśuddhikantham, or Kanthamuttamam), Pūrṇakaṁ, *Ājñā*, Kāka-puttaṁ, Śṛṅgātaṁ, Kāmarūpa, Pūrṇagiri, Mahā-vyoma, Śaktirūpa. But, as the author says, in the Vedas (that is, Yoga-cūdamanī, Yogaśikha Upaniṣads, and others) we read of only six Cakras—namely, those italicized in the above list, and described in the works here translated—and so it is said: "How can there be any Siddhi for a man who knows not the six Adhvās, the sixteen Ādhāras, the

---

[1] Brahmānanda-Śvāmī, a native of Palghat, in the Madras Presidency, late Guru of H. H. the late Mahārajā of Kashmir. The work is printed at Jummoo.

[2] I am not sure that the author himself was aware of this in all cases. He may have been quoting himself from some lists without other knowledge on the subject. The list has, to my eyes, in some respects an uncritical aspect—*e.g.*, apart from bracketed notes in the text, Kāma-rūpa and Pūrṇa-giri are Pīṭhas, the others, Jālaṁdhara and Auddīyāṇa, not being mentioned. The last quotation he makes draws a distinction between the Cakras and Ādhāras.

three Liṅgas and the five (elements) the first of which is Ether?" [1]

I have already pointed out that the positions of the Cakras generally correspond to spinal centres of the anatomical divisions of the vertebræ into five regions, and it has been stated that the Padmas or Cakras correspond with various plexuses which exist in the body surrounding those regions. Various suggestions have been here made. The Author of the work cited [2] identifies (commencing with the Mūlādhāra and going upwards) the Cakras with the sacral, prostatic, epigastric, cardiac, laryngeal (or pharyngeal), and cavernos plexuses, and the Sahasrāra with the Medulla. In passing it may be noted that the last suggestion cannot in any event be correct. It is apparently based on verse 120 of chapter V of the Śiva-Saṁhitā.[3] But this work does not in my opinion support the suggestion. Elsewhere the Author cited rightly identifies mount Kailāsa with the Sahasrāra, which is undoubtedly the upper cerebrum. The anatomical position of the Medulla is below that assigned to the Ājñā-Cakra. Professor Sarkar's work contains some valuable appendices by Dr. Brojendranath Seal on, amongst others, Hindu ideas concerning plant and animal life, physiology, and biology, including accounts of the nervous system in

---

[1] The six Adhvās are Varṇa, Pada, Kalā, Tattva, Bhuvana and Mantra. The sixteen Ādhāras are named in the commentary to verse 33 of the text, the elements are also described in the text. The three Liṅgas are Svayaṁbhu, Bānā and Itara also dealt with in the text.

[2] "The Positive Background of Hindu Sociology," by Professor Benoy Kumar Sarkar.

[3] P. 54 of the translation of Srīśh-Candra-Vasu, to which I refer because the author cited does so. The rendering, however, does not do justice to the text, and liberties have been taken with it. Thus, a large portion has been omitted without a word of warning, and at p. 14 it is said, that Kuṇḍalinī is "of the form of electricity". There is no warrant for this in the text, and Kuṇḍalinī is not, according to the Śāstra, mere electricity.

Caraka and in the Tantras.[1] After pointing out that the cerebo-spinal axis with the connected sympathetic system contains a number of ganglionic centres and plexuses (Cakras, Padmas), from which nerves (Nāḍī, Sirā, and Dhamanī) radiate over the head, trunk, and limbs, the latter says, as regards the ganglionic centres and plexuses consisting of the sympathetic spinal system:

"Beginning with the lower extremity, the centres and plexuses of the connected spinal and sympathetic systems may be described as follows:

"(1) The Ādhāra-Cakra, the sacro-coccygeal plexus with four branches, nine Angulis (about six inches and a half) below the solar plexus (Kaṇḍa, Brahmagranthi); the source of a massive pleasurable æsthesia; voluminous organic sensations of repose. An inch and a half above it, and the same distance below the membrum virile (Mehana), is a minor centre called the Agni-śikhā. (2) The Svādhiṣṭhāna-Cakra, the sacral plexus, with six branches (Dalāni—petals) concerned in the excitation of sexual feelings, with the accompaniments of lassitude, stupor, cruelty, suspicion, contempt.[2] (3) The Nābhi-kaṇḍa (corresponding to the solar plexus, Bhānu-bhavanam), which forms the great junction of the right and left sympathetic chains (Piṅgalā and Iḍā) with the cerebro-spinal axis. Connected with this is the Maṇipūraka, the lumbar plexus, with connected sympathetic nerves, the ten branches[3] of which are concerned in the

[1] Both the work of Professor Sarkar and the Appendices of Dr. Seal are of interest and value, and gather together a considerable number of facts of importance on Indian Geography, Ethnology, Mineralogy, Zoology, Botany and Hindu Physiology, Mechanics, and Acoustics. These Appendices have since been republished separately as a work entitled "Positive Sciences of the Hindus".

[2] These and other Vṛttis, as they are called, are enumerated in the "Introduction to Tantra-Śāstra".

[3] That is, petals.

production of sleep and thirst, and the expressions of passions like jealousy, shame, fear, stupefaction. (4) The Anāhata-Cakra, possibly the cardiac plexus of the sympathetic chain with twelve branches, connected with the heart, the seat of the egoistic sentiments, hope, anxiety, doubt, remorse, conceit, egoism, etc. (5) The Bhāratī-Ṣthāna,[1] the junction of the spinal cord with the medulla oblongata, which, by means of nerves like the pneumogastric, etc., regulate the larynx and other organs of articulation. (6) The Lalanā-Cakra, opposite the uvula, which has twelve leaves (or lobes), supposed to be the tract affected in the production of ego-altruistic sentiments and affections, like self-regard, pride, affection, grief, regret, respect, reverence, contentment, etc. (7) The sensori-motor tract, comprising two Cakras: (*a*) the Ājñā-Cakra (*lit.*, the circle of command over movements) with its two lobes (the cerebellum); and (*b*) the Manas-Cakra, the sensorium, with its six lobes (five special sensory for peripherally initiated sensations, and one common sensory for centrally initiated sensations, as in dreams and hallucinations). The Ājñāvahā-Nāḍīs, efferent or motor nerves, communicate motor impulses to the periphery from this Ājñā-Cakra, this centre of command over movement; and the afferent or sensory nerves of the special senses, in pairs, the Gandhavahā-Nāḍī (olfactory sensory), the Rūpavahā-Nāḍī (optic), the Śabdavahā-Nāḍī (auditory), the Rasavahā-Nāḍī (gustatory), and the Sparśavahā-Nāḍī (tactile), come from the periphery (the peripheral organs of the special senses) to this Manas-Cakra, the sensory tract at the base of the brain. The Manas-Cakra also receives the Manovahā-Nāḍī, a generic name for the channels along which centrally initiated presentations (as in dreaming or hallucination) come to the

[1] This is a name for the Viśuddha-Cakra as abode of the Goddess of Speech (Bhāratī).

sixth lobe of the Manas-Cakra. (8) The Soma-Cakra, a sixteen-lobed ganglion, comprising the centres in the middle of the cerebrum, above the sensorium; the seat of the altruistic sentiments and volitional control—*e.g.*, compassion, gentleness, patience, renunciation, meditativeness, gravity, earnestness, resolution, determination, magnanimity, etc. And lastly, (9) the Sahasrāra-Cakra, thousand-lobed, the upper cerebrum with its lobes and convolutions, the special and highest seat of the Jīva, the soul."[1]

Then, dealing with the cerebro-spinal axis and the heart, and their respective relations to the conscious life, the Author cited says:

"Vijñāna-bhikṣu, in the passage just quoted, identifies the Manovahā-Nāḍī (vehicle of consciousness) with the cerebro-spinal axis and its ramifications, and compares the figure to an inverted gourd with a thousand-branched stem hanging down. The Suṣuṁnā, the central passage of the spinal cord, is the stem of this gourd (or a single branch). The writers on the Yoga (including the authors of the various Tāntrik systems), use the term somewhat differently. On this view, the Manovahā-Nāḍī is the channel of the communication of the Jīva (soul) with the Manas-Cakra (sensorium) at the base of the brain. The sensory currents are brought to the sensory ganglia along afferent nerves of the special senses. But this is not sufficient for them to rise to the level of discriminative consciousness. A communication must now be established between the Jīva (in the Sahasrāra-Cakra, upper cerebrum) and the sensory currents received at the sensorium, and this is done by means of the Manovahā-Nāḍī. When sensations are centrally initiated, as

[1] The author cited refers to the Jñāna-Saṁkalinī-Tantra, Saṁhitā-ratnākara, and for functions of Ājñāvahā-Nāḍī and Manovahā-Nāḍī to Śaṁkara Miśra's Upaskāra.

in dreams and hallucinations, a special Nāḍī (Svapnavahā-Nāḍī), which appears to be only a branch of the Manovahā-Nāḍī, serves as the channel of communication from the Jīva (soul) to the sensorium. In the same way, the Ājñāvahā-Nāḍī brings down the messages of the soul from the Sahasrāra (upper cerebrum) to the Ājñā-Cakra (motor tract at the base of the brain), messages which are thence carried further down, along efferent nerves, to various parts of the periphery. I may add that the special sensory nerves, together with the Manovahā-Nāḍī, are sometimes generally termed Jñānavahā-Nāḍī—*lit.*, channel of presentative knowledge. There is no difficulty so far. The Manovahā-Nāḍī and the Ājñāvahā connect the sensory-motor tract at the base of the brain (Manas-Cakra and Ājñā-Cakra) with the highest (and special) seat of the soul (Jīva) in the upper cerebrum (Sahasrāra), the one being the channel for carrying up the sensory and the other for bringing down the motor messages. But efforts of the will (Ājñā, Prayatna) are conscious presentations, and the Manovahā-Nāḍī must therefore co-operate with the Ājñāvahā in producing the consciousness of effort. Indeed, attention, the characteristic function of Manas, by which it raises sense-presentation to the level of discriminative consciousness, implies effort (Prayatna) on the part of the soul (Ātmā, Jīva), an effort of which we are conscious through the channel of the Manovahā-Nāḍī. But how to explain the presentation of effort in the motor nerves? Śaṁkara-Miśra, the author of the Upaskāra on Kaṇāḍa's Sūtras, argues that the Nāḍīs (even the volitional or motor nerves) are themselves sensitive, and their affections are conveyed to the sensorium by means of the nerves of the (inner) sense of touch (which are interspersed in minute fibrillæ among them). The consciousness of effort, then, in any motor nerve, whether Ājñāvahā (volitional motor) or Prāṇa-vahā (automatic motor, depends on the tactile nerves or nerves of organic sensation mixed up with it. Thus the assimilation of food and drink by the automatic activity of the Prāṇas implies an (automatic) effort (Prayatna) accompanied by a vague organic consciousness, which is due to the fact that minute fibres of the inner touch-sense are interspersed with the machinery of the automatic nerves (the Prāṇavahā-Nāḍīs)."

To a certain extent the localizations here made must be tentative. It must, for instance, be a matter of opinion whether the throat centre corresponds with the carotid, laryngeal, or pharyngeal, or all three; whether the navel centre corresponds with the epigastric, solar, or lumbar, the Ājñā with the cavernous plexus, pineal gland, pituitary body, cerebellum, and so forth. For all that is known to the contrary each centre may have more than one of such correspondences. All that can be said with any degree of certainty is that the four centres, above the Mūlādhāra, which is the seat of the presiding energy, have relation to the genito-excretory, digestive, cardiac, and respiratory functions, and that the two upper centres (Ājñā and Sahasrāra) denote various forms of cerebral activity, ending in the repose of pure Consciousness. The uncertainty which prevails as regards some of those matters is indicated in the Text itself, which shows that on various of the subjects here debated differing opinions have been expressed as individual constructions of statements to be found in the Tantras and other Śāstras.

There are, however, if I read them correctly, statements in the above-cited accounts with which, though not uncommonly accepted, I disagree. It is said, for instance, that the Ādhāra Cakra *is* the sacro-coccygeal plexus, and that the Svādhiṣṭhāna *is* the sacral plexus, and so forth. This work, however, not to mention others, makes it plain that the Cakras are in the Suṣuṁnā. Verse 1 speaks of the

"Lotuses inside the Meru (spinal column); and as the Suṣumnā supports these (that is, the lotuses) She must needs be within the Meru." This is said in answer to those who, on the strength of a passage in the Tantra-cūḍāmani, erroneously suppose that Suṣumnā is outside the Meru. In the same way the Commentator refutes the error of those who, relying on the Nigama-tattva-sāra, suppose that not only Suṣumnā, but Iḍā, and Piṅgalā, are inside the Meru. Verse 2 says that inside Vajrā (which is itself within Suṣumnā) is Citriṇī, on which the lotuses are strung as it were gems, and which like a spider's thread pierces all the lotuses which are within the backbone. The Author in the same place combats the view, based on the Kalpa-Sūtra, that the lotuses are within Citriṇī. These lotuses are in the Suṣumna; and as Citriṇī is within the latter, she pierces but does not contain them. Some confusion is raised by the statement in v. 51, that the lotuses are in or on the Brahma-Nāḍī. But by this is meant appertaining to this Nāḍī, for they are in Suṣumnā, of which the Brahma-Nāḍī is the central channel. The commentator Viśvanātha, quoting from the Māyā-Tantra, says that all the six lotuses are attached to the Citriṇī Nāḍī (Citriṇī-grathitaṁ). One conclusion emerges clearly from all this, namely, that the Lotuses are in the vertebral column in Suṣumnā, and not in the nerve plexuses which surround it. There in the spinal column they exist as extremely subtle vital centres of Prāṇa-Śakti and centres of consciousness. In this connection I may cite an extract from an article on the "Physical Errors of Hinduism,"[1] for which I am indebted to Professor Sarkar's work: "It would indeed excite the surprise of our readers to hear that the Hindus, who would not even touch a dead body, much less dissect it, should possess any anatomical knowledge at all. . . . It is the Tantras that furnish us

[1] Published in Vol. XI, pp. 436-440, of the *Calcutta Review*.

with some extraordinary pieces of information concerning the human body. . . . But of all the Hindu Śāstras extant, the Tantras lie in the greatest obscurity. . . . The Tāntrik theory, on which the well-known Yoga called 'Ṣaṭcakra-bheda' is founded, supposes the existence of six main internal organs, called Cakras or Padmas, all bearing a special resemblance to that famous flower, the lotus. These are placed one above the other, and connected by three imaginary chains, the emblems of the Ganges, the Yamunā, and the Saraswatī. . . . Such is the obstinacy with which the Hindus adhere to these erroneous notions, that, even when we show them by actual dissection the non-existence of the imaginary Cakras in the human body, they will rather have recourse to excuses revolting to common sense than acknowledge the evidence of their own eyes. They say, with a shamelessness unparalleled, that these Padmas exist as long as a man lives, but disappear the moment he dies."[1] This, however, is nevertheless quite correct, for conscious and vital centres cannot exist in a body when the organism which they hold together dies. A contrary conclusion might indeed be described as "shameless" stupidity.[2]

The Author of the work from which this citation is made says that, though these Cakras cannot be satisfactorily identified, the Tāntriks must nevertheless have obtained their knowledge of them by dissection. By this he must refer to the physical regions which correspond on the gross plane to, and are governed by, the Cakras proper, which as subtle, vital, and conscious centres in the spinal cord are invisible

[1] "Physical Errors of Hinduism," *Calcutta Review*, Vol. XI, pp. 436-440.

[2] This reminds one of the story of a materialistic doctor who said he had done hundreds of *post-mortem* examinations, but had never yet discovered the trace of a soul.

to any but a Yogī's vision,[1] existing when the body is alive and disappearing when vitality (Prāṇa) leaves the body as part of the Liṅga-śarīra.

It is a mistake, therefore, in my opinion, to identify the Cakras with the physical plexuses mentioned. These latter are things of the gross body, whereas the Cakras are extremely subtle vital centres of various Tāttvik operations. In a sense we can connect with these subtle centres the gross bodily parts visible to the eyes as plexuses and ganglia. But to connect or correlate and to identify are different things. Indian thought and the Sanskrit language, which is its expression, have a peculiarly penetrative and comprehensive quality which enables one to explain many ideas for which, except by paraphrase, there is no equivalent meaning in English. It is by the Power or Śakti of the Ātmā or Consciousness that the body exists. It is the collective Prāṇa which holds it together as an individual human unit, just as it supports the different Principles and Elements (Tattva) of which it is composed. These Tattvas, though they pervade the body, have yet various special centres of operation. These centres, as one might otherwise suppose, lie along the axis, and are the Sūkṣma-Rūpa, or subtle forms of that which exists in gross form (Sthūla-Rūpa) in the physical body which is gathered around it. They are manifestations of Prāṇa-Śakti or Vital Force. In other words, from an objective standpoint the subtle centres, or Cakras, vitalize and control the gross bodily tracts which are indicated by the various regions of the vertebral column and the ganglia, plexuses, nerves, arteries, and organs, situate in these respective regions. It is only therefore (if at all) in the sense of being the gross outer

[1] So it is said: Tāni vastūni tanmātrādīnī pratyakṣaviṣayāni (Such things as the Tanmātra and others are subject to immediate perception by Yogins only). A Yogī "sees" the Cakras with his mental eye (Ājñā). In the case of others they are a matter of inference (Anumāna).

representatives of the spinal centres that we can connect the plexuses and so forth with the Cakras spoken of in the Yoga books. In this sense only the whole tract, which extends from the subtle centre to the periphery, with its corresponding bodily elements, may be regarded as the Cakra. As the gross and subtle are thus connected, mental operation on the one will affect the other. Certain forces are concentrated in these Cakras, and therefore and by reference to their function they are regarded as separate and independent centres. There are thus six subtle centres in the cord with grosser embodiments within the cord itself, with still grosser sheaths in the region pervaded by the sympathetics Iḍā and Piṅgalā, and other Nāḍīs. Out of all this and the gross compounded elements of the body are fashioned the organs of life, the vital heart of which is the subtle Cakra by which they are vivified and controlled. The subtle aspects of the six centres according to Tāntrik doctrine must not be overlooked whilst attention is paid to the gross or physiological aspect of the body. As previously and in the Commentary to the thirty-fifth verse of the Ānandalaharī explained, there are six Devas—*viz.*, Śaṁbhu, Sadāśiva, Īśvara, Viṣṇu, Rudra, Brahmā—whose abodes are the six Lokas or regions: *viz.*, Maharloka, Tapaloka, Janaloka, Svarloka, Bhuvarloka, and Bhūrloka (the Earth). It is these Divinities who are the forms of Consciousness presiding over the Ṣaṭcakra. In other words, Consciousness (Cit) as the ultimate experiencing principle, pervades and is at base all being. Every cell of the body has a consciousness of its own. The various organic parts of the body which the cells build have not only particular cell-consciousness, but the consciousness of the particular organic part which is other than the mere collectivity of the consciousness of its units. Thus there may be an abdominal consciousness. And the consciousness of such bodily region is its Devatā—

that is, that aspect of Cit which is associated with and informs that region. Lastly, the organism as a whole has its consciousness, which is the individual Jīva. Then there is the subtle form or body of these Devatās, in the shape of Mind—supersensible "matter" (Tanmātra); and sensible "matter"—namely, ether, air, fire, water, earth, with their centres at the Ājñā, Viśuddha, Anāhata, Maṇipūra, Svādhiṣṭhāna and Mūlādhāra. Of these six Tattvas, not only the gross human body, but the vast Macrocosm, is composed. The six Cakras are therefore the divine subtle centres of the corresponding physical and psychical sheaths. The seventh or supreme centre of Consciousness is Parama-Śiva, whose abode is Satyaloka, the Cosmic aspect of the Sahasrāra in the human body. The Supreme, therefore, descends through its manifestations from the subtle to the gross as the six Devas and Śaktis in their six abodes in the world-axis, and as the six centres in the body-axis or spinal column. The special operation of each of the Tattvas is located at its individual centre in the microcosm. But, notwithstanding all such subtle and gross transformations of and by Kula-Kuṇḍalinī, She ever remains in Her Brahman or Svarūpa aspect the One, Sat, Cit, and Ānanda, as is realized by the Yogī when drawing the Devī from Her world-abode in the earth centre (Mūlādhāra) he unites Her with Parama-Śiva in the Sahasrāra in that blissful union which is the Supreme Love (Ānanda).

In a similar manner other statements as regards these Cakras should be dealt with, as, for instance, those connected with the existence of the "Petals" the number of which in each case has been said to be determined by characteristics of the gross region which the particular Cakra governs. The centres are said to be composed of petals designated by certain letters. Professor Sarkar [1] expresses the opinion that these

[1] *Op. cit.*, p. 292.

petals point to either the nerves which go to form a ganglion or plexus, or the nerves distributed from such ganglion or plexus. I have been told that the disposition of the Nāḍīs at the particular Cakra in question determines the number of its petals.[1] In the five lower Cakras their characteristics are displayed in the number and position of the Nāḍīs or by the lobes and sensory and motor tracts of the higher portions of the cerebro-spinal system. As I have already explained, the Cakra is not to be identified with the physical ganglia and plexuses, though it is connected with, and in a gross sense represented by them. The lotuses with these petals are within the Suṣumnā and they are there represented as blooming upon the passage through them of Kuṇḍalī. The letters are on the petals.

The letters in the six Cakras are fifty in number—namely, the letters of the Sanskrit alphabet less Kṣa, according to the Kamakāla-mālinī-Tantra cited in v. 40, or the second or cerebral La (*ib.*). All these letters multiplied by 20 exist potentially in the Sahasrāra, where they therefore number 1,000 giving that Lotus its name. There are, on the other hand, 72,000 Nāḍīs which rise from the Kaṇḍa. Further, that these letters in the Cakras are not gross things is shown by vv. 28 and 29, which say that the vowels of the Viśuddha are visible to the enlightened mind (Dīpta-buddhi) only—that is, the Buddhi which is free of impurity resulting from worldly pursuits, as the effect of the constant practice of Yoga. Verse 19 and other verses speak of the letters there mentioned as being coloured. Each object of perception, whether gross or subtle, has an aspect which corresponds to each of the senses. It is for this reason that the Tantra

[1] See my "Introduction to Tantra Śāstra". My reference there to the lotus as a plexus of Nāḍīs is to the gross sheath of the subtle centre, which gross sheath is said to contain the determinant, though in another sense it is the effect, of the characteristics of the subtle centre.

correlates sound, form and colour. Sound produces form, and form is associated with colour. Kuṇḍalī is a form of the Supreme Śakti who maintains all breathing creatures. She is the source from which all sound or energy, whether as ideas or speech, manifests. That sound or Mātṛkā when uttered in human speech assumes the form of letters and prose and verse, which is made of their combinations. And sound (Śabda) has its meaning—that is, the objects denoted by the ideas which are expressed by sound or words. By the impulse of Icchā-Śakti acting through the Prāṇa-vāyu (vital force) of the Ātmā is produced in the Mūlādhāra the sound power called Parā, which in its ascending movement through other Cakras takes on other characteristics and names (Paśyantī and Madhyamā), and when uttered by the mouth appears as Vaikharī in the form of the spoken letters which are the gross aspect of the sound in the Cakras themselves (see vv. 10 and 11). Letters when spoken are, then, the manifested aspect in gross speech of the subtle energy of the Śabdabrahman as Kuṇḍalī. The same energy which produces these letters manifesting as Mantras produces the gross universe. In the Cakras is subtle Śabda in its states as Parā, Paśyantī, or Madhyamā-Śakti, which when translated to the vocal organ assumes the audible sound form (Dhvani) which is any particular letter. Particular forms of energy of Kuṇḍalī are said to be resident at particular Cakras, all such energies existing in magnified form in the Sahasrāra. Each manifested letter is a Mantra, and a Mantra is the body of a Devatā. There are therefore as many Devatās in a Cakra as there are petals which are surrounding (Āvaraṇa) Devatās or Śaktis of the Devatā of the Cakra and the subtle element of which He is the presiding Consciousness. Thus, Brahmā is the presiding Consciousness of the Mūlādhāra lotus, indicated by the Bindu of the Bīja La (Laṁ), which is the body of the earth Devatā; and around and associated with these are subtle forms of the Mantras, which constitute the petals and the bodies of associated energies. The whole human body is in fact a Mantra, and is composed of Mantras. These sound powers vitalize, regulate, and control, the corresponding gross manifestations in the regions surrounding them.

Why, however, particular letters are assigned to particular Cakras is the next question. Why, for instance, should Ha be in the Ājñā and La in the Mūlādhāra? It is true that in some places in the Tantras certain letters are assigned to particular elements. Thus, there are certain letters which are called Vāyava-Varṇa, or letters pertaining to the Vāyu-Tattva; but an examination of the case on this basis fails to account for the position of the letters as letters which are assigned to one element may be found in a Cakra the predominant Tattva of which is some other element. It has been said that in the utterance of particular letters the centres at which they are situated are brought into play, and that this is the solution of the question why those particular letters were at their particular centre. A probable solution is that given by me in my "Śakti and Śākta".[1] Apart from this one can only say that it is either Svabhāva or the nature of the thing, which in that case is as little susceptible of ultimate explanation as the disposition in the body of the gross organs themselves; or the arrangement may be an artificial one for the purpose of meditation, in which case no further explanation is necessary.

The four Bhāvas, or states of sound, in the human body are so called as being states in which sound or movement is produced or becomes, evolving from Parā-Śakti in the body of Īśvara to the gross Vaikharī-Śakti in the body of Jīva. As already stated, in the bodily aspect (Adhyātma) the

[1] See Chapter, "Kuṇḍalī-yoga".

Kāraṇa-Bindu resides in the Mūlādhāra centre, and is there known as the Śakti-Piṇḍa [1] or Kuṇḍalinī. [2] Kuṇḍalī is a name for Śabda-brahman in human bodies. The Ācārya, speaking of Kuṇḍalinī, says: "There is a Śakti called Kuṇḍalinī who is ever engaged in the work of creating the universe. He who has known Her never again enters the mother's womb as a child or suffers old age." That is, he no longer enters the Saṁsāra of world of transmigration. [3] This Kāraṇa-Bindu exists in a non-differentiated condition. [4]

The body of Kuṇḍalī is composed of the fifty letters or sound-powers. Just as there is an apparent evolution [5] in the cosmic body of Īśvara, represented in the seven states preceding

---

[1] She is so called because all the Śaktis are collected or "rolled into one mass" in Her. Here is the Kendra (centre) of all the Śaktis. The Svacchanda as also the Śāradā says:

> Piṇḍaṁ Kuṇḍalinī-śaktiḥ
> Padaṁ haṁsaḥ prakīrtitaḥ
> Rūpaṁ bindur iti khyataṁ
> Rūpātītas tu cinmayaḥ.

[Kuṇḍalinī-Śakti is Piṇḍa; Hamsaḥ is Pada; Bindu is Rūpa, but Cinmaya (Cit) is formless]: The first, as potentiality of all manifested power, is in the Mūlādhāra-Cakra; the second, as Jīvātmā, is in Anāhata, where the heart beats, the life-pulse. Bindu, the causal form body, as Supreme Śakti, is in Ājñā, and the formless Consciousness passing through Bindu Tattva manifesting as Haṁsa, and again resting as Kuṇḍalinī, is in the Brahma-randhra (see Tīkā of first Saṁketah of Yoginīhṛdaya-Tantra).

[2] Adhyātmaṁ tu kāraṇa-binduḥ śaktipiṇḍa-kuṇḍalyādi-śabdavācyo mūlādhārasthaḥ (Bhāskararāya, Comm. Lalitā, v. 132).

[3] "Śaktiḥ kuṇḍalinīti viśva-jananavyāpārabaddholyamāṁ
Jñātvā itthaṁ na punar viśanti jananīgarbhe 'rbhakatvaṁ narāḥ
ityādirītyācāryair vyavahṛitaḥ (*ib.*)."

[4] So 'yam avibhāgāvasthaḥ kāraṇa-binduḥ (*ib.*).

[5] Vikāra or Vikṛti is something which is really changed, as curd from milk. The former is a Vikṛti of the latter. Vivarta is apparent but unreal change, such as the appearance of what was and is a rope as a snake. The Vedānta-sāra thus musically defines the two terms:

> Satattvato 'nyathāprathā vikāra ityudīritaḥ
> Atattvato 'nyathāprathā vivarta ityudāhṛitaḥ.

from Sakala-Parameśvara to Bindu, so there is a similar development in the human body in Kuṇḍalī who is the Īśvarī, therein. There evolved the following states, corresponding with the cosmic development—*viz.*, Śakti, Dhvani, Nāda, Nirodhikā, Ardhendu, Bindu. These are all states of Kuṇḍalī Herself in the Mūlādhāra, and are known as Parā sound. Each one of the letters composing the body of Kuṇḍalī exists in four states as Parā-Śakti, or in the succeeding states of sound, Paśyanti, Madhyamā, and Vaikharī to which reference is later made. The first is a state of differentiated sound, which exists in the body of Īśvara; the second and third as existing in the body of Jīva are stages towards that complete manifestation of differentiated sound in human speech which is called Vaikharī-Bhāva. In the cosmic aspect these four states are Avyakta, Īśvara, Hiraṇya-garbha and Virāt. The Artha-sṛṣṭi (object creation) of Kuṇḍalinī are the Kalās, which arise from the letters such as the Rudra and Viṣṇu-Mūrtis and their Śaktis, the Kāmas and Ganeśas and their Śaktis, and the like. In the Sakala-Parameśvara or Śabda-brahman in bodies—that is, Kuṇḍalinī-Śakti—the latter is called Cit-Śakti or Śakti simply, "when Sattva enters"—a state known as the Paramakāsāvasthā. When She into whom Sattva has entered is next "pierced" by Rajas, She is called Dhvani, which is the Akṣarāvasthā. When She is again "pierced" by Tamas, She is called Nāda. This is the Avyaktāvasthā, the Avyakta-Nāda which is the Para-bindu. Again, She in whom Tamas abounds is, as Rāghava-Bhatta says, called Nirodhika; She in whom Sattva abounds is called Ardhendu; and the combination of the two (Icchā and Jñāna) in which Rajas as Kriyā-Śakti works is called Bindu. Thus it has been said: "Drawn by the force of Icchā-Śakti (will), illumined by Jñāna-Śakti (knowledge), Śakti the Lord appearing as male creates (Kriyā-Śakti, or action)."

When the Kāraṇa-Bindu "sprouts" in order to create the three (Bindu, Nāda, and Bīja) there arises that unmanifested Brahman-word or Sound called the Śabdabrahman (Sound Brahman).[1] It is said: "From the differentiation of the Kāraṇa-Bindu arises the unmanifested 'Sound' which is called Śabdabrahman by those learned in Śruti."[2] It is this Śabdabrahman which is the immediate cause of the universe, which is sound and movement manifesting as idea and language. This sound, which is one with the Kāraṇa-Bindu, and is therefore all-pervading, yet first appears in man's body in the Mūlādhāra. "It is said in the Mūlādhāra in the body the 'air' (Prāṇa-vāyu) first appears. That 'air' acted upon by the effort of a person desiring to speak, manifests the all-pervading Śabda-brahman."[3] The Śabdabrahman which is in the form of the Kāraṇa-Bindu when it

---

[1] Ayaṁ eva ca yadā kārya-bindvādi-trayajananonmukho bhidyate, taddaśāyāṁ avyakatah śabda-brahmābhidheyo ravas tatrotpadyate (*ib.*).

When this (Kāraṇa-bindu) inclines to produce the three Bindus the first of which is Kārya-bindu and bursts or divides itself (Bhidyate, then at that stage there arises the indistinct (Avyakta) sound (Ravạ) which is called Śabdabrahman.

[2] Tadapyuktaṁ:

> Bindos tasmād bhidyamānād avyaktātmā ravo 'bhavat,
> Sa ravah śruti-sampannaih śabda-brahmeti gīyate (*ib.*).

So it has been said: From the bursting Bindu there arises the indistinct sound which is called Śabdabrahman by those versed in Śruti.

[3] So 'yam ravah kāraṇa-bindu-tādātmyāpannatvāt sarvagato 'pi vyañjaka-yatna-saṁskṛta-pavanavaśāt prāṇināṁ mūlādhāra eva abhivyajyate. Taduktam:

> Dehe 'pi mūlādhāre 'smin samudeti samīraṇah,
> Vivakṣoricchayotthena prayatnena susamskṛtah.
> Sa vyañjayati tatraiva śabda-brahmāpi sarvagaṁ (*ib.*).

This sound again being one with the Kāraṇa-bindu and, therefore, everywhere, manifests itself in the Mūlādhāra of animals, being led there by the air purified by the effort made by the maker of the sound. So it is said: In the body also in the Mūlādhāra air arises; this (air) is purified by the effort and will of the person wishing to speak and manifests the Śabda which is everywhere.

remains motionless (Niṣpanda) in its own place (that is, in Kuṇḍalī, who is Herself in the Mūlādhāra) is called Parā-Śakti of speech. The same Śabdabrahman manifested by the same "air" proceeding as far as the navel, united with the Manas, possessing the nature of the manifested Kārya Bindu with general (Sāmānya-spanda) motion, is named Paśyantī speech.[1] Paśyantī, which is described as Jñānātmaka and Bindvātmaka (in the nature of Cit and Bindu), extends from the Mūlādhāra to the navel, or, according to some accounts, the Svādiṣṭhāna.

Next, the Śabdabrahman manifested by the same "air" proceeding as far as the heart, united with the Buddhi, possessing the nature of the manifested Nāda and endowed with special motion (Viśeṣa-spanda) is called Madhyamā speech.[2] This is Hiraṇyagarbha sound, extending from the region of Paśyantī to the heart. Next,[3] the same Śabdabrahman manifested by the same air proceeding as far as

---

[1] Tad idaṁ kāraṇa-bindvātmakaṁ abhivyaktaṁ śabda-brahma svapratiṣṭhatayā niṣpandaṁ tadeva ca parā vāg ityucyate. Atha tadeva nābhi-paryantamāgacchatā tena pavanenābhivyaktaṁ vimarśar-ūpeṇa manasā yuktaṁ sāmānya-spanda-prakāśarūpa-kārya-bindumayaṁ sat paśyantī vāg ucyate (*ib.*).

This evolved Śabdabrahman which is one with the Kāraṇa-bindu when it is in itself and vibrationless (motionless) is called Parā-Vāk; when that again is, by the same air going up to the navel, further evolved and united with mind, which is Vimarśa then it becomes Kārya-bindu slightly vibrating and manifest. It is there called Paśyantī Vāk.

[2] Atha tad eva śabda-brahma tenaiva vāyunā hṛdaya-paryantamabhivyajyamānaṁ niścayātmikayā buddhyā yuktaṁ viśeṣa-spanda-prakāśarūpanādamayaṁ sat madhyamā-vāg ityucyate (*ib.*).

Thereafter the same Śabdabrahman as it is led by the same air to the heart is in a state of manifestation and united with Buddhi which never errs and becomes possessed of Nāda whose vibration is perceptible. It is called Madhyamā-Vāk.

[3] Atha tad eva vadana-paryantaṁ tenaiva vāyunā kaṇṭhādi-sthāneṣvabhivyajyamānaṁ akārādi-varṇarūpaṁ para-śrotrā-grahaṇa-yogyaṁ spaṣṭatara-prakāśa-rūpa-bījātmakaṁ sat vaikharī-vak ucyate (*ib.*).

the mouth, developed in the throat, etc., articulated and capable of being heard by the ears of others, possessing the nature of the manifested Bīja with quite distinct articulate (Spaṣtatara) motion, is called Vaikharī speech.[1] This is the Virāt state of sound, so called because it " comes out ".

This matter is thus explained by the Ācārya: " That sound which first arises in the Mūlādhāra is called Parā; next Paśyantī; next, when it goes as far as the heart and is joined to the Buddhi, it is called ' Madhyamā '." This name is derived from the fact that She abides " in the midst ". She is neither like Paśyantī nor does She proceed outward like Vaikharī, with articulation fully developed. But She is in the middle between these two.

The full manifestation is Vaikharī of the man wishing to cry out. In this way articulated sound is produced by air.[2] The Nityā-Tantra also says: " The Parā form rises in the Mūlādhāra produced by 'air'; the same 'air' rising upwards,

---

Thereafter the same (Śabda-brahman) when led by the same air to the mouth is in a state of manifestation, in the throat and other places and becomes capable of hearing by others, being more manifest as the letters A and others. It is then called Vaikharī-Vāk.

[1] That is Śabda in its physical form. Bhāskararāya, in the commentary to the same verse (132) of the Lalitā, gives the following derivations. Vi=much; khara=hard. According to the Saubhāgya-Sudhodaya, Vai=certainly; kha=cavity (of the ear); ra=to go or enter. But according to the Yoga-Śāstras, the Devī who is in the form of Vaikharī (Vaikharī-rūpī) is so called because she was produced by the Prāṇa called Vikhara.

[2] Taduktamācāryaih:

> Mūlādhārāt prathamaṁ udito yaś ca bhāvah parākhyah,
> Paścāt paśyanty atha hṛdayago buddhiyug madhyamākhyah.
> Vaktre vaikhary atha rurudiśor asya jantoh suṣumnā,
> Baddhas tasmāt bhavatī pavanapreritā varṇasaṁjñā (Bhāskararāya, *op. cit.*).

So it has been said by the great teacher (Śaṁkara: Prapañcasāra II. 44): When the child wishes to cry the first state of sound attached to the Suṣumnā as it arises in the Mūlādhāra is called Parā, driven

manifested in the Svādhiṣṭhāna, attains the Paśyantī [1] state. The same slowly rising upwards and manifested in the Anāhata united with the understanding (Buddhi), is Madhyamā. Again rising upwards, and appearing in the Viśuddha, it issues from the throat as Vaikharī." [2] As the Yogakuṇḍalī-Upaniṣad [3] says: "That Vāk (power of speech) which sprouts in Parā gives forth leaves in Paśyantī, buds forth in Madhyamā, and blossoms in Vaikharī. By reversing the above order sound is absorbed. Whosoever realizes the great Lord of Speech (Vāk) the undifferentiated illuminating Self is unaffected by any word, be it what it may."

Thus, though there are four kinds of speech, gross-minded men (Manuṣyāh sthūladṛśah) [4] who do not understand the first three (Parā, etc.), think speech to be

---

(upward) by air, it next becomes Paśyantī and in the heart united with Buddhi it gets the name of Madhyamā and in the mouth it becomes Vaikharī and from this arise the letters of the alphabet.

[1] Bhāskararāya cites Her other name Uttīrṇā (rise up) and the Saubhāgya-Sudhodaya, which says: "As She sees all in Herself, and as She rises (Uttīrṇā) above the path of action, this Mother is called Paśyantī and Uttīrṇā.

[2] Nityā-tantre 'pi:

> Mūlādhāre samutpannah parākhyo nāda-saṁbhavah,
> Sa evordhvaṁ tayā nītah svādhiṣṭhāne vijṛṁbhitah.
> Paśyantyākhyāṁ avāpnoti tathaivhrdhvaṁ śanaih śanaih,
> Anāhate buddhi-tattvasameto madhyamābhidhah,
> Tathā tayordhvaṁ nunnah san viśuddhau kanṭhadeśatah,
> Vaikharyākhya ityādi (Bhāskararāya, *op. cit.*).

The Nityā-tantra also says: From the Mūlādhāra first arises sound which is called Parā. The same led upwards becomes manifest in the Svādhiṣṭhāna and gets the name of Paśyantī. Gently led upward again in the same manner to the Anāhata (in the heart) it becomes united with Buddhi-tattva and is called Madhyamā and led up in the same manner to the Viśuddhi in the region of the throat it gets the name of Vaikharī and so forth.

See also Ch. II, Prapañcasāra-Tantra, Vol. III of Tāntrik Texts, ed. A. Avalon.

[3] Ch. III.

[4] That is, men who see and accept only the gross aspect of things.

Vaikharī alone,[1] just as they take the gross body to be the Self, in ignorance of its subtler principles. Śruti says: "Hence men think that alone to be speech which is imperfect"—that is, imperfect in so far as it does not possess the first three forms.[2] Śruti also says:[3] "Four are the grades of speech—those Brāhmaṇās who are wise know them: three are hidden and motionless; men speak the fourth." The Sūta-Saṁhitā also says: "Apada (the motionless Brahman) becomes Pada (the four forms of speech), and Pada may become Apada. He who knows the distinction between Pada[4] and Apada, he really sees (*i.e.*, himself becomes) Brahman."[5]

Thus, the conclusions of Śruti and Smṛti are that the "That" (Tat) in the human body has four divisions (Parā, etc.). But even in the Parā form the word Tat only denotes the Avyakta with three Guṇas, the cause of Parā, and not the unconditioned Brahman who is above Avyakta. The word "Tat" which occurs in the transcendental sayings means the Śabdabrahman, or Īśvara endowed with the work of creation, maintenance, and "destruction," of the Universe. The same word also indicates indirectly

---

[1] Itthaṁ caturvidhāsu mātṛkāsu parādi-trayaṁ ajānanto manuṣyāh sthūladṛśo vaikharīṁ eva vācaṁ manvate (Bhāskararāya, *ib.*).

[2] Tathā ca śrutih: Tasmād yadvāco 'nāptam tanmanuṣyā upajīvanti iti, anāptaṁ apūrṇaṁ tisṛbhir virahitaṁ ityartha iti vedabhāṣhye.

[3] Śrutyantare 'pi:

Catvāri vākparimitā padānī, tāni vidur brāhmaṇā yet manīṣinah.
Guhā trīṇi nihitā neṅgayanti, turīyaṁ vāco manuṣyā vadanti (*ib.*).

[4] The Pada, or word, is that which has a termination. Pāṇini says (Sūtra I, iv, 14): "That which ends in Sup (nominal endings) and in Tin (verbal terminations) is called Pada." Again, the Sup (termination) has five divisions.

[5] Bhāskararāya, *loc. cit.*

(Lakṣanayā) the unconditioned of supreme Brahman who is without attributes. The relation between the two Brahmans is that of sameness (Tādātmya). Thus, the Devī or Śakti is the one consciousness-bliss (Cidekarasarūpiṇī)—that is, She is ever inseparate from Cit. The relation of the two Brahmans is possible, as the two are one and the same. Though they appear as different (by attributes), yet at the same time they are one.

The commentator cited then asks, How can the word Tat in the Vaikharī form indicate Brahman and replies that it only does so indirectly. For sound in the physical form of speech (Vaikharī) only expresses or is identified with the physical form of Brahman (the Virāt), and not the pure Supreme Brahman.

The following will serve as a summary of correspondences noted in this and the previous Chapter. There is first the Nirguṇa-Brahman, which in its creative aspect is Saguṇa Śabdabrahman, and assumes the form of Parabindu, and then of the threefold (Tri-bindu); and is the four who are represented in the sense above stated by the four forms of speech, sound or state (Bhāva).

The causal (Kāraṇa) or Supreme Bindu (Para-bindu) is unmanifest (Avyakta), undifferentiated Śiva-Śakti, whose powers are not yet displayed, but are about to be displayed from out the then undifferentiated state of Mūlaprakṛti. This is the state of Supreme Speech (Parā-Vāk), the Supreme Word or Logos, the seat of which in the individual body is the Mūlādhāra-Cakra. So much is clear. There is, however, some difficulty in co-ordinating the accounts of the threefold powers manifesting upon the differentiation of the Great Bindu (Mahā-bindu). This is due in part to the fact that the verses in which the accounts appear are not always to be read in the order of the words (Śabda-krama), but according to the actual order in fact, whatever that may be

(Yathāsaṁbhavaṁ).[1] Nextly, there is some apparent variance in the commentaries. Apart from names and technical details, the gist of the matter is simple and in accordance with other systems. There is first the unmanifested Point (Bindu), as to which symbol St. Clement of Alexandria says[2] that if from a body abstraction be made of its properties, depth, breadth, and length, that which remains is a point having position, from which, if abstraction be made of position,[3] there is the state of primordial unity. There is one Spirit, which appears three-fold as a Trinity of Manifested Power (Śakti). As so manifesting, the one (Śiva-Śakti) becomes twofold, Śiva and Śakti, and the relation (Nāda) of these two (Tayor mithah samavāyah) makes the threefold Trinity common to so many religions. The One first moves as the Great Will (Icchā), then as the Knowledge or Wisdom (Jñāna) according to which Will acts, and then as Action (Kriyā). This is the order of Śaktis in Īśvara. So, according to the Paurāṇik account, at the commencement of creation Brahmā wakes. The Saṁskāras then arise in His mind. There arises the Desire to create (Icchā-Śakti); then the Knowledge (Jñāna-Śakti) of what He is about to create; and lastly, the Action (Kriyā) of creation. In the case of Jīva the order of Jñāna, Icchā, Kriyā. For He first considers or knows something. Informed by such knowledge, He wills and then acts. The

---

[1] As pointed out by the author of Prāṇa-toṣiṇī, p. 2 when citing the verse from the Gorakṣa Saṁhitā:

> Icchā kriyā tathā jñānaṁ gaurī brāhmī tu vaiṣṇavī,
> Tridhā śaktih sthitā yatra tarparaṁ jyotir Oṁ iti.

According to this account of the Devas of different Ādhāras of Prāṇa-Śakti upāsanā the order is (according to sequence of words): Icchā=Gaurī; Kriyā=Brāhmī; Jñāna= Vaiśṇavi.

[2] Stromata, Book V, Ch. II, in Vol. IV, Antenicene Library. So also in "Les Mystāres de la Croix," an eighteenth-century mystical work we read: "Ante omina punctum exstitit; non mathematicum sed diffusivuṁ."

[3] See "Garland of Letters" or Studies in the Mantra-Śāstra.

three powers are, though counted and spoken of as arising separately, inseparable and indivisible aspects of the One. Wherever there is one there is the other, though men think of each separately and as coming into being—that is, manifested in time—separately.

According to one nomenclature the Supreme Bindu becomes threefold as Bindu (Kārya), Bīja, Nāda. Though Śiva is never separate from Śakti, nor Śakti from Śiva, a manifestation may predominantly signify one or another. So it is said that Bindu is in the nature of Śiva (Śivātmaka) and Bīja of Śakti (Śaktyātmaka), and Nāda is the combination of the two (Tayor mithah samavāyah). These are also called Mahābindu (Parābindu), Sitabindu (White Bindu), Ṣonabindu (Red Bindu), and Miśrabindu (Mixed Bindu). These are supreme (Parā), subtle (Sūkṣma), gross (Sthūla). There is another nomenclature—*viz.*, Sun, Fire, and Moon. There is no question but that Bīja is Moon, that from Bīja issues the Śakti Vāmā, from whom comes Brahmā, who are in the nature of the Moon and Will-Power (Icchā-Śakti).[1] Icchā-Śakti in terms of the Guṇas of Prakṛti is Rajas Guṇa, which impels Sattva to self-display. This is Paśyantī Śabda, the seat of which is in the Svādhiṣṭhāna Cakra. From Nāda similarly issue Jyeṣthā Śakti and Viṣṇu, and from Bindu Raudrī and Rudra, which are Madhyamā and Vaikharī Śabda, the seats of which are the Anāhata and Viśuddha Cakras respectively. According to one account[2] Bindu is "Fire" and Kriyā-Śakti (action), and Nāda is "Sun" and Jñāna-Śakti, which in terms of the

---

[1] Raudrī bindos tato nādāj jyeṣthā bījād ajāyata
Vāmā tābhyah samutpannā rudrabrahmaramādhipāh
Saṁjnānecchākriyātmāno vahnīndvarka-svarūpinah.
(Śāradā Tilaka, Ch. I.)

[2] Yoginīhṛdaya Tantra: Commentary already cited referring to Saubhāgya-Sudhodaya and Tattvasandoha. See also Tantrāloka, Ch. VI.

Guṇas are Tamas and Sattva respectively.[1] Rāghava-bhatta, however, in his Commentary on the Śāradā, says that the Sun is Kriyā because, like that luminary, it makes all things visible, and Jñāna is Fire because knowledge burns up all creation. When Jīva through Jñāna knows itself to be Brahman it ceases to act, so as to accumulate Karma, and attains Liberation (Mokṣa). It may be that this refers to the Jīva, as the former represents the creation of Īśvara.

In the Yoginīhṛdaya-Tantra it is said that Vāmā and Icchā-Śakti are in the Paśyantī body; Jñāna and Jyeṣṭhā are called Madhyamā; Kriyā-Śakti is Raudrī; and Vaikharī is in the form of the universe.[2] The evolution of the Bhāvas is given in the Śāradā-Tilaka[3] as follows: the all-pervading Śabdabrahman or Kuṇḍalī emanates Śakti, and then follow Dhvani, Nāda, Nirodhikā, Ardhendu, Bindu. Śakti is Cit with Sattva (Paramākāśāvasthā); Dhvani is Cit with Sattva and Rajas (Akṣarāvasthā); Nāda is Cit with Sattva, Rajas, Tamas. (Avyaktavastha); Nirodhika is the same with abundance of Tamas (Tamah-prācuryāt); Ardhendu the same with abundance of Sattva; and Bindu the combination of the two. This Bindu is called by the different names of Parā and the rest, according as it is in the different centres, Mūlādhāra and the rest. In this way Kuṇḍalī, who is Icchā, Jñāna, Kriyā, who is both in the form of consciousness

---

[1] The following shows the correspondence according to the texts cited:

Bīja Ṣoṇabindu	Śakti, Moon, Vāmā, Brahmā, Bhāratī, Icchā, Rajas, Paśyantī, Svādhiṣṭhāna,
Nāda Miśrabindu	Śiva-Śakti, Sun, Jyeṣṭhā, Viṣṇu, Viśvambhara, Jñāna, Sattva, Madhyamā, Anāhata.
Bindu Sitabindu	Śiva, Fire, Raudrī, Rudra, Rudrāṇi, Kriyā, Tamas, Vaikharī, Viśuddha.

[2] Icchā-śaktis tathā Vāmā paśyantī-vapuṣā sthitā,
Jnāna-śaktis tathā Jyeṣṭhā madhyamā vāg udīritā
Kriyā-śaktis tu Raudrīyaṁ vaikharī viśvavigraha.
(Cited under v. 22, Comm. Kāmakalāvilāsa.)

[3] Chap. I.

(Tejorūpā) and composed of the Guṇas (Gunātmikā), creates the Garland of Letters (Varṇamālā).

The four Bhāvas have been dealt with as coming under Nāda, itself one of the following nine manifestations of Devī.

Paṇḍit Anantakṛṣṇa-Śāstrī, referring to Lakṣmīdhara's commentary on v. 34 of Ānandalaharī, says:[1]

"'Bhagavatī is the word used in the text to denote Devī. One that possesses Bhaga is called Bhagavatī (feminine). Bhaga signifies the knowledge of (1) the creation, (2) destruction of the universe, (3) the origin of beings, (4) the end of beings, (5) real knowledge or divine truth, and (6) Avidyā, or ignorance. He that knows all these six items is qualified for the title Bhagavān. Again, Bha = 9. "Bhagavatī" refers to the nine-angled Yantra (figure) which is used in the Candrakalā-vidya.'

"According to the Āgamas, Devī has nine manifestations which are:

"1. Kāla group—lasting from the twinkling of an eye to the Pralaya time. The sun and moon are included in this group. TIME.

"2. Kula group—consists of things which have form and colour. FORM.

"3. Nāma group—consists of things which have name. NAME.

"4. Jñāna group—Intelligence. It is divided into two branches: Savikalpa (mixed and subject to change), and Nirvikalpa (pure and unchanging). CIT.

"5. Citta group—consists of (1) Ahaṁkāra (egoism), (2) Citta, (3) Buddhi, (4) Manas, and (5) Unmanas. MIND.

"6. Nāda group—consists of (1) Rāga (desire),[2] (2) Icchā (desire[2] strengthened, or developed desire),

[1] Anantakṛṣṇa Śāstrī, *op. cit.*, pp. 63-66.

[2] Rāga should be translated as "interest," as in Rāga-kañcuka. Icchā is the will towards action (Kriyā) in conformity therewith. Desire is a gross thing which comes in with the material world.

(3) Kṛti (action, or active form of desire), and (4) Prayatna (attempt made to achieve the object desired). These correspond, in order, to (1) Parā (the first stage of sound, emanating from Mūlādhāra), (2) Paśyantī (the second stage), (3) Madhyamā (the third stage), and (4) Vaikharī (the fourth stage of sound as coming out of the mouth). SOUND.

"7. Bindu group—consists of the six Cakras from Mūlādhāra to Ājñā. PSYCHIC ESSENCE, THE SPIRITUAL GERM.[1]

"8. Kalā group—consists of fifty letters from Mūlādhāra to Ājñā. KEYNOTES.[2]

"9. Jīva group—consists of souls in the bondage of matter.

"The Presiding Deities or Tattvas of the four constituent parts of Nāda are Māyā, Śuddha-vidyā, Maheśa, and Sadāśiva. The Commentator deals with this subject fully, quoting extracts from occult works. The following is a translation of a few lines from Nāma-kalā-vidyā,[3] a work on phonetics, which will be of interest to the reader:

"'Parā is Ekā (without duality); its opposite is the next one (Paśyanti); Madhyamā is divided into two, gross and subtle forms; the gross form consists of the nine groups of letters; and the subtle form is the sound which differentiates the nine letters. . . One is the cause, and the other the effect; and so there is no material difference between the sound and its gross forms.'

---

[1] I cite the passage as written, but these terms are not clear to me.

[2] I do not know what the Paṇḍit means by this term.

[3] "This work is not easily available to Paṇḍits or scholars; we do not find this name in any of the catalogues prepared by European or Indian scholars. The make-secret policy has spoiled all such books. Even now, if we find any MS. dealing with occult matters in the houses of any ancient Paṇḍits, we will not be allowed even to see the book; and actually these works have for a long time become food for worms and white ants," (Anantakṛṣṇa-Śāstrī)

"Com. 'Ekā': When the three Guṇas, Sattva, Rajas, and Tamas, are in a state of equilibrium (Sāṁya), that state is called Parā. Paśyantī is the state when the three Guṇas become unequal (and consequently produce sound). The next stage is called Madhyamā; the subtle form of this is called Sūkṣma-madhyamā, and the second and gross form is called Sthūla-madhyamā, which produces nine distinct forms of sound represented by nine groups of letters; *viz.*, अ (and all the other vowels), क (Kavarga, 5 in number), च (Cavarga, 5), ट (Ṭavarga, 5), त (Tavarga, 5), प (Pavarga, 5), य (Ya, Ra, La and Va), श (Śa, Ṣa, Sa and Ha), and क्ष (Kṣa). These letters do not in reality exist, but represent only the ideas of men. Thus all the forms and letters originate from Parā, and Parā is nothing but Caitanya (Consciousness).

"The nine groups or Vyūhas (manifestations of Devī) above enumerated are, again, classed under the following three heads: (1) Bhoktā (enjoyer)—comprises No. 9, Jīva-vyūha. (2) Bhogya (objects of enjoyment)—comprises, groups Nos. 1, 2, 3, 5, 6, 7, and 8. (3) Bhoga (enjoyment)—comprises No. 4, Jñāna-vyūha.

"The above is the substance of the philosophy of the Kaulas as expounded by Śrī Śaṁkarācārya in this śloka of Ānandalaharī (No. 34). In commenting on this, Lakṣmīdhara quotes several verses from the Kaula-Āgamas, of which the following is one:

"'The blissful Lord is of nine forms. This God is called Bhairava. It is He that confers enjoyment (bliss) and liberates the souls (from bondage). His consort is Ānandabhairavī, the ever-blissful consciousness (Caitanya). When these two unite in harmony, the universe comes into existence.'

"The Commentator remarks here that the power of Devī predominates in creation, and that of Śiva in dissolution."

VI

PRACTICE (YOGA: LAYA-KRAMA)

Yoga is sometimes understood as meaning the result and not the process which leads to it. According to this meaning of the term, and from the standpoint of natural dualism, Yoga has been described to be the union of the individual spirit with God.

But if Jīva and Paramātmā are really one, there can be no such thing in an Advaitic system as union, which term is strictly applicable to the case of the coming together of two distinct beings. Samādhi (ecstasy) consists in the realization that the Jīvātmā *is* Paramātmā; and Yoga means, not this realization, but the *means* by which it is attained. Yoga is thus a term for those physical and psychical processes which are used to discover man's inner essence, which is the Supreme.

It is thus not a result, but the *process*, method, or practice, by which this result is attained. This result is possible, according to Advaita-Vedānta, because pure Cit, as the essential being of every Jīva, is not in itself fettered, but appears to be so. Were Ātmā as such not truly free, Liberation (Mokṣa) would not be possible. Liberation or Mokṣa therefore is potentially in the possession of every Jīva. His identity with Paramātmā exists now as then, but is not realized owing to the veil of Māyā, through which Jīvātmā and Paramātmā appear as separate. As ignorance of the identity of the Jīvātmā and Paramātmā is due to Avidyā, the realization of such identity is attained by Vidyā or Jñāna.

The latter alone can immediately produce Liberation (Sadyomukti). Jñāna is used in a twofold sense—namely, Svarūpa-Jñāna and Kriyā-Jñāna. The first is Pure Consciousness, which is the end and aim of Yoga; the second is those intellective processes which are the means taken to acquire the first. Jñāna considered as means or mental action (Mānasī-Kriyā) is an intellective process that is the discrimination between what is and what is not Brahman; the right understanding of what is meant by Brahman, and the fixing of the mind on what is thus understood until the Brahman wholly and permanently occupies the mind to the displacement of all else Mind is then absorbed into Brahman as pure Consciousness, which alone remains; this is realization or the attainment of the state of pure consciousness, which is Jñāna in its Svarūpa sense. Liberating Yoga short of perfect Jñāna effects what is called Kramamukti—that is, the Yogī attains Sāyujya or union with Brahman in Satya-loka, which is thence perfected into complete Mukti through the Devatā with whom he is thus united. What the Siddha (complete) Jñānayogī or Jīvanmukta himself accomplishes in this life is thereafter attained as the sequel to Brahma-sāyujya. But man has not only intellect. He has feeling and devotion. He has not only these, but has a body. Other processes (Yogas) are therefore associated with and in aid of it, such as those belonging to worship (Upāsanā) and the gross (Sthūla-Kriyā) and subtle processes (Sūkṣma-Kriyā) of Haṭhayoga.

Mind and body are the instruments whereby the ordinary separatist worldly experience is had. As long, however, as they are so used they are impediments in the way of attainment of the state of pure Consciousness (Cit). For such attainment all screenings (Āvaraṇa) of Cit must be cleared away. Yoga therefore is the method whereby mental intellection and feeling (Citta-vṛtti) and Prāṇa are first controlled and then stayed.[1] When the Citta, Vṛtti, and Prāṇa are stilled, then Cit or Paramātmā stands revealed. It supervenes without further effort on the absorption of matter and mind into the primordial Power (Śakti) whence they sprang, of whom they are manifested forms, and who is Herself as Śiva one with Him who is Śiva or Consciousness. Yoga thus works towards a positive state of pure consciousness by the negation of the operation of the principle of unconsciousness which stands in the way of its uprising. This pruning action is well illustrated by the names of a Śakti which in this work is variously described as Nibodhikā and Nirodhikā. The first means the Giver of Knowledge, and the second That which obstructs—that is, obstructs the affectation of the mind by the objective world through the senses. It is by the prohibition of such impressions that the state of pure consciousness arises. The arising of such state is called Samādhi—that is, the ecstatic condition in which the "equality" that is identity of Jīvātmā and Paramātmā is realized. The experience is achieved after the absorption (Laya) of Prāṇa and Manas and the cessation of all ideation (Saṁkalpa). An unmodified state (Samarasatvam) is thus produced which is the natural state (Sahajāvasthā) of the Ātmā. Until then there is that fluctuation and modification (Vṛtti) which is the mark of the conditioned consciousness, with its self-diremption of "I" and "Thou". The state of Samādhi is "like that of a grain of salt, which mingled in water becomes one with it".[2] It is, in the words of the Kulārṇava-Tantra, "that form

---

[1] The Tattva (Reality) is revealed when all thought is gone (Kulārṇava-Tantra, IX, 40.)

[2] Haṭha-yoga-pradīpikā, IV, 5-7. The same simile is used in the Buddhist Demchog Tantra. See Vol. VII, Tāntrik Texts.

of contemplation (Dhyāna) in which there is neither 'here' nor 'not here,' in which there is illumination and stillness as of some great ocean, and which is the Void Itself."[1]

The all-knowing and venerable Teacher has said, "One who has attained complete knowledge of the Ātmā reposes like the still waters of the deep" (v. 31). The Māyā-Tantra defines Yoga as the unity of Jīva and Paramātmā (v. 51); that by which oneness is attained with the Supreme (Paramātmā), and Samādhi, or ecstasy, in this unity of Jīva and Ātmā (*ib.*).[2] Others define it as the knowledge of the identity of Śiva and Ātmā. The Āgamavādīs proclaim that the knowledge of Śakti (Śaktyātmakaṁ jñānaṁ) is Yoga. Other wise men say that the knowledge of the "Eternal Puruṣa" (Purāṇa-Puruṣa) is Yoga, and others, again, the Prakṛti-vādīs, declare that the knowledge of the union of Śiva and Śakti is Yoga (*ib.*). All such definitions refer to one and the same thing—the realization by the human spirit that it is in essence the Great Spirit, the Brahman, who as the Ruler of the worlds is known as God. As the Haṭha-yoga-pradīpikā says:[3] "Rājayoga, Samādhi, Unmanī,[4] Manonmanī,[4] Amaratvaṁ (Immortality), Śūnyāśūnya (void yet non-void),[5] Paramapada[6] (the Supreme State), Amanaska (without Manas—suspended operation of mental functioning),[7] Advaita (non-dual),

---

[1] IX, 9.

[2] As water poured into water the two are undistinguishable (Kularṇava-Tantra, IX, 15).

[3] Ch. IV, vv. 3, 4.

[4] State of mindlessness. See Nāda-bindu Up.

[5] See Haṭha-yoga-pradīpikā, IV, v. 37. The Yogī, like the Consciousness with which he is one, is beyond both.

[6] The root pad="to go to," and Padam therefore is that to which one has access (Comm. on v. 1, Ch. IV, of Haṭha-yoga-pradīpikā).

[7] See Maṇḍala-brāhmaṇa Up., II, III.

Nirālaṁba (without support—*i.e.*, detachment of the Manas from the external world),[1] Nirañjana (stainless),[2] Jīvanmukti (liberation in the body), Sahajāvasthā (natural state of the Ātmā), and Turīya (Fourth State), all mean one and the same thing—that is, the cessation of both mental functioning (Citta) and action (Karma), on which there arises freedom from alternating joy and sorrow and a changeless (Nirvikāra) state. This on the dissolution of the body is followed by bodiless (Videha-kaivalya) or supreme Liberation (Paramamukti), which is the permanent state (Svarūpāvasthānaṁ). Whilst the aim and the end of Yoga is the same, the methods by which it is attained vary.

There are, it is commonly said, four forms of Yoga, called Mantra-yoga, Haṭha-yoga, Laya-yoga, and Rāja-yoga.[3] These are all various modes of practice (Sādhana) whereby the feelings and intellectual activities of the mind (Citta-vṛtti) are brought into control and the Brahman is in various ways realized (Brahmasākṣātkāra). Each of these forms has the same eight subservients, which are called the "eight limbs" (Aṣṭāṅga). Each of these has the same aim—namely, the experience which is realization of Brahman; they differ, however, as to the means employed and, it is said, in degree of result. The Samādhi of the first has been described as Mahābhāva, of the second as Mahābodha, of the third as

[1] This is the Nirālaṁbapurī referred to in the Text.

[2] Añjana=Māyopādhi (the Upādhi, or apparently limiting condition produced by Māyā, or appearance); therefore Nirañjana=destitute of that (Tadrahitaṁ), or Śuddham (pure)—that is, the Brahman. Comm. Haṭha-yoga-pradīpikā IV, v. 1.

[3] Varāha-Upaniṣad, Ch. V, II; Yoga-tattva Up. A useful analysis of Yoga will be found in Rajendra Ghose's "Śaṁkara and Rāmānuja". Mention is also made of a threefold division corresponding to the three Vaidik Kāṇdas, *viz.*, Karma-Yoga (Karma-Kāṇda), Bhakti-Yoga (Upāsanā-Kāṇda), Jñāna or Rāja-Yoga (Jñāna-Kāṇda). Karma-Yoga is good action without desire for its fruit. Bhakti-Yoga is devotion to God.

Mahā-laya, and by Rāja-Yoga and Jñāna-Yoga, it is said, the liberation called Kaivalyamukti is obtained.

It is to be noted, however, that in the estimation of the practitioners of Kuṇḍalī Yoga it is the highest Yoga in which a perfect Samādhi is gained by the union with Śiva of both mind and body, as hereafter described. In Rāja- and Jñāna-Yoga intellective processes are the predominant where they are not the sole means employed. In Mantra-Yoga, worship and devotion predominate. In Haṭha-Yoga there is more stress on physical methods, such as breathing. Each, however, of these Yogas employs some methods of the others. Thus, in Haṭha-Laya-Yoga there is Kriyā-jñāna. But whereas the Jñāna-Yogī attains Svarūpa-Jñāna by his mental efforts without rousing Kuṇḍalinī, the Haṭhayogī gets this Jñāna through Kuṇḍalinī Herself. For Her union with Śiva in the Sahasrāra brings, and in fact is, Svarūpa-Jñāna.

It will be convenient, therefore, to deal with the general subservients (Aṣṭāṅga) which are common to all forms of Yoga, and then follow with an account of Mantra and the lower Haṭha-yogas as a preliminary to that form of Laya-yoga which is the subject of this work, and includes within itself elements to be found both in Mantra and such Haṭha-yogas.

The pre-requisites of all Yoga are the eight limbs or parts, Yama, Niyama, and others. Morality, religious disposition and practice, and discipline (Sādhana), are essential pre-requisites of all Yoga which has as its aim the attainment of the Supreme Experience.[1] Morality (Dharma) is the expression of the true nature of being. The word Dharma,

---

[1] There are forms of Yoga, such as that with the elements giving "powers" (Siddhi) over them, to which different considerations apply. This is a part of Magic, and not of religion. So the uniting of Prāṇa with the Tejas-Tattva in the navel (Āgneyī-dhāraṇā-mudra) is said to secure immunity from fire.

which includes both ethics and religion, but has also a wider context, comes from the root *dhri*, to sustain, and is therefore both the sustainer and the act of sustaining. The Universe is sustained (Dhāryate) by Dharma, and the Lord who is its Supreme Sustainer is embodied in the eternal law and is the Bliss which its fulfilment secures. Dharma is thus the law governing the universal evolution, or the path of outgoing (Pravṛtti), and involution, or the path of return (Nivṛtti).[1] And only those can attain the liberation to which the latter path leads who by adherence to Dharma co-operate in the carrying out of the universal scheme. For this reason it is finely said, "Doing good to others is the Supreme Duty" (Paropakāro hi paramo dharmah).

In this scheme the Jīva passes from Śabda-vidyā, with its Tapas involving egoism and fruit attained through the "Path of the God," its Karma (rites), which are either Sakama (with desire for fruit) or Niṣkāma (disinterested), to Brahma-vidyā (knowledge of the Brahman) or Theosophy as taught by the Upaniṣads. This transition is made through Niṣkāma-Karma. By Sakāma-Karma is attained the "Path of the Fathers" (Pitṛ), Dharma, Artha (wealth), Kāma (desire and its fulfilment). But Niṣkāma-Karma produces that purity of mind (Citta-śuddhi) which makes man competent for Brahma-vidyā, or Theosophy, which leads to, and in its completest sense is, Liberation (Mokṣa).

It is obvious that before the pure blissful state of the Ātmā can be attained the Jīva must first live that ordered life which is its proper expression on this plane.

---

[1] This grand concept, therefore, is a name for *all* those laws (of which "religion" is but one) which hold the universe together. It is the inherent law of all manifested being. It is thus the Law of Form, the essence of which is beyond both Dharma or Adharma. As pain follows wrong-doing, the Vaiśeṣika-Darśana describes Dharma as "that by which happiness is attained in this and the next world, and birth and suffering are brought to an end (Mokṣa-dharma)".

To use theological language, only those who follow Dharma can go to its Lord. The disorder of an immoral life is not a foundation on which such a Yoga can be based. I do not use the term "immorality" in the absurdly limited meaning which ordinary English parlance gives it, but as the infringement of all forms of moral law. All such infringements are founded on selfishness. As the object of Yoga is the surpassing of the limited self even in its more ordered manifestation, its doctrines, clearly presuppose the absence of a state governed by the selfishness which is the grossest obstacle to its attainment. The aim of Yoga is the achievement of complete detachment from the finite world and realization of its essence. In a life governed by Dharma, there is that natural attachment to worldly objects and sense of separateness even in acts of merit which must exist until by the absorption of Manas the Unmanī or mindless state is attained. Where, however, there is unrighteousness (Adharma), attachment (Rāga) exists in its worst and most injurious form, and the sense of separateness (Dvaitabhāva) which Yoga seeks to overcome is predominantly present in sin. The body is poisoned by the secretion of passions, poisons, and vitality or Prāṇa is lessened and injured. The mind under the influence of anger,[1] lust, malice, and other passions, is first distracted, and then, on the principle what a man thinks that he "becomes," is centred on, and is permanently moulded into and becomes, the expression of Adharma (unrighteousness) itself. In such a case the Jīva is not merely bound to the world by the Māyā which affects both him and the virtuous Sakāma-Sādhaka, but suffers Hell (Naraka), and "goes down" in the scale of Being.

Dharma in its devotional aspect is also necessary. Desire to achieve the highest aim of Yoga can only spring from

[1] According to Indian notions, anger is the worst of sins.

a religious disposition, and such a disposition and practice (Sādhana) furthers the acquisition of those qualities which Yoga requires. Indeed, by persevering devotion to the Mother, Samādhi may be achieved.

Therefore is it that the Commentator in v. 50 of the first of these works says:

"He alone whose nature has been purified by the practice of Yama and Niyama and the like (referring to the Sādhana hereinafter described) will learn from the mouth of the Guru the means whereby the way to the great Liberation is discovered."

He adds, however, that the practice of Yama and the like is only necessary for those whose minds are disturbed by anger, lust, and other evil propensities. If, however, a man through merit acquired in previous births is by good fortune of a nature which is free of these and other vices, then he is competent for Yoga without this preliminary preparation.

All forms of Yoga, whether Mantra, Haṭha, or Rāja, have the same eight limbs (Astāṅga) or preparatory subservients: Yama, Niyama, Āsana, Prāṇāyāma, Pratyāhāra, Dhāraṇā, Dhyāna, and Samādhi.[1] Yama is of ten kinds: avoidance of injury to all living creatures (Ahiṁsā); truthfulness (Satyaṁ); restraint from taking what belongs to another, or covetousness (Āsteyaṁ); sexual continence in mind, speech, or body (Brahmacarya);[2] forbearance, the

[1] Varāha Up., Ch. V. The preliminaries are necessary only for those who have not attained. For those who have, Niyama, Āsana, and the like, are needless. Kulārṇava-Tantra, XI, 28, 29.

[2] As the Haṭha-yoga-pradīpikā says: "He who knows Yoga should preserve his semen. For the expenditure of the latter tends to death, but there is life for him who preserves it."

Evaṁ saṁrakṣayet binduṁ mrityuṁ jayati yogavit.
Maraṇaṁ bindupātena jīvanaṁ bindudhāraṇāt.

See also Yogatattva Up., which says that Haṭha-yoga secures such personal beauty to the Yogī that all women will desire him, but they

bearing patiently of all things pleasant or unpleasant (Kṣamā); fortitude in happiness or unhappiness (Dhṛtī); mercy, kindliness (Dayā); simplicity (Ārjavaṁ); moderation[1] in and regulation[2] of diet (Mitāhāra), suited to the development of the Sattvaguṇa; and purity of body and mind (Śaucaṁ). The first form of purity is the external cleansing of the body, particularly dealt with by Haṭha-yoga (*v. post*); and the second is gained through the science of the Self (Adhyātma-vidyā).[3]

Niyama is also of ten kinds: Austerities, such as fasts and the like, in the nature of purificatory actions (Tapah); contentment with that which one has unasked (Saṁtoṣa); belief in Veda (Āstikyam); charity (Dānaṁ)—that is gifts to the deserving of what one has lawfully acquired; worship of the Lord or Mother (Īśvara-pūjaṇaṁ) according to His or Her various forms; hearing of Śāstric conclusion, as by study of the Vedānta (Siddhānta-vākya-śravaṇaṁ); modesty and shame felt in the doing of wrong actions (Hrī); a mind rightly directed towards knowledge revealed and practice enjoined by the Śāstra (Mati); recitation of Mantra (Japa);[4]

---

must be resisted. And see also v. 90, which shows the connection between semen, mind, and life. In the early stages of Haṭha-yoga Sādhana the heat goes upwards, the penis shrinks, and sexual powers are largely lost. Coition with emission of semen at this stage is likely to prove fatal. But a Siddha regains his sexual power and can exercise it. For if as is said fire and the other elements cannot hurt him, what can a woman do? Presumably, however, the dictum cited applies, for continence must in all cases tend to strength and longevity. It may, however, be that the physical perfection assumed negatives the ill effects observed in ordinary men.

[1] Yoga-yājñavalkya (Ch. I) says: "32 mouthfuls for householder, 16 for a forest recluse, and 8 for a Muni."

[2] For foods detrimental to Yoga, see Yoga-tattva Up., Yoga-kuṇḍalī Up.

[3] Śāṇḍilya Up., Ch. I; see also Maṇḍala-brāhmaṇa Up.

[4] Which is either spoken (which, again, is loud or soft) or mental (Śāṇḍilya-Up.).

and Homa sacrifice (Hutaṁ)[1]—that is, religious observances in general (Vrata). The Pātañjala-Sūtra mentions only five Yamas—the first four and freedom from covetousness (Aparigraha). Ahimsā is the root of those which follows. Śaucaṁ, or cleanliness, is included among the Niyama. Five of the latter are stated—namely, cleanliness (Śaucaṁ), contentment (Saṁtoṣa), purificatory action (Tapah), study of the Scriptures leading to liberation (Svādhyāya), and devotion to the Lord (Īśvara-praṇidhāna).[2]

The statement of such obvious truths would hardly be necessary were it not that there are still some who see in all Yoga mere "Shamanism," feats of breathing, "acrobatic posturing," and so forth. On the contrary, no country since the Middle Ages and until our own has laid greater stress on the necessity of the association of morality and religion with all forms of human activity, than India has done.[3]

The practice of Yama and Niyama leads to renunciation of, and detachment from, the things of this world and of the next,[4] arising from the knowledge of the permanent

---

[1] See Ch. I, vv. 16, 17, Haṭha-yoga-pradīpikā, and p. 123, Sanskrit Text, post. The Śāṇḍilya Up., Ch. I, gives Vrata as the last, which is described as the observance of actions enjoined and refraining from actions prohibited. See also Ch. V, Varāha Up.

[2] Patañjali's Yoga-Sūtra, Ch. II, 30, 32.

[3] So, as was the case in our Mediæval guilds, religion inspires Indian Art; and Indian speculation is associated with religion as was the Western scholastic philosophy. In modern times in the West, the relevancy of religion in these matters has not been generally considered to be apparent, craftsmanship in the one case and intelligence in the other being usually thought to be sufficient.

[4] Such as the Sudhā (nectar) which is gained in the heavens (Haṭha-yoga-pradīpikā, Comm. to v. 9, Ch. I). Renunciation may doubtless be practised by giving up what one wants, but renunciation or abandonment (Tyāga) here means the *want of desire* of enjoyment (Tyāgah=bhogecchābhāvah) (*ib.*). Those who seek the joys of any heaven can never attain the end of monistic Yoga.

and impermanent, and intense desire for and incessant striving after emancipation, which characterizes him who is Mumukṣu, or longs for Liberation.

Yama and Niyama are the first two of the eight accessories of Yoga (Aṣṭāṅga-yoga). These accessories or limbs may be divided into five exterior methods [1] (Bahiraṅga), chiefly concerned with the subjugation of the body, and three inner methods [2] (Antaraṅga), or states affecting the development of the mind.

Attention is paid to the physical body, which is the vehicle of the Jīva's existence and activity. Purity of mind is not possible without purity of the body in which it functions and by which it is affected. Purity of mind is here used in the Hindu sense. According to English parlance, such purity merely connotes absence of irregular sexual imaginations. This, though creditable, particularly in a civilization which almost seems designed to fan every desire, is yet obviously insufficient for the purpose in hand. Proper thought and conduct in all its forms is but the alphabet of a school in which they are merely the first steps to the conquest of greater difficulties to follow. What is here meant is that state of the mind or approach thereto which is the result of good functioning, clear thinking, detachment, and concentration. By these the Manas is freed of all those mental modifications (Vṛtti) which enshroud the Ātmā from Itself. It is turned inward on the Buddhi which becomes dissolved (Laya) in Prakṛti, and the Ātma-tattva or Brahman.

Provision therefore is made in respect both of Āsana (posture) and Prāṇāyāma or breath development, both of which are shortly dealt with later in connection with Haṭha-yoga, of which they are particular processes. Pratyāhāra

[1] Yama, Niyama, Āsana, Prāṇāyāma, Pratyāhāra.

[2] Dhyāna, Dhāraṇā, Samādhi which is both incomplete (Savikalpa or Saṁprajñāta) and complete (Nirvikalpa or Asaṁprajñāta).

is the restraint of and subjection of the senses to the mind, which is thereby steadied.[1] The mind is withdrawn from the objects of the senses. The mind is by nature unsteady, for it is at every moment being affected by the sight, sounds, and so forth, of external objects which Manas through the agency of the senses (Indriyas) perceives. It must therefore be detached from the objects of the senses, withdrawn from whatsoever direction it may happen to tend, freed from all distraction, and kept under the control of the dominant self. Steadiness (Dhairya) therefore is the aim and result of Pratyāhāra.[2] The three processes known as the "inner limbs" (Antaraṅga)—namely, Dhāraṇā, Dhyāna, and Savikalpa-Samādhi—complete the psychic and mental discipline. These are concentration of the mind on an object; unity of the mind with its object by contemplation; resulting in the last or consciousness of the object only. The first is the "holding by"—that is, fixing the Citta, or thinking principle, on a particular object of thought or concentration (Dhāraṇā). The mind, having been drawn away from the objects of the senses by Pratyāhāra, is fixed on one object, such as the Devatās of the Bhūtas, alone. Uniform contemplation on the subject which the Citta holds in Dhāraṇā is Dhyāna (meditation). Dhyāna has been defined to be the state of the Antahkaraṇa (mind) of those whose Caitanya holds to and is occupied by the thought of one object, having

---

[1] See Gheraṇḍa-Saṁhitā, Fourth Upadeśa; Śāṇḍilya Up., Ch. I; Amṛtanāda Up.; Maṇḍala-brāhmaṇa Up., First Brāhmaṇa. The Śāradā-Tilaka defines Pratyāhāra as "the forcible obstruction of the senses wandering over their objects" (Indriyānāṁ vicaratāṁ viṣayeṣu balād āharaṇaṁ tebhyah pratyāhārah vidhīyate). The Śāṇḍilya Up. (*loc. cit.*) speaks of five kinds of Pratyāhāra, the last of which is Dhārāṇa on eighteen important points of the body.

[2] Śāṇḍilya Up., Ch. I; Amṛtanāda Up.; Maṇḍala-brāhmaṇa Up., First Brāhmaṇa.

first cast away thought of all other objects.[1] Through Dhyāna is acquired the quality of mental realization (Pratyakṣa).[2] It is of two kinds: Saguṇa, or meditation of a form (Mūrti); and Nirguṇa, in which the self is its own object.

Samādhi or ecstasy has been defined to be the identification of Manas and Ātmā as salt in water,[3] that state in which all is known as one (equal)[4] and the "nectar of equality" (oneness).[5] Complete Samādhi is thus the state of Parā-saṁvit or Pure Consciousness. Of Samādhi there are two degrees, in the first of which (Savikalpa) the mind in a lesser degree, and in the second (Nirvikalpa) in a complete degree, continuously and to the exclusion of all other objects, assumes the nature and becomes one with the subject of its contemplation.

There are in Advaita-Vedanta three states (Bhūmikā) of Saṁprajñāta (Savikalpa) Samādhi—namely, Ṛtaṁbharā, Prajñālokā, Praśānta-vāhitā.[6] In the first the content of the mental Vṛtti is Saccidānanda. There is still a separate knower. The second is that in which every kind of Āvaraṇa (screening) is cast away, and there is Sākṣātkāra Brahmajñāna passing into the third state of Peace in which the mind is void of all Vṛtti and the self exists as the Brahman alone;[7] "On which being known everything is known"

---

[1] Vijātīya-pratyaya-tiraskāra-pūrvaka-sajātīya-vṛttikābhih, nirantara (vyāpti-viṣayīkṛta-caitanyaṁ yasya, tat tādṛśaṁ cittaṁ antahkaraṇaṁ yeśām (Comm. on v. 35 of the Triśatī, on the title of the Devī as Ekāgra-citta-nirdhyātā).

Those from whose Citta or Antahkaraṇa (inner sense) have been removed all impressions of a conflicting nature and are constantly realizing or experiencing Caitaṇya.

[2] Śāṇḍilya Up., Ch. I; Maṇḍala-brāhmaṇa Up., First Brāhmaṇa.

[3] Varāha Up., Ch. II.

[4] Amṛtanāda Up.

[5] Yogakuṇḍalī Up., Ch. III.

[6] Comm. v. 35 of Triśatī.

[7] Comm. *ibid.*, Manaso vṛttiśūnyasya brahmākāratayā sthitih. The mind has always Vṛtti (modifications)—that is, Guṇa. If the Jīva's mind is freed of these, he is Brahman.

(Yasmin vijñāte sarvaṁ idaṁ vijñātaṁ bhavati.) Entrance is here made into Nirvikalpa-Samādhi by Rāja-yoga.

These three—Dhāraṇā, Dhyāna, Savikalpa-Samādhi—called Saṁyama, are merely stages in the mental effort of concentration, though, as later stated, according to the Haṭha-yoga aspect, they are progressions in Prāṇāyāma, each stage being a longer period of retention of Prāṇa.[1] Thus by Yama, Niyama, Āsana, the body is controlled; by these and Prāṇāyāma the Prāṇa is controlled; by these and Pratyāhāra the senses (Indriyas) are brought under subjection. Then through the operation of Dhāraṇā, Dhyāna and the lesser Samādhi (Savikalpa or Saṁprajñāta), the modifications (Vṛtti) of the Manas cease and Buddhi alone functions. By the further and long practice of dispassion or indifference to both joy and sorrow (Vairāgya) Buddhi itself becomes Laya, and the Yogī attains the true unmodified state of the Ātmā, in which the Jīva who is then pure Buddhi is merged in Prakṛti and the Brahman, as salt in the waters of ocean and as camphor in the flame.

Passing then to the processes[2] peculiar to the different Yogas, Mantra-yoga comprises all those forms of Sādhana in which the mind is controlled by means of its own object—that is, the manifold objects of the world of name and form (Nāma-rūpa). The whole universe is made up of names and forms (Nāma-rūpātmaka) which are the objects (Viṣaya) of the mind. The mind is itself modified into the form of that which it perceives. These modifications are called its Vṛtti, and the mind is not for one moment devoid of ideas and feelings. It is the feeling or intention

[1] See Yoga-tattva-Upaniṣad.

[2] See two publications by the Śrī Bhārata-dharma-mahāmaṇḍala—Mantra-yoga and Haṭha-yoga in the Dharma-Pracāra Series (Benares). The latter in a short compass explain the main essentials of each of the four systems.

(that is, Bhāva) with which an act is done which determines its moral worth. It is on this Bhāva that both character and the whole outlook on life depend. It is sought therefore to render the Bhāva pure. As a man who falls on the ground raises himself by means of the same ground, so to break worldly bonds the first and easiest method is to use those bonds as the means of their own undoing.[1] The mind is distracted by Nāma-rūpa, but this Nāma-rūpa may be utilized as the first means of escape therefrom. In Mantra-yoga, therefore, particular form of Nāma-rūpa, productive of pure Bhāva, is given as the object of contemplation. This is called Sthūla or Saguṇa-Dhyāna of the five Devatās, devised to meet the requirements of different natures. Besides the ordinary "eight limbs" (Aṣṭāṅga)[2] common to all forms of Yoga, certain modes of training and worship are prescribed. In the latter material media are utilized as the first steps whereby the formless One is by Jñāna-yoga attained—such as images (Mūrti),[3] emblems (Liṅga, Sālagrāma), pictures (Citra), mural markings (Bhitti-rekhā), Maṇḍalas and Yantras (diagrams),[4] Mudrās,[5] Nyāsa.[6] With this the prescribed Mantra is said (Japa) either aloud or softly only. The source of all Bīja-Mantras (Seed-Mantra), the Praṇava (Oṁ), or Brahman, is the articulate equivalent of that primal "Sound" which issued from the first vibration of the Guṇas of Mūlaprakṛti,

---

[1] This is an essentially Tāntrik principle. See Kulārṇava, Ch. II.

[2] *Vide ante*, p. 192.

[3] "The Deva of the unawakened (Aprabuddha) is in Images; of the Vipras in Fire; of the wise in the Heart. The Deva of those who know the Ātmā is everywhere." (Kulārṇava-Tantra, IX, 44) "O Beautiful-Eyed! Not in Kailāsa, Meru, or Mandara, do I dwell. I am there where the knowers of the Kula doctrine are." (*ib.*, v. 94).

[4] See "Introduction to Tantra-Śāstra".

[5] *Ib.* These ritual Mudrās are not to be confused with the Yoga Mudrās later described.

[6] See "Introduction to Tantra-Śāstra".

and the other Bīja-Mantras are the same equivalents of the various Saguṇa forms, Devas and Devīs, which thereafter appeared when Prakṛti entered the Vaiśaṁyāvastā state. In Mantra-yoga the state of Samādhi is called Mahābhāva. This is the simplest form of Yoga practice, suited for those whose powers and capacities are not such as to qualify them for either of the other methods.

Haṭha-yoga comprises those Sādhanas, or prescribed methods of exercise and practice, which are concerned primarily with the gross or physical body (Sthūla-śarīra). As the latter is connected with the superphysical or subtle body (Sūkṣma-śarīra), of which it is the outer sheath, control of the gross body affects the subtle body with its intellection, feelings, and passions. In fact, the Sthūla-śarīra is expressly designed to enable the Sūkṣma-śarīra to work out the Karma it has incurred. As the former is constructed according to the nature of the latter, and both are united and interdependent, it follows that operation in and upon the gross body affects the subtle body; the physical processes of this Yoga have been prescribed for particular temperaments, in order that, that physical body being first mastered, the subtle body with its mental functioning may be brought under control.[1] These merely physical processes are auxiliary to others. As the Kulārṇava-Tantra says:[2] "Neither the lotus seat nor fixing the gaze on the tip of the nose are Yoga. It is the identity of Jīvātmā and Paramātmā, which is Yoga." The special features of this Yoga may be first contrasted with Mantra-yoga. In the latter there is concern with things outside the physical body, and special attention is given to outward observances of ceremonials. Due regard must be paid to the laws of the caste and stages

[1] See the short summary of the Haṭha-yoga Saṁhitā given in the Dharma-Pracāra Series (Śrī Bhārata-dharma-mahā-maṇḍala, Benares).

[2] IX, 30.

of life (Varṇāśrama-Dharma), and the respective duties of men and women (Kula-Dharma). So the Mantra which is given to the male initiate may not be given to a woman. Nor is the Mantra given to a Brāhmaṇa suitable for a Śūdra. The objects of contemplation are Devas and Devīs in their various manifestations and concrete symbols, and the Samādhi called Mahā-bhāva is attained by contemplation of and by means of Nāma-rūpa. In Haṭha-yoga, on the other hand, the question of the fitness or otherwise of a novice is determined from the physical point of view, and rules are prescribed to procure and increase health and to free the body of disease. In Haṭha-yoga, contemplation is on the "Light," and the Samādhi called Mahā-bodha is attained by the aid of control of breath and other vital Vāyus (Prāṇāyāma), whereby the mind is also controlled. As already observed, Āsana and Prāṇāyāma, which are parts of Haṭha-yoga, are also parts of Mantra-yoga. Those who practise the latter will derive benefit from taking advantage of some of the other exercises of Haṭha-yoga, just as the followers of the latter system will be helped by the exercises of Mantra-yoga.

The word Haṭha is composed of the syllables Ha and Ṭha, which mean the "Sun" and "Moon"—that is, the Prāṇa and Apāna Vāyus. In v. 8 of the Ṣat-cakra-nirūpaṇa it is said that the Prāṇa (which dwells in the heart) draws Apāna (which dwells in the Mūlādhāra), and Apāna draws Prāṇa, just as a falcon attached by a string is drawn back again when he attempts to fly away. These two by their disagreement prevent each other from leaving the body, but when they are in accord they leave it. Both their union or Yoga in the Suṣumnā and the process leading thereto is called Prāṇāyāma. Haṭha-yoga or Haṭha-vidya is therefore the science of the Life-Principle,[1] using that

[1] See section on "Power as Life" (Prāṇa-Śakti) in "The World As Power".

word in the sense of the various forms of vital Vāyu into which Prāṇa is divided. Prāṇa in the body of the individual is a part of the Universal Breath (Prāṇa), or the "Great Breath". An attempt, therefore, is first made to harmonize the individual breath, known as Piṇda or Vyaṣti-Prāṇa, with the cosmic or collective breath, or the Brahmāṇḍa or Samaṣti-Prāṇa. Strength and health are thereby attained. The regulation of the harmonized breath helps the regulation and steadiness of mind, and therefore concentration.

In correspondence with the threefold division Ādhyātma, Ādhibhūta, Ādhidaiva, Mind (Manas), Prāṇa (vitality), and Vīrya (semen), are one. Therefore the subjection of Manas causes the subjection of Prāṇa or Vāyu and Vīrya. Similarly, by controlling Prāṇa, Manas and Vīrya are automatically controlled. Again, if the Vīrya is controlled, and the substance which under the influence of sexual desire develops into gross seed,[1] is made to flow upwards (Ūrdhvaretas), control is had over both Manas and Prāṇa. With Prāṇāyāma the semen (Śukra) dries up. The seminal force ascends and comes back as the nectar (Amṛta) of Śiva-Śakti.

Prāṇāyāma is recognized as one of the "limbs" of all the (Aṣtāṅga) forms of Yoga. But whereas it is used in Mantra-, Laya- and Rāja-Yoga, as an auxiliary, the Haṭha-yogī as such regards this regulation and Yoga of breath as the chief means productive of that result (Mokṣa), which is the common end of all schools of Yoga. This school, proceeding on the basis that the Vṛtti or modification of the mind

[1] According to Hindu ideas semen (Śukra) exists in a subtle form throughout the whole body. Under the influence of the sexual will it is withdrawn and elaborated into a gross form in the sexual organs. To be ūrdhvaretas is not merely to prevent the emission of gross semen already formed but to prevent its formation as gross seed, and its absorption in the general system. The body of a man who is truly ūrdhvaretas has the scent of a lotus. A chaste man where gross semen has formed may, on the other hand, smell like a buck goat.

always follows Prāṇa,[1] and on the sufficiency of that fact, held that by the aid of the union of Ha and Ṭha in the Suṣumnā, and the leading of the combined Prāṇas therein to the Brahma-randhra, Samādhi was attained. Though the reciprocal action of matter and mind is common knowledge, and bodily states influence psychic or mental states as the latter the former, the Haṭha-yoga method is preponderantly a physical one, though the gross physical acts of the preparatory stages of this Yoga are succeeded by Kriyā-jñāna and subtle vital processes which have Prāṇa as their subject.

Under the heading of gross physical training come provisions as to the place of residence, mode of life as regards eating, drinking, sexual function, exercise, and so forth.

The practice and exercises connected with Haṭha-yoga are divided into seven parts or stages—namely, cleansing (Śodhana) by the six processes (Ṣaṭ-karma); the attainment of strength or firmness (Dṛḍhatā) by bodily postures (Āsana); of fortitude (Sthiratā) by bodily positions (Mudrā); of steadiness of mind (Dhairya) by restraint of the senses (Pratyāhāra); of lightness (Lāghavā) by Prāṇāyāma; of realization (Pratyakṣa) by meditation (Dhyāna); and of detachment (Nirliptatva) in Samādhi.

Those who suffer from inequality of the three "humours"[2] are required to practise the "six acts" (Ṣaṭ-karma) which purify the body and facilitate Prāṇāyāma. For others who are free from these defects they are not necessary in such case, and according to some teachers the practice of Prāṇāyāma alone is sufficient. These form the first steps in the Haṭha-yoga. On this cleansing (Śodhana)

---

[1] Citta has two causes—Vāsanā and Prāṇa. If one is controlled, then both are controlled (Yoga-Kuṇḍalī Up., Ch. I).

[2] Vāta, Kapha and Pitta. These will be found described in my Introduction to the Prapañcasāra-Tantra, Vol. III of Tāntrik Texts, and "The World As Power".

of the body and Nāḍīs, health is gained, the internal fire is rendered more active, and restraint of breath (Kuṁbhaka) is facilitated. Recourse is also had, if necessary, to Oṣadhi-yoga, in which herbal preparations are administered to cure defective health.

Cleansing (Śodhana) is effected by the six processes known as the Ṣaṭ-karma. Of these, the first is Dhauti, or washing, which is fourfold, or inward washing (Antar-dhauti), cleansing of the teeth, etc. (Danta-dhauti), of the "heart," that is throat and chest (Hṛd-dhauti) and of the anus (Mūla-dhauti). Antar-dhauti is also fourfold—namely, Vāta-sāra, by which air is drawn into the belly and then expelled; Vāri-sāra, by which the body is filled with water, which is then evacuated by the anus[1]; Vahni-sāra, in which the Nābhi-granthi is made to touch the spinal column (Meru); and Bahiṣkṛta, in which the belly is by Kākini-mudrā[2] filled with air, which is retained half a Yāma,[3] and then sent downward. Danta-dhauti is fourfold, consisting in the cleansing of the root of the teeth and tongue, the ears, and the "hollow of the skull" (Kapāla-randhra). By Hṛd-dhauti phlegm and bile are removed. This is done by a stick (Danta-dhauti) or cloth (Vāso-dhauti) pushed into the throat, or swallowed, or by vomiting (Vamana-dhauti). Mūla-dhauti is done to cleanse the exit of the Apānavāyu,

---

[1] The intestines are depleted of air and then by the action of the anal muscles water is sucked in. It naturally flows in to fill the void created by the depletion of air in the intestines. Another feat which I have seen is the drawing in of air and fluid into the urethra, and out again. Apart from its suggested medical value as a lavement of the bladder it is a mudrā used in sexual connection whereby the Haṭha-yogī sucks into himself the forces of the woman without ejecting any of his force or substance—a practice which (apart from any other ground) is to be condemned as injurious to the woman who "withers" under such treatment.

[2] Gheraṇḍa-Saṁhitā, Third Upadeśa (v. 86); see also Haṭha-yoga-pradīpikā, II, 21-38.

[3] A Yāma is three hours.

either with the middle finger and water or the stalk of a turmeric plant.

Vasti, the second of the Ṣaṭ-karma, is twofold, and is either of the dry (Śuṣka) or watery (Jala) kind. In the second form the Yogī sits in the Utkatāsana[1] posture in water up to the navel, and the anus is contracted and expanded by Aśvinī-Mudrā; or the same is done in the Paścimottānāsana,[2] and the abdomen below the navel is gently moved. In Neti the nostrils are cleansed with a piece of string. Lāulikī is the whirling of the belly from side to side (see Plate X). In Trātaka the Yogī, without winking, gazes at some minute object until the tears start from his eyes. By this the "celestial vision" (Divya-Dṛṣṭi) so often referred to in the Tāntrik-Upāsanā is acquired. Kapālabhāti is a process for the removal of phlegm, and is threefold: Vāta-krama, by inhalation and exhalation; Vyūtkrama, by water drawn through the nostrils and ejected through the mouth; and Śitkrama, the reverse process.

These are the various processes by which the body is cleansed and made pure for the Yoga practice to follow.

Āsana, or posture, is the next, and when the Ṣaṭ-karma are dispensed with, is the stage of Haṭha-yoga.

Dṛḍhatā, or strength or firmness, the acquisition of which is the second of the above-mentioned processes, is attained by Āsana.

The Āsanas are postures of the body. The term is generally described as modes of seating the body, but

[1] Gheraṇḍa-Saṁhitā, Second Upadeśa (v. 23). That is, squatting resting on the toes, the heels off the ground, and buttocks resting on heels. A Haṭha-yogī can, it is said, give himself a natural enema by sitting in water and drawing it up through the anus. The sphincter muscles are opened and shut, and suction established.

[2] *Ibid.*, v. 20.

the posture is not necessarily a sitting one; for some Āsanas are done on the belly, back, hands, etc. It is said [1] that the Āsanas are as numerous as living beings, and that there are 8,400,000 of these; 1,600 are declared to be excellent, and out of these thirty-two are auspicious for men, which are described in detail. Two of the commonest of these are Mukta-padmāsana [2] (the loosened lotus seat), the ordinary position for worship, and Baddha-padmāsana.[3] Kuṇḍalī-yoga is ordinarily done in an Āsana and Mudrā in which the feet press upon the region of the genital centre and close the anal aperture, the hands closing the others—nostrils, eyes, ears, mouth (Yoni-mudrā). The right heel is pressed against the anus and the left against the region of the genital centre and in order to close the aperture of the penis, it is contracted and withdrawn into the pubic arch so that it is no longer seen.[4] The tongue is turned back in Khecarī Mudrā so as to close the throat also where these two Mudrās are combined.

There are certain other Āsanas which are peculiar to the Tantras, such as Muṇḍāsana, Citāsana and Śavāsana,

---

[1] Gheraṇḍa-Saṁhitā, Second Upadeśa. In the Śiva-Saṁhitā (Ch. III, vv. 84-91) eighty-four postures are mentioned, of which four are recommended—*viz.*, Siddhāsana, Ugrāsana, Svastikāsana and Padmāsana. Another account given me added four more—Baddha-padmāsana, Trikoṇāsana, Mayūrāsana, Bhujaṅgāsana.

[2] The right foot is placed on the left thigh, the left foot on the right thigh, and the hands are crossed and placed similarly on the thighs; the chin is placed on the breast, and the gaze fixed on the tip of the nose (see also Śiva-Saṁhitā, Ch. I, v. 52).

[3] The same, except that the hands are passed behind the back, and the right hand holds the right toe and the left hand the left toe. By this, increased pressure is placed on the Mūlādhāra, and the nerves are braced with the tightening of the body. The position is figured in Plate XVII.

[4] Some Yogīs can make both the penis and testes disappear in the pubic arch so that the body has the appearance of that of a woman.

in which skulls, the funeral pyre, and a corpse,[1] respectively, form the seat of the Sādhaka. These, though they have other ritual and magical objects, also form part of the discipline for the conquest of fear and the attainment of indifference, which is the quality of a Yogī. And so the Tantras prescribe as the scene of such rites the solitary mountain-top, the lonely empty house and riverside, and the cremation ground. The interior cremation ground is there where the Kāmik or desire body and its passions are consumed in the fire of knowledge.[2]

Patañjali, on the subject of Āsana, merely points out what are good conditions, leaving each one to settle the details for himself according to his own requirements.

Āsana is an aid to clear and correct thought. The test of suitability of Āsana is that which is steady and pleasant, a matter which each will settle for himself. Posture becomes perfect when effort to that end ceases, so that there is no more movement of the body.[3] The Rajo-Guṇa, the action of which produces fickleness of mind, is restrained. A suitable steady Āsana produces mental equilibrium. Haṭha-yoga,

---

[1] In successful Śavāsana the Devī, it is said, appears to the Sādhaka. In Śava-sādhana the Sādhaka sits astride on the back of a corpse (heading the north), on which he draws a Yantra and then does Japa of Mantra with Ṣodhānyāsa and Pūjā on its head. A corpse is selected as being a pure form of organized matter, since the Devatā which is invoked into it is the Mahā-vidyā whose Svarūpa is Nirguṇa-brahman, and by such invocation becomes Saguṇa. The corpse is free from sin or desire. The only Vāyu in it is the Dhanaṁjaya, " which leaves not even a corpse ". The Devatā materializes by means of the corpse. There is a possession of it (Āveśa)—that is, entry of the Devatā into the dead body. At the conclusion of a successful rite, it is said, that the head of the corpse turns round, and, facing the Sādhaka, speaks, bidding him name his boon, which may be spiritual or worldly advancement as he wishes. This is part of Nīla Sādhana done by the " Hero " (Vīra), for it and Śavāsana are attended by many terrors.

[2] As the Yogakuṇḍalī-Upaniṣad says (Ch. III), the outer burning is no burning at all.

[3] Pātanjala-Yogasūtra, 46, 47 (Sthira-sukhaṁ āsanaṁ).

however, prescribes a very large number of Āsanas, to each of which a peculiar effect is ascribed. These are more in the nature of a gymnastic than an Āsana in its sense of a seated posture. Some forms of this gymnastic are done seated, but others are not so, but standing upright, bending, lying down, and standing on the head. This latter is Vṛkṣāsana. Thus, again, in Cakrāsana the Yogi stands and bends and touches his feet with his hand, a familiar exercise, as is also Vāma-dakṣiṇa-pādāsana, a kind of goose step, in which, however, the legs are brought up to right angles with the body. These exercises secure a fine physical condition and freedom from disease.[1] They also bring different portions of the body into such a position as to establish a direct contact of Prāṇa-vāyu between them. They are also said to assist in Prāṇāyāma, and to help to effect its object, including the rousing of Kuṇḍalinī. The author of the work last cited says [2] that as among the Niyamas the most important is Ahimsā, and among Yamas Mitāhāra, or a moderate diet (a significant choice), so is Siddhāsana (in which the Mūlādhāra is firmly pressed by the heel and the Svādhiṣṭhāna region by the other foot) among the Āsanas. (See Plates XI, XII). Mastery of this helps to secure the Unmanī Avasthā, and the three Bandhas (*v. post*) are achieved without difficulty.

Sthiratā, or fortitude, is acquired by the practice of the Mudrās.[3] The Mudrā dealt with in works of Hatha-yoga are positions of the body.[4] They are gymnastic, health-giving, and destructive of disease and of death, such as the

---

[1] See Ch. II of Gheraṇḍa-Saṁhitā, and Haṭha-yoga-pradīpikā, I, vv. 19-35; Śāṇḍilya-Upaniṣad, Ch. I.

[2] Ch. I, v. 39.

[3] According to the Commentary on the Haṭha-yoga-pradīpikā (Ch. IV, v. 37), Mudrā is so called because it removes pain and sorrow (Mudrayati kleśaṁ iti mudrā). See Ch. III of Gheraṇḍa-Saṁhitā.

[4] Gheraṇḍa-Saṁhitā, Third Upadeśa.

Jālaṁdhara [1] and other Mudrās. They also preserve from injury by fire, water, or air. Bodily action and the health resulting therefrom react upon the mind, and by the union of a perfect mind and body, Siddhi is by their means attained. The Mudrā is also described as the key for opening of the door of Kuṇḍalinī-Śakti. It is not (as I understand it) that all keys are necessarily to be employed in each case, but only such as are necessary to accomplish the purpose in that particular case; what is necessary in one case may not be necessary in another. The Gheraṇḍa-Saṁhitā describes a number of Mudrās, of which (with the eight Āsanas mentioned at p. 203) ten are said to be of importance in Kuṇḍalī Yoga, of which Khecarī is the chief as Siddhāsana is chief amongst Āsanas. In Yoni-mudrā, the Yogī in Siddhāsana stops with his fingers the ears, eyes, nostrils, and mouth, so as to shut out all external impressions. As already stated he presses with his heel the Sīvanī or centre of the perinæum thus closing the anal aperture and withdrawing the penis into the pubic arch. (See Plate XV.) He inhales Prāṇa-vāyu by Kākinī-mudrā,[2] and unites it with Apānavāyu. Meditating in their order upon the six Cakras, he arouses the sleeping Kula-kuṇḍalinī by the Mantra "Huṁ Haṁsah"[3]. With

[1] *Ibid.*, v. 12.

[2] The lips are formed to resemble the beak of a crow, and the air gently drawn in (Gheraṇḍa-Saṁhitā, III, 86, 87).

[3] Hūm is called Kūrca-Bīja. Huṁ is Kavaca-Bīja="May I be protected." Hūṁ stands for Kāma (desire) and Krodha (anger). Kāma here means creative will (Sṛṣṭi) and Krodha its reverse, or dissolution (Laya). So-called "angry" Devatās are not angry in the ordinary sense, but are then in that aspect in which they are Lords of Dissolution, an aspect which seems angry or terrible to the worldly minded. It is said of the Tarā-mantra that the Hūṁ in it is the sound of the wind as it blew with force on the Cola lake to the west of Meru what time She manifested. Haṁsah=Prakṛti (Sah) and Puruṣa (Haṁ) or Jīvātmā. This Mantra is used in taking Kuṇḍalinī up, and So'haṁ (He I am) in bringing Her down. Haṁ also=Sun (Sūrya), and Sah=Moon (Indu)=Kāma=Icchā.

"Haṁ," or the Sun, heat is produced, and this heat is made to play on Kuṇḍalī-Śakti. By "Sah" the Kāma or will (Icchā) is made active. The vital air (Vāyu) in the Mūlādhāra is in the form of both Moon and Sun (Soma-sūrya-rūpī). With "Haṁsah" She is roused, Ham rousing Her with his heat, and Sah lifting Her upwards. He raises Her to the Sahasrāra; then deeming himself pervaded with the Śakti, and in blissful union (Saṅgama) with Śiva, he meditates upon himself as, by reason of that union, Bliss Itself and the Brahman.[1] Aśvinī-mudrā consists of the repeated contraction and expansion of the anus for the purpose of Śodhanā, or of contraction to restrain the Apānavāyu in Ṣaṭ-cakra-bheda. Śakti-cālana employs the latter Mudrā, which is repeated until Vāyu manifests in the Suṣumnā. Śakti-cālana is the movement of the abdominal muscle from left to right and right to left; the object being to arouse Kuṇḍalinī by this spiraline movement. The process is accompanied by inhalation and the union of Prāṇa and Apāna whilst in Siddhāsana.[2]

Yoni-mudrā is accompanied by Śakti-calana Mudrā,[3] which should be well practised first before the Yoni-mudrā is done. The rectal muscle is contracted by Aśvinī-mudrā until the Vāyu enters the Suṣumnā, a fact which is indicated by a peculiar sound which is heard there.[4] And with the Kuṁbhaka the Serpent goes upwards to the Sahasrāra roused by the Mantra "Hūṁ Haṁsah". The Yogī should then think himself to be pervaded with Śakti and in a state of blissful union (Saṅgama) with Śiva. He then contemplates:

---

[1] Gheraṇḍa-Saṁhitā, Third Upadeśa.

[2] *Ibid.*, vv. 37, 49, 82.

[3] *Ibid.*, III, vv. 49-61.

[4] Haṭha-yoga-pradīpikā, Commentary to Ch. II, v. 72.

"I am the Bliss Itself," "I am the Brahman".[1] Mahāmudrā[2] and Mahā-vedha are done in conjunction with Mahā-bandha, already described. In the first the Yogī presses the Yoni (Mūlādhāra) with the left heel, and, stretching out the right leg, takes hold of the two feet with both hands. (See Plate XVI.) Jālaṁdhara-Bandha is then done. When Kuṇḍalinī is awakened, the Prāṇa enters the Suṣumnā, and Iḍā and Piṅgala, now that Prāṇa has left them, become lifeless. Expiration should be done slowly, and the Mudrā should be practised an equal number of times on the left and right side of the body. This Mudrā, like other Haṭha-yoga-Mudrās, is said to ward off death and disease. In Mahā-vedha[3] the Yogī assumes the Mahā-bandha posture, and, concentrating his mind, stops by methods already described the upward and downward course of the Prāṇa. Then, placing the palms of his hands on the ground, he taps the ground with his buttocks (Sphic),[4] and the "Moon," "Sun," and "Fire"—that is, Iḍā, Piṅgalā, and Suṣumnā—become united upon the entry of the Prāṇa into the latter Nāḍī. Then the body assumes a death-like aspect, which disappears with the slow expiration which follows. According to another mode of rousing Kuṇḍalinī, the Yogī seated in Vajrāsana takes firm hold of his feet a little above the ankles, and slowly taps the Kanda (*v. post*) with them. Bhastrikā-Kuṁbhaka is done and the abdomen is contracted.[5]

---

[1] The Mantra Haṁsah is the breath held in Kuṁbhaka.

[2] Gheraṇḍa-Saṁhitā, III, 37-42. The Yoni-mudrā "which detaches the Manas from the objective world," is described in the Comm. to v. 36, *post*.

[3] *Ibid.*, v. 25. *et seq.*

[4] See as to this tapping Plate IX which shows the position of the ground before or after it has been tapped.

[5] Gheraṇḍa-Saṁhitā, Ch. III, v. 114 *et seq.*

The Khecarī-Mudrā,[1] which, as well as the Yoni-Mudrā, as referred to in the text translated, is the lengthening of the tongue until it reaches the space between the eyebrows. It is then turned back in the throat, and closes the exit of the breath previously inspired. The mind is fixed in the Ājñā [2] until with Siddhi this "path of the upward Kuṇḍalī" (Ūrdha-kuṇḍalinī) conquers the whole universe, which is realized in the Yogī's body as not different from Ātmā.[3] It is said that sometimes the *frænum* is cut but others can do the Mudrā without doing a physical injury which interferes with the putting out and withdrawing the tongue without manual help. In Śāṁbhavī-Mudrā the mind is kept free from Vṛtti or functioning in Siddhāsana.

The term Mudrā also includes [4] what are called Bandha (bindings), certain physical methods of controlling Prāṇa. Three important one's which are referred to in the texts here translated are Uḍḍiyāna, Mūla and Jālaṁdhara.[4] (See Plates XI, XII, XIV.) In the first, the lungs are emptied

[1] So called, according to the Dhyāna-bindu Up., because Citta moves in Kha (Ākāśa) and the tongue through this Mudrā enters Kha.

[2] Gheraṇḍa-Saṁhitā, Ch. III, vv. 25-27. Suspension of breath and insensibility result, so that the Yogī may be buried in the ground without air, food, or drink, as in the case of the Yogī spoken of in the accounts of Dr. McGregor and Lieut. A. H. Boileau, cited in N. C. Paul's "Treatise on the Yoga Philosophy," p. 46. In Ch. IV, v. 80, of the Haṭha-yoga-pradīpikā, it is said that concentration between the eyebrows is the easiest and quickest way of attainment of Unmanī Avasthā. See Śāṇḍilya Up., Ch. I; Dhyāna-bindu Up.

[3] Yoga-kuṇḍalī Up., Ch. II.

[4] *Ib.*, Ch. III, vv. 55-76. There is also the Mahā-Bandha. (See Plate XIII) Ch. II, v. 45, says that Jālaṁdhara should be done at the end of Pūraka; and Uḍḍiyāṇa-Bandha at the end of Kuṁbhaka and beginning of Rechaka. See also Yoga-kuṇḍalī Up., Ch. I. *Ib.*, Ch. III, v. 57; Yoga-tattva Up., Dhyāna-bindu Up. The Varāha Up., Ch. V, says that as Prāṇa is always flying up (Uḍḍiyāṇa), so this Bandha, by which its flight is arrested, is called Uddīyāṇa-Bandha. Yoga-kuṇḍalī Up., Ch. I, says, because Prāṇah uddīyate (goes up the Suṣumnā) in this Bandha, it is called Uḍḍiyāṇa.

by a strong expiration, and drawn against the upper part of the thorax, carrying the diaphragm along with them, and Prāṇa is made to rise and enter the Suṣumnā. Through Mūla-Bandha (see Plate XIV) the Prāṇa and Apāna unite [1] and go into the Suṣuṁnā. Then the inner "sounds" are heard, that is, a vibration is felt, and Prāṇa and Apāna, uniting with Nāda of the cardiac Anāhata-Cakra, go to the heart, and are thereafter united with Bindu in the Ājñā. In Mūla-Bandha the perinæal region (Yoni) is pressed with the foot, the rectal muscle contracted (by Aśvinī-Mudrā), and the Apāna drawn up.[2] The natural course of the Apāna is downwards, but by contraction at the Mūlādhāra it is made to go upwards through the Suṣumnā when it meets Prāṇa. When the latter Vāyu reaches the region of fire below the navel,[3] the fire becomes bright and strong, being fanned by Apāna. The heat in the body then becomes very powerful, and Kuṇḍalinī, feeling it, awakes from Her sleep "just as a serpent struck by a stick hisses and straightens itself". Then it enters the Suṣumnā. Jālaṁdhara-Bandha is done by deep inspiration and then contraction of the thoracic region (wherein is situated the Viśuddha-Cakra), the chin being held firmly pressed against the root of the neck at a distance of about four fingers (Aṅguli) from the heart. This is said to bind the sixteen Ādhāras,[4] or vital centres, and the nectar (Pīyūṣa) which flows from the cavity above the palate,[5]

---

[1] The Śāṇḍilya Up., Ch. I, defines Prāṇāyāma to be the union of Prāṇa and Apāna. Nāda and Bindu are thus united.

[2] See Āgama-kalpadruma, cited in notes to v. 50, *post*, comm., and Dhyāna-bindu Up. The Yoga-kuṇḍalī Up., Ch. I, says that the downward tendency of Apāna is forced up by bending down.

[3] Vahner maṇḍalaṁ trikoṇaṁ nābher adhobhāge (Haṭha-yoga-pradīpikā, *ib*. v. 66).

[4] See Commentary, *post*, v. 33.

[5] The "Moon" is situate in the palatal region near Ājñā. Here is the Soma-Cakra under the Ājñā, and from the Soma-Cakra comes a

and is also used to cause the breath to become Laya in the Suṣumnā. If the thoracic and perinæal regions are simultaneously contracted, and Prāṇa is forced downward and Apāna upward, the Vāyu enters the Suṣumnā.[1] This union of the three Naḍīs, Iḍā, Piṅgala and Suṣumnā, may be also effected by the Mahā-Bandha,[2] which also aids the fixation of the mind in the Ājñā. Pressure is done on the perinæal region between the anus and penis with the left heel, the right foot being placed on the left thigh. Breath is inspired and the chin placed firmly on the root of the neck that is top of the breast-bone as in Jālaṁdhara (see position in Plate XVI) or alternatively the tongue is pressed firmly against the base of the front teeth; and while the mind is centred on the Suṣumnā the Vāyu is contracted. After the breath has been restrained as long as possible, it should be expired slowly. The breath exercise should be done first on the left and then on the right side. The effect of this Bandha is to stop the upward course of the breath through all the Nāḍīs except the Suṣumnā.

As the Dhyāna-bindu Upaniṣad says, the Jīva oscillates up and down under the influence of Prāṇa and Apāna and is never at rest, just as a ball which is hit to the earth with the palm of the hand uprises again, or like a bird which, tied to its perch by a string, flies away and is drawn back again.

---

stream of nectar which, according to some, has its origin above. It descends to the "Sun" near the navel, which swallows it. By the process of Viparīta-karaṇa these are made to change positions, and the internal fire (Jāṭharāgni) is increased. In the Viparīta position the Yogī stands on his head.

[1] Haṭha-yoga-pradīpikā, II, vv. 46, 47; Yoga-tattva Up., Dhyāna-bindu Up. Yoga-kuṇḍalī Up. (Ch. I) says that the contraction of the upper part of the body is an impediment to the passage of the Vāyu upwards.

[2] Dhyāna-bindu Up., *ib.*, III, v. 19, done in conjunction with Mahā-mudrā and Mahā-vedha, described *post*; *ib.*, v. 25, and Yoga-tattva Upaniṣad.

These movements, like all other dualities, are stayed by Yoga, which unites the Prāṇas.

When the physical body has been purified and controlled, there follows Pratyāhāra to secure steadiness (Dhairya), as already described. With this the Yogī passes from the physical plane, and seeks to acquire the equipoise of, and control over, the subtle body. It is an advanced stage in which control is acquired over mind and body.

From the fifth or Prāṇāyāma arises lightness (Lāghava) —that is, the levitation or lightening of the body.

The air which is breathed through the mouth and nostrils is material air (Sthūla-Vāyu). The breathing is a manifestation of a vitalizing force called Prāṇa-Vāyu. By control over the Sthūla-Vāyu, the Prāṇa-Vāyu (Sūkṣma-Vāyu or subtle air) is controlled; the process concerned with this is called Prāṇāyāma.

Prāṇāyāma is frequently translated "breath control". Having regard to the processes employed, the term is not altogether inappropriate if it is understood that "breath" means not only the Sthūla but the Sūkṣma-Vāyu. But the word does not come from Prāṇa (breath) and Yama (control), but from Prāṇa and Āyāma, which latter term, according to the Amarakośa, means length, rising, extensity, expansion;[1] in other words, it is the process whereby the ordinary and comparatively slight manifestation of Prāṇa is lengthened and strengthened and developed. This takes place firstly in the Prāṇa as it courses in Iḍā and Piṅgalā, and then by its transference to the Suṣumnā, when it is said to bloom (Sphurati)[2] or to display itself in its fulness. When the body has been purified by constant practice, Prāṇa forces its way with ease

[1] Dairghyaṁ āyāma ārohah pariṇāho viśālatā (Amarakośa Dictionary).

[2] Comm. Haṭha-yoga-pradīpikā, III, v. 27.

through Suṣumnā in their middle.[1] From being the small path of daily experience, it becomes the "Royal Road"[2] which is the Sūṣumnā. Thus, Sūrya-bheda Kuṁbhaka is practised until Prāṇa is felt to pervade the whole of the body from head to toe; Ujjāyī until the breath fills the body from throat to heart; and in Bhastrā the breath is inhaled and exhaled again and again rapidly, as the blacksmith works his bellows. The breath is controlled only in the sense that it is made the subject of certain initial processes. These processes, however, do not control in the sense of confine, but expand. The most appropiate term, therefore, for Prāṇāyāma is "breath control and development," leading to the union of Prāṇa and Apāna. Prāṇāyāma is first practised with a view to control and develop the Prāṇa. The latter is then moved into Suṣumnā by the stirring of Kuṇḍalinī, who blocks the entry (Brahma-dvāra) thereto. With the disappearance of Prāṇa therefrom, Iḍā and Piṅgalā "die,"[3] and the Prāṇa in Suṣumnā by means of the Śakti-Kuṇḍalinī pierces the six Cakras which block the passage in the Brahmanāḍī, and eventually becomes Laya in the Great Breath which is the final end and aim of this process.

Prāṇāyāma[4] should be practised according to the instructions laid down by the Guru, the Sādhaka living on a nutritious but moderate diet, with his senses under control. As already stated, mind and breath react upon one another,

[1] Śāṇḍilya Up., Ch. I.

[2] Pānasya śūnyapadavī tathā rājapathāyate (*ib.*, vv. 2, 3).

[3] That is, they are relaxed and devitalized, as every part of the body is from which the Prāṇa-Śakti is withdrawn.

[4] The Śāṇḍilya Up., Ch. I says: "As lions, elephants. and tigers are gradually tamed, so also the breath when rightly managed comes under control; else it kills the practitioner." It should not, therefore, be attempted without instruction. Many have injured themselves and some have died through mistakes made in the processes, which must be adapted to the needs of each person. Hence the necessity for an experienced Guru.

and when the latter is regulated so is the mind, and therefore rhythmic breathing is sought. This Prāṇāyāma is said to be successful only when the Nāḍīs are purified, for unless this is so the Prāṇa does not enter the Suṣumnā.[1] The Yogī, assuming the Padmāsana posture, inhales (Pūraka) and exhales (Recaka) alternately through the left (Īḍā) and right (Piṅgalā) nostrils, retaining the breath meanwhile (Kuṁbhaka) for gradually increasing periods. The Devatās of these elements of Prāṇāyāma are Brahmā, Rudra, and Viṣṇu.[2] The Prāṇa enters Suṣumnā, and if retained sufficiently long goes, after the piercing of the Cakras, to the Brahma-randhra. The Yoga manuals speak of various forms of Prāṇāyāma according as commencement is made with Recaka or Pūraka, and according as the breath is suddenly stopped without Pūraka and Recaka. There are also various forms of Kuṁbhaka, such as Sahita-Kuṁbhaka, which resembles the first two above mentioned, and which should be practised until the Prāṇa enters the Suṣumnā; and Kevala, in which the breath is restrained without Pūraka and Recaka.[3] Then there are others which cure excess of Vāta, Pitta, and Kapha,[4] and the diseases arising therefrom; and Bhastrā, which is an important Kuṁbhaka, as it operates in the case of all three Doṣas,[4] and aids the

---

[1] Haṭha-yoga-pradīpikā, Ch. II, vv. 1-6.

[2] Dhyāna-bindu Up., and see Amṛtanāda Up., Varāha Up., Ch. V. Maṇḍala-brāhmaṇa Up.

[3] The Śāṇḍilya Up., Ch. I, says that by Kevala, the knowledge of Kuṇḍalī arises, and man becomes Ūrdhva-retas—that is, his seminal energy goes upward instead of developing into the gross seed which is thrown by Apāna downwards. Bindu (seminal energy) must be conquered, or the Yoga fails. As to the Bhedas associated with Sahita, see Ch. I, Yoga-kuṇḍalī-Upaniṣad.

[4] See Introduction to Prapañcasāra-Tantra, Tāntrik Texts, Vol. III, p. 11, *et seq.*

Prāṇa to break through the three Granthis, which are firmly placed in the Suṣumnā.[1]

It will be observed that all the methods previously and subsequently described practically subserve one object, of making the Prāṇa enter Suṣumnā, and then become Laya in the Sahasrāra after Prāṇa-Devatā-Kuṇḍalinī has pierced the intervening Cakras; for when Prāṇa flows through the Suṣumnā the mind becomes steady. When Cit is absorbed in Suṣumnā, Prāṇa is motionless.[2] This object colours also the methods Pratyāhāra, Dhāraṇā, Dhyāna, and Samādhi; for whereas in the Rāja-yoga aspect they are various mental processes and states, from the Haṭha-yoga point of view, which is concerned with "breathing," they are progressions in Prāṇāyāma. Therefore it is that some works describe them differently to harmonize them with the Haṭha theory and practice, and explain them as degrees of Kuṁbhaka varying according to the length of its duration.[3] Thus if the Prāṇa is retained for a particular time it is called Pratyāhāra, if for a longer time it is called Dhāraṇā, and so on until Samādhi is attained, which is equivalent to its retention for the longest period.[4]

All beings say the Ajapā-Gāyatrī,[5] which is the expulsion of the breath by Haṁ-kāra, and its inspiration by Sah-kāra, 21,600 times a day. Ordinarily the breath goes forth a distance of 12 fingers' breadth, but in singing, eating, walking, sleeping, coition, the distances are 16, 20, 24, 30, and 36 breadths, respectively. In violent exercise these distances are exceeded, the greatest distance being 96 breadths.

---

[1] Haṭha-yoga-pradīpikā, II, 44-75.

[2] Yoga-kuṇḍalī Up., Ch. I.

[3] See Yoga-Sūtra, ed. Manilal Nabhubhai Dvivedi, Ap. VI.

[4] See comm. to Haṭha-yoga-pradīpikā, Ch. II, v. 12.

[5] This is the Mantra-Haṁsah manifested by Prāṇa. See Dhyāna-bindu Up. Haṁsah is Jīvātmā, and Paramahaṁsa is Paramātmā. See Haṁsa-Upaniṣad.

Where the breathing is under the normal distance, life is prolonged. Where it is above that, it is shortened. Pūraka is inspiration, and Recaka expiration. Kuṁbhaka is the retention of breath between these two movements. Kuṁbhaka is, according to the Gheraṇḍa-Saṁhitā, of eight kinds: Sahita, Sūrya-bheda, Ujjāyī, Śītalī, Bhastrikā, Bhrāmarī, Mūrcchā, and Kevalī. Prāṇāyāma similarly varies. Prāṇāyama awakens Śakti, frees from disease, produces detachment from the world and bliss. It is of varying values, *viz.*, best (Uttama), middling (Madhyama), and inferior (Adhama). The value is measured by the length of the Pūraka, Kuṁbhaka, and Recaka. In Adhama Prāṇāyāma it is 4, 16, and 8 respectively = 28. In Madhyama it is double of that, *viz.*, 8, 32, 16 = 56. In Uttama it is double of the last, *viz.*, 16, 64, 32 respectively = 112. The number given is that of the recitations of the Praṇava-Mantra. The Sādhaka passes through three different stages in his Sādhana which are similarly named. In Adhama perspiration is produced, in Madhyama tremor, and Uttama done for a 100 times is said to result in levitation.

It is necessary that the Nāḍī should be cleansed, for air does not enter those which are impure. Months or years may be spent in the preliminary process of cleansing the Nāḍīs. The cleansing of the Naḍī (Nāḍī-śuddhi) is either Samanu or Nirmanu—that is, with or without the use of Bīja-Mantra. According to the first form, the Yogī in Padmāsana does Guru-nyāsa according to the directions of the Guru. Meditating on "Yaṁ," he does Japa through Iḍā of the Bīja 16 times, Kuṁbhaka with Japa of Bīja 64 times, and then exhalation through the solar Nadī and Japa of Bīja 32 times. Fire is raised from Maṇipūra and united with Pṛthivī. Then follows inhalation by the solar Nādī with the Vahni-Bīja 16 times, Kuṁbhaka with 64 Japa of the Bīja, followed by exhalation through the lunar

Nāḍī and Japa of the Bīja 32 times. He then meditates on the lunar brilliance, gazing at the tip of the nose, and inhales by Iḍā with Japa of the Bīja "Thaṁ" 16 times. Kuṁbhaka is done with the Bīja "Vaṁ" 64 times. He then thinks of himself as flooded by nectar, and considers that the Nāḍīs have been washed. He exhales by Piṅgalā with 32 Japa of the Bīja "Laṁ," and considers himself thereby strengthened. He then takes his seat on a mat of Kuśa grass, a deerskin, etc., and, facing east or north, does Prāṇāyāma. For its exercise there must be, in addition to Nāḍī-Śuddhi (purification of "nerves"), consideration of proper place, time, and food. Thus, the place should not be so distant as to induce anxiety, nor in an unprotected place, such as a forest, nor in a city or crowded locality, which induces distraction. The food should be pure and of a vegetarian character. It should not be too hot or too cold, pungent, sour, salt or bitter. Fasting, the taking of one meal a day and the like are prohibited. On the contrary, the Yogī should not remain without food for more than one Yāma (three hours). The food taken should be light and strengthening. Long walks and other violent exercise should be avoided as also—certainly in the case of beginners—sexual intercourse. The stomach should only be half filled. Yoga should be commenced, it is said, in spring or autumn. As stated, the forms of Prāṇāyāma vary. Thus, Sahita, which is either with (Sagarbha) or without (Nirgarbha) Bīja, is, according to the former form, as follows: The Sādhaka meditates on Vidhi (Brahmā), who is full of Rajoguṇa, red in colour, and the image of A-kāra. He inhales by Iḍā, in six measures (Mātrā). Before Kuṁbhaka he does the Uḍḍiyāṇa-Bandha-Mudrā. Meditating on Hari (Viṣṇu) as Sattvamaya and the black Bīja U-kāra, he does Kuṁbhaka with 64 Japa of the Bīja; then, meditating on Śiva as Tamomaya and his white Bīja Ma-kāra, he exhales through Piṅgalā with 32 Japa of the Bīja; then, inhaling by Piṅgalā he does Kuṁbhaka, and exhales by Iḍā with the same Bīja. The process is repeated in the normal and reversed order.

Dhyāna, or meditation, is, according to the Gheraṇḍa-Saṁhitā, of three kinds: (1) Sthūla, or gross; (2) Jyotih; (3) Sūkṣma, or subtle.[1] In the first form the Devatā is brought before the mind. One form of Dhyāna for this purpose is as follows: Let the Sādhaka think of the great Ocean of nectar in his heart. In the middle of that Ocean is the Island of Gems, the shores of which are made of powdered gems. The island is clothed with a Kadaṁba forest in yellow blossom. This forest is surrounded by Mālati, Campaka, Pārijāta, and other fragrant trees. In the midst of the Kadaṁba forest there rises the beautiful Kalpa tree laden with fresh blossom and fruit. Amidst its leaves the black bees hum and the Koel birds make love. Its four branches are the four Vedas. Under the tree there is a great Maṇḍapa of precious stones, and within it a beautiful couch, on which let him picture to himself his Iṣṭa-devatā. The Guru will direct him as to the form, raiment, Vāhana, and the title of the Devatā.

Jyotir-dhyāna is the infusion of fire and life (Tejas) into the form so imagined. In the Mūlādhāra lies the snake-like Kuṇḍalinī. There the Jīvātmā, as it were the tapering flame of a candle, dwells. The Sādhaka then meditates upon the Tejomaya (Light) Brahman, or, alternatively, between the eyebrows on the Praṇavātmaka flame (the light which is Oṁ) emitting its lustre.

---

[1] Gheraṇḍa-Saṁhitā, Sixth Upadeśa. It is said by Bhāskararāya, in the Lalitā (v. 53), that there are three forms of the Devī which equally partake of both the Prakāṣa and Vimarśa aspects—*viz.*, the physical (Sthūla), the subtle (Sūkṣma), and the supreme (Para). The physical form has hands, feet, etc., the subtle consists of Mantra, and the supreme is the Vāsanā, or, in the technical sense of the Mantra Śāstra, own form. The Kulārṇava-Tantra divides Dhyāna into Sthūla and Sūkṣma (IX, 3) beyond which, it says, is Samādhi.

Sūkṣma-dhyāna is meditation on Kuṇḍalinī with Śāṁbhavī-Mudrā after She has been roused. By this Yoga (*vide post*) the Ātmā is revealed (Ātma-sākṣātkāra).

Lastly, through Samādhi the quality of Nirliptatva, or detachment, and thereafter Mukti (Liberation) is attained.

This Samādhi-Yoga is, according to the Gheraṇḍa-Saṁhitā, of six kinds:[1] (1) Dhyāna-yoga-samādhi, attained by Śāṁbhavī-Mudrā,[2] in which, after meditation on the Bindu-Brahman and realization of the Ātmā (Ātmā-pratyakṣa), the latter is resolved into the Mahākāśa or the Great Ether. (2) Nāda-Yoga, attained by Khecarī-Mudrā,[3] in which the tongue is lengthened until it reaches the space between the eyebrows, and is then introduced in a reversed position into the mouth. This may be done with or without cutting of the *frænum.* (3) Rasānanda-Yoga, attained by Kuṁbhaka,[4] in which the Sādhaka in a silent place closes both ears and does Puraka and Kumbhaka until he hears Nāda in sounds varying in strength from that of the cricket's chirp to that of the large kettledrum. By daily practice the Anāhata sound is heard, and the Light (Jyotih) with the Manas therein is seen, which is ultimately dissolved in the supreme Viṣṇu. (4) Laya-siddhi-Yoga accomplished by the celebrated Yoni-Mudrā already described.[5] The Sādhaka, thinking of himself as Śakti and Paramātma as Puruṣa, feels himself in union (Saṅgama) with Śiva, and enjoys with Him the bliss which is Śṛṅgāra-rasa,[6] and becomes

[1] Seventh Upadeśa.

[2] *Ibid.*, Third Upadeśa, v. 65 *et seq.*

[3] *Ibid.*, v. 25 *et seq.*

[4] *Ibid.*, Fifth Upadeśa, v. 77 *et seq.*

[5] In the Lalitā (v. 193) the Devī is addressed as Layakarī—the cause of Laya or absorption.

[6] Śṛṅgāra is the love sentiment or sexual passion and sexual union. Here Śṛṅgāra-rasa is the cosmic root of that. The first of the eight or nine Rasas (sentiments)—*viz.*, Śṛṅgāra, Vīra (heroism), Karuṇa (compassion), Adbhūta (wondering), Hāsya (humour), Bhayānaka (fear),

Bliss itself, or the Brahman. (5) Bhakti-Yoga, in which meditation is made on the Iṣṭa-devatā with devotion (Bhakti) until, with tears flowing from the excess of bliss, the ecstatic condition is attained.[1] (6) Rāja-Yoga, accomplished by aid of the Manomūrcchā Kuṁbhaka. Here the Manas, detached from all worldly objects, is fixed between the eyebrows in the Ājñā-Cakra, and Kuṁbhaka is done. By the union of the Manas with the Ātmā, in which the Jñānī sees all things, Rāja-yoga-samādhi is attained.

The Haṭha-yoga-pradīpikā says that on perfection being attained in Haṭha the body becomes lean and healthy, the eyes are bright, the semen is concentrated, the Nāḍīs are purified, the internal fire is increased, and the Nāda sounds above-mentioned are heard.[2] These sounds (Nāda) issue from Anāhata-Cakra in the cardiac region, for it is here that the Śabda-Brahman manifested by Vāyu and in association with Buddhi, and of the nature of manifested Nāda endowed with a special motion (Viśeṣa-Spanda), exists as Madhyamā speech. Though sound (Śabda) is not distinct and heard by the gross senses until it issues in the form of Vaikharī speech, the Yogī is said to hear this subtle Nāda when, through the various Bandhas and Mudrās described, Prāṇa and Apāna have united in the Suṣumnā. This combined Prāṇa and Nāda proceed upwards and unite with Bindu.

There is a particular method by which Laya (absorption) is said to be attained by hearing the various bodily sounds.[3] The Yogī in Muktāsana and with Śaṁbhavī-Mudrā

Bībhatsa (disgust), Raudra (wrath), to which Mammata-bhatta, author of the Kāvyaprakāśa, adds Śānti (peace). What the Yogī enjoys is that supersensual bliss which manifests on the earthly plane as material Śṛṅgāra.

[1] *Ibid.*, Fifth Upadeśa, v. 82.

[2] Ch. II, v. 78.

[3] As the Nādabindu Up. says, the sound controls the mind which roves in the pleasure-garden of the senses.

concentrates on the sounds heard in the right ear; then after closing the sense apertures by Ṣaṇmukhī-Mudrā and after Prāṇāyāma a sound is heard in the Suṣumnā. In this Yoga there are four stages. When the Brahma-granthi has been pierced, the sweet tinkling sound of ornaments is heard in the ethereal void (Śūnya) of the heart; in the second stage the Prāṇa united with Nāda pierces the Viṣṇu-granthi. In this, the further void (Ati-śūnya) of the thoracic region, sounds are heard like those of a kettle-drum. In the third stage a drum-like sound (Mardala) is heard in the Ājñā or Mahā-śūnya, the seat of all powers (Siddhis). Then the Prāṇa, having forced the Rudra-granthi or Ājñā, goes to the abode of Īśvara. On the insetting of the fourth stage, when the Prāṇa goes to Brahma-randhra, the fourth or Niṣpatti state occurs. During the initial stages the sounds are loud, and gradually become very subtle. The mind is kept off all external objects, and is centred first on the loud and then on the subtle sounds. The mind thus becomes one with Nāda, on which it is fixed. Nāda is thus like a snare for catching a deer, for like a hunter it kills the mind. It first attracts it and then slays it. The mind absorbed in Nāda is freed from Vṛttis.[1] The Antahkaraṇa, like a deer, is attracted to the sound of the bells, and, remaining immovable, the Yogī like a skilful archer kills it by directing his breath to the Brahma-randhra through the Suṣumnā, which becomes one with that at which it is aimed. Cit exists within these sounds, which are its Śaktis, and by union with Nāda the self-effulgent Caitanya (Consciousness) is said to be attained. As long as sound is heard the Ātmā is with Śakti. The Laya

[1] As the Amṛtanāda-Upaniṣad says (v. 24), the Akṣara (imperishable) is that which is Aghoṣa (without sound), which is neither vowel nor consonant and is not uttered.

state is soundless.[1] There are also other methods[2] by which Laya is achieved, such as Mantra-Yoga, on the recitation of Mantras according to a particular method.

Laya-Yoga is the third and higher form of Haṭha-Yoga, which, in connection with other auxiliary Haṭha processes, is the subject-matter of the works here translated. Both Saccidānanda or Śiva and Saccidānanda or Śakti are present in the body, and Laya-Yoga consists in the control of Citta-vṛtti by merging the Prakṛti-Śakti in the Puruṣa-Śakti according to the laws which govern the Piṇḍa (individual—Vyaṣṭi) and Brahmāṇḍa (cosmic—Samaṣṭi) bodies and thereby gaining Liberation (Mokṣa).

As in the case of the preceding systems, Laya-Yoga has special features of its own.[3] Speaking in a general way, ordinary Haṭha-Yoga is specially, though not exclusively, concerned with the physical body, its power and functions, and affects the subtle body through the gross body; Mantra-Yoga is specially, though not exclusively, concerned with the forces and powers at work outside, though affecting the body. Laya-Yoga deals with the supersensible Pīṭhas (seats or centres) and the supersensible forces and functions of the inner world of the body. These Pīṭhas, or seats of the Devatās, are the Cakras already described, ranging from the Sahasrāra, the abode of the unattached (Nirlipta) Saccidānandamaya Paramātmā, to the Mūlādhāra, the seat of Prakṛti-Śakti, called Kula-kuṇḍalinī in the Yoga-Śāstras. The object of this Yoga is therefore to take and merge this Śakti in Puruṣa when Samādhi is attained. In Haṭha-Yoga the contemplation of "Light" is in particular prescribed, though, as already

---

[1] Haṭha-yoga-pradīpikā, Ch. IV, vv. 65-102.

[2] Amṛtanāda-Upaniṣad, Ch. IV, v. 66, says that Śiva has given out a quarter of a crore (2,500,000) of ways for the attainment of Laya, though Nāda is the best of them all.

[3] See Dharma-Pracāra Series, 9.

stated, its Dhyāna is threefold. In Mantra-Yoga the material forms in which Spirit clothes Itself are contemplated. After Prakṛti-Śakti in the form of Kula-kuṇḍalinī has, according to this method of Laya-Yoga, been roused by constant practice, its reflection is manifested as a Light between the eyebrows, which when it is fixed by practice and contemplation becomes the subject of Bindu-dhyāna. Kuṇḍalī is aroused by various Haṭha and other processes hereafter described. Methods are followed which are common to all the systems, such as Yama, Niyama, Āsana, though only a limited number of these and of the Mudrās of Haṭha-Yoga are used. These belong to the physical processes (Sthūla-Kriyā), and are followed by Prāṇāyāma,[1] Pratyāhāra, Dhāraṇā, Dhyāna (on Bindu), which are super-physical exercises (Sūkṣma-Kriyā). In addition to these are certain features peculiar to this Yoga. There are, besides those already noted, Svarodaya, or the science relating to the Nāḍīs; Pañca tattva Cakra, Sūkṣma prāṇa, and the like inner forces of nature; and the Laya-Kriyā, leading through Nāda and Bindu to the Samādhi, which is called Mahā-laya.

The hearing of the Nāda sounds is included under Pratyāhāra, and under Dhāraṇā the rousing of Kuṇḍalī. As Japa, or recitation of Mantra, is the chief element in Mantra-yoga, and Prāṇāyāma in the ordinary Haṭha-Yoga, so Dhāraṇā is, with the last as a preliminary, the most important part of Laya-yoga. It is to be observed, however, that Prāṇāyāma is only a preliminary method to secure mastery of the breath. It is the lower door at which the already perfect in this matter need not enter. Some processes described are for practice (Sādhana) only. An expert (Siddha) can, it is said, raise and lower Kuṇḍalī-Śakti within an hour.

---

[1] Of the several forms of Prāṇāyāma given in Haṭha-Yoga, it is said that only two are employed in Laya-Yoga.

It is said that as Ananta, the Lord of Serpents, supports the whole universe, so is Kuṇḍalinī, " by whom the body is supported,"[1] the support of all Yoga practice,[2] and that " as one forces open a door with a key," so the Yogī should force open the door of liberation (Mokṣa), by the aid of Kuṇḍalinī[3] (the coiled one), who is known by various names, such as the Śakti, Īṣvarī (Sovereign Lady), Kutilāṅgī (the crooked one), Bhujaṅgī (serpent), Arundhatī (unstayable helper to good action).[3] This Śakti is the Supreme Śakti (Parā-śakti) in the human body, embodying all powers and assuming all forms. Thus the sexual force is one of such powers and is utilized. Instead, however, of descending into gross seminal fluid, it is conserved as a form of subtle energy, and rises to Śiva along with Prāṇa. It is thus made a source of spiritual life instead of one of the causes of physical death. With the extinction of sexual desire, mind is released of its most powerful bond.[4]

She the " Serpent Power " sleeps coiled up in the Mūlādhāra, closing with Her mouth the entry to the Suṣumnā called the " door of Brahman " (Brahmadvāra). She sleeps above what is called the Kanda or Kanda-yoni, which is four fingers in length and breadth, and is covered by a " soft

---

[1] Varāha-Upaniṣad, Ch. V.

[2] Haṭha-yoga-pradīpikā, Ch. III, v. 1: Sarveṣāṁ yoga-tantrāṇāṁ tathādhārā hi Kuṇḍalī.

[3] Haṭha-yoga-pradīpikā, Ch. III, v. 105:

> Udghātayet kapāta tu yathā kuñcikayā hathāt.
> Kuṇḍalinyā tathā yogī mokṣadvāraṁ vibhedayet.

The same verse occurs in Ch. III, v. 5, of the Gherāṇḍa-Saṁhitā.

The Yoga-kuṇḍalī Up., Ch. I, calls Sarasvatī Arundhatī, saying that it is by arousing Her that Kuṇḍalī is aroused. When Kuṇḍalī wishes to go up nothing can stop Her. Therefore She is called Arundhatī, which is also the name of a Nāḍī.

[4] Yoga-Kuṇḍali Upaniṣad Ch. I.

white cloth " that is, membrane like the egg of a bird. It is generally described as being two fingers (Anguli) above the anus (Guda) and two fingers below the penis (Meḍhra).[1] From this Kaṇḍa spring the 72,000 Nāḍīs which here both unite and separate. Kula-kuṇḍalinī is the Śabda-Brahman, and all Mantras are Her manifestations (Svarūpa-vibhūti). For this reason one of the names of this, the Mantra-devatā, whose substance is " letters " is Mātṛkā—that is, the Genetrix of all the universes. She is Mātṛkā, for She is the Mother of all and not the child of any. She is the World-consciousness (Jagaccaitanya), the Virāṭ consciousness of the world as a whole.[2] Just as in space sound is produced by movements of air, so also in the ether within that Jīva's body currents flow, owing to the movements of the vital air (Prāṇa-vāyu), and its inward and outward passage as inhalation and exhalation. Verse 12 describes Kuṇḍalinī as the revered supreme Parameśvari (Sovereign Lady), the Omnipotent Kalā [3] in the form of Nāda-Śakti. She, the subtlest of the subtle, holds within Herself the mystery of creation,[4] and the stream of Ambrosia which flows from the attributeless Brahman. By Her radiance the universe is illumined, and by it eternal consciousness is awakened [5]—that is She both binds as Creatrix

[1] As given by Yājñavalkya, cited in Commentary to v. 113, Ch. III, of Haṭha-yoga-pradīpikā, which also refers to the Gorakṣa-śataka. The verse itself appears to fix its position as between the penis and navel (Nābhi), twelve fingers (Vitasti) above the Mūla-sthāna. Kaṇḍa is also applied to the seat of Prāṇa, the heart (see Ṣatcakra-nirūpaṇa, v. 8.)

[2] See " Principles of Tantra," Chs. XI, XII, *et seq.* It is because She is Mantra-devatā that She is roused by Mantra.

[3] See " Garland of Letters " as to the Kalās.

[4] She is creation itself (Sṛṣṭi-rūpā), vv. 10, 11, *post*; in Her are creation, maintenance, and dissolution, Sṛṣṭi-sthiti-layātmikā, *ib.*

[5] For She is also beyond the universe (Viśvātītā) and is Consciousness itself (Jñānarūpā), *ib.* As such She is thought of as going upward, as in descending She creates and binds.

(Avidyā-Śakti) and is the means as Vidyā-Śakti whereby Liberation may be attained. For this reason it is said in the Haṭha-yoga-pradīpikā that She gives liberation to Yogīs and bondage to the ignorant. For he who knows Her knows Yoga, and those who are ignorant of Yoga are kept in the bondage of this worldly life. As vv. 10 and 11 of the Ṣatcakra-nirūpaṇa say: "She, the World-charmer is lustrous as lightning; her sweet murmur is like the indistinct hum of swarms of love-mad bees.[1] She is the source of all Speech. It is She who maintains all the beings of the world by means of inspiration and expiration,[2] and shines in the hollow of the Mūla lotus like a chain of brilliant lights." Mantras are in all cases manifestations (Vibhūti) of Kula-kuṇḍalinī Herself, for She is all letters and Dhvani[3] and the Paramātmā Itself. Hence Mantras are used in the rousing of Kuṇḍalinī. The substance of Mantras is the Eternal Śabda or Consciousness, though their appearance and expression is in words. Words in themselves seem lifeless (Jada), but the Mantra power which they embody is Siddha—that is, the truth and capable of teaching it, because it is a manifestation of Caitanya, which is Satya Itself. So Veda, which is the formless (Amūrti) Brahman in Veda-form (Vedamūrti), is the self-illumined Principle of Experience[4] (Cit) itself, and is displayed in words (Siddha-śabda) which are without human authorship

---

[1] Viśvanātha the Commentator says that She makes this sound when awakened. According to the Commentator Śaṁkara, this indicates the Vaikharī state of Kuṇḍalinī.

[2] Thus, Prāṇa and Apāna are declared to be the maintainers of animate being (v. 3, *post*).

[3] See "Principles of Tantra," Ch. XI, and XII.

[4] Veda is one with Caitanya. As Śaṁkara says (comm. Triśatī, v. 19), dealing with the Pañcadaśi-Mantra: Sarve vedā yatrā ekam bhavanti, etc. Śrutyā vedasya ātmabhedena svaprakāśatayā.

(Apauruṣeyā),[1] incessantly revealing knowledge [2] of the nature of Brahman, or Pure Being, and of Dharma,[3] or those principles and laws, physical and psychical and spiritual, by which the universe is sustained (Dhāryate). And so the Divine Mother is said to be Brahman-knowledge (Brahma-vidyā) in the form of that immediate experience [4] which is the fruit of the realization of the great Vedāntic sayings (Mahā-vākya).[5] As, notwithstanding the existence of feeling-consciousness in all things, it does not manifest without particular processes, so, although the substance of Mantras is feeling-consciousness that feeling-consciousness is not perceptible without the union of the Sādhaka's Śakti (derived from Sādhana) with Mantra-Śakti. Hence it has been said in the Śāradā-Tilaka: "Although Kula-kuṇḍalinī whose substance is Mantras, shines brilliant as lightning in the Mūlādhāra of every Jīva, yet it is only in the lotuses of the hearts of Yogīs that She reveals Herself and dances in Her own joy. (In other cases, though existing in subtle form), She does not reveal Herself. Her substance is all Vedas, all Mantras, and all Tattvas. She is the Mother of the three forms of energy, 'Sun,' 'Moon,' and 'Fire,' and Śabda-Brahman Itself." Kuṇḍalinī is therefore the mightiest manifestation of creative power in the human

---

[1] And because it is without such authorship and is "heard" only, it is called Śruti ("what is heard"): Śruyate eva na tu kena cit kriyate (Vācaspati-Miśra in Sāṁkhya-Tattva Kaumudī); and see the Yāmala cited in Prāṇatoṣiṇī, 19: "Veda is Brahman; it came out as His breathing."

[2] The term Veda is derived from the root *vid*, to know.

[3] Veda, according to Vedānta, is that word without human authorship which tells of Brahman and Dharma: Dharma-brahma-pratipādakaṁ apauruṣeyaṁ vākyaṁ.

[4] Sākṣātkāra—that is, Nirvāṇa Experience (Aparokṣa-jñāna) as opposed to indirect (parokṣa) or merely intellectual knowledge.

[5] Vedānta-mahāvākyajanya-sākṣātkārarūpa-brahmavidyā (Śaṁkara's Comm. on Triśatī, v. 8). The Vedānta here means Upaniṣad, and not any particular philosophy so called.

body. Kuṇḍalī is the Śabda-Brahman—that is, Ātmā as manifested Śakti—in bodies, and in every power, person, and thing. The Six Centres and all evolved therefrom are Her manifestation. Śiva "dwells" in the Sahasrāra. The latter is the upper Śrī-Cakra, as the six centres are the lower. Yet Śakti and Śiva are one. Therefore the body of Kuṇḍalinī-Śakti consists of eight parts (Aṅgas)—namely, the six centres of psychic and physical force, Śakti and Sadāśiva Her Lord.[1] In the Sahasrāra Kuṇḍalī is merged in the Supreme Ātma-Śakti. Kuṇḍalinī is the great Prāṇa-devatā or Lord of Life which is Nādātmā, and if Prāṇa is to be drawn up through the "middle path," the Suṣumnā, towards the Brahma-randhra, it must of necessity pierce the lotuses or Cakras which bar the way therein. Kuṇḍalinī being Prāṇa-Śakti, if She is moved Prāṇa is moved.

The Āsanas, Kuṁbhakas, Bandhas, and Mudrās, are used to rouse Kuṇḍalinī, so that the Prāṇa withdrawn from Iḍā and Piṅgalā may by the power of its Śakti, after entry into the Suṣumnā or void (Śūnya), go upwards towards the Brahma-randhra.[2] The Yogī is then said to be free of the active Karma, and attain the natural state.[3] The object, then, is to devitalize the rest of the body by getting the Prāṇa from Iḍā and Piṅgalā into Suṣumnā, which is for this reason regarded as the most important of all the Nāḍīs and "the delight of the Yogī," and then to make it ascend through the lotuses which "bloom" on its approach. The body on each side of the spinal column is devitalized, and the whole current of Prāṇa thrown into that column. The

---

[1] See Lakṣmīdhara's Comm. on v. 9, "Saundaryalahari," p. 28. Diṇḍima on v. 35, *ib.*, p. 67, says that the eight forms are the six ("Mind" to "Earth"), the Sun and Moon.

[2] Haṭha-yoga-pradīpikā, Ch. IV, v. 10.

[3] *Ib.*, v. 11; upon what follows refer also to Ch. IV, *ib. passim.*

Manonmanī state is said to arise with the dissolution (Laya) of Prāṇa, for on this ensues Laya of Manas. By daily practising restraint of Prāṇa in Suṣumnā the natural effort of the Prāṇa along its ordinary channels is weakened and the mind is steadied. For when there is movement (Pari-spanda) of Prāṇa there is movement of mind; that is, it feeds upon the objects (Viṣaya) of the objective world.

But when Prāṇa is in Suṣumnā "there is neither day nor night," for "Suṣumnā devours time".[1] When there is movement of Prāṇa (Prāṇa-spanda), there is no cessation of Vṛtti (mind functioning). And, as the Yoga-vāśiṣṭha says, so long as Prāṇa does not cease to exist there is neither Tattva-jñāna nor destruction of Vāsanā, the subtle cause of the will towards life which is the cause of rebirth. For Tattva-jñāna, or supreme knowledge, is the destruction of both Citta and Vāsanā.[2] Restraint of breath also renders the semen firm. For the semen fluctuates as long as Prāṇa does so. And when the semen is not steady the mind is not steady.[3] The mind thus trained detaches itself from the world. These various results are said to be achieved by rousing Kuṇḍalinī, and by the subsequent process for which She is the "key". "As one forces open a door with a key, so the Yogī should force open the door of Liberation by Kuṇḍalinī."[4] For it is She who sleeps in the Mūlādhāra, closing with Her mouth the channel (Suṣumnā) by which ascent may be made to the Brahmarandhra. This must be opened when the Prāṇa naturally enters into it. "She, the 'young widow,' is to be despoiled forcibly." It is prescribed that there shall be daily

---

[1] Haṭha-yoga-pradīpikā, Ch. IV, vv. 16 and 17, Commentary thereto.

[2] *Ib.*, vv. 19-21, and Commentary (Tattva-jñānam mano-nāśo vāsanā-kṣaya eva ca).

[3] See *ante*, and Varāha Up., Ch. V.

[4] *Ib.*, Ch. III, v. 106. See Bhūta-Śuddhi-Tantra cited under v. 50, *post*.

practice, with a view to acquiring power to manipulate this Śakti.[1]

It generally takes years from the commencement of the practice to lead the Śakti to the Sahasrāra, though in exceptional cases it may be done in a short time.[2] At first She can only be led to a certain point, and then gradually higher. He who has led Her to a particular centre can reach the same centre more easily at the next attempt. But to go higher requires further effort. At each centre a particular kind of bliss (Ānanda) is experienced, and particular powers, such as the conquest of the elementary forms of sensible matter (Bhūta) are, it is said, gained, until at the Ājñā centre the whole universe is experienced. In the earlier stages, moreover, there is a natural tendency of the Śakti to return. In the continued practice facility and greater control are gained. Where the Nāḍīs are pure it is easy to lead Her down even from the Śahasrāra. In the perfection of practice the Yogī can stay as long as he will in the Sahasrāra, where the bliss is the same as that experienced in Liberation (subject in this case to return), or he may transfer himself into another body, a practice known to both the Indian and Tibetan Tantras, in the latter of which it is called Phowa.

The principle of all the methods to attain Samādhi is to get the Prāṇa out of Iḍā and Piṅgalā. When this is achieved these Nāḍīs become "dead," because vitality has gone out of them. The Prāṇa then enters the Suṣumnā and, after piercing by the aid of Kuṇḍalinī the six Cakras in the Suṣumnā, becomes Laya or absorbed in the Sahasrāra. The means to this end, when operating from the Mūlādhāra, seem to vary in detail, but embody a common principle—namely, the forcing of Prāṇa downward and

---

[1] Haṭha-yoga-pradīpikā, Ch. III, v. 112 *et seq.*

[2] As related by a Yogī from Girnar speaking of his own case.

Apāna upwards[1] (that is, the reverse of their natural directions) by the Jālaṁdhāra and Mūla-Bandha, or otherwise, when by their union the internal fire is increased. The position seems to be thus similar to a hollow tube in which a piston is working at both ends without escape of the central air, which thus becomes heated. Then the Serpent Force, Kuṇḍalinī, aroused by the heat thus generated, is aroused from Her potential state called "sleep," in which She lies curled up; She then hisses and straightens Herself, and enters the Brahma-dvāra, or enters into the Suṣumnā, when by further repeated efforts the Cakras in the Suṣumnā are pierced. This is a gradual process which is accompanied by special difficulties at the three knots (Granthis) where Māyā-Śakti is powerful, particularly the abdominal knot, the piercing of which may, it is admitted, involve considerable pain, physical disorder, and even disease. As already explained, these "knots" are the points at which converge the Cakras of each of the three groups. Some of the abovementioned processes are described in the present work, to which we now proceed, and which on this matter may be summarized as follows:

The preliminary verse (and in the reference to the verses I include the Commentary) says that only those who are acquainted with the Six Lotuses can deal with them; and the first verse says that Yoga by means of the method here described cannot be achieved without knowledge of the Cakras and Nāḍīs. The first verse says that Brahman will be realized. The next question is, How is this effected? The Commentator in the preliminary verse says that the very merciful Pūrṇānanda-Svāmī, being wishful to rescue the world sunk in the mire of misery, has undertaken the task firstly of instructing it as regards the union of the

---

[1] See Varāha-Upaniṣad, Ch. III.

Śakti-Kuṇḍalinī with the vital centres, or Cakras, and secondly of imparting that knowledge of Brahman (Tattva-jñāna) which leads to Liberation. The former—that is, knowledge concerning the Cakras, and so forth—is the " first shoot " of the Yoga plant. Brahman, as the Commentator says, is the Supreme Consciousness which arises upon the acquisition of knowledge. The first cause of such knowledge is an acquaintance with and practice of the Tāntrik Yoga Sādhana which is concerned with the Cakras, Nāḍīs, and Kuṇḍalinī; the next cause is the realization of that Sādhana by the rousing of Kuṇḍalinī; and the final result is experience as Brahman, which is the effect of the action of Kuṇḍalinī, who is the Śakti or power of Will (Icchā), Action (Kriyā), and Knowledge (Jñāna), and exists in forms both subtle and gross. Mind is as much one of the forms of Kuṇḍalī as is that which is called " matter ". Both are equally products of Prakṛti-Śakti, which is a grosser form of the Nādamayī-Śakti. Kuṇḍalī takes the form of the eight Prakṛtis.[1] The Power which is aroused is in itself (Svarūpa) Consciousness, and when aroused and taken to the upper cerebral centre is the giver of true knowledge (Svarūpa-Jñāna), which is the Supreme Consciousness.

The arousing of this force is achieved both by will and mind power (Yoga-bala), accompanied by suitable physical action. The Sādhaka [2] seats himself in the prescribed Āsana and steadies his mind by the Khecarī-Mudrā, in which concentration is between the eyebrows. Air is inhaled (Pūraka) and then retained (Kuṁbhaka). The upper part of the body is then contracted by Jālaṁdhara-Bandha,[3] so that the upward breath (Prāṇa) is checked. By this

[1] Śāṇḍilya-Upaniṣad, Ch. I; Yogakuṇḍalī Up., Ch. I.

[2] The account here given follows and amplifies the text. The Commentary to v. 50, *post*.

[3] *Vide ante* and Dhyāna-bindu Up.

contraction the air so inhaled is prevented from escape. The air so checked tends downwards. When the Yogī feels that the air within him, from the throat to the belly, is tending downwards through the channels in the Nāḍīs, the escape or Vāyu as Apāna is again checked by the Mūla-Bandha and Aśvinī-Mudrā, in which the anal muscle is contracted. The air (Vāyu) thus stored becomes an instrument by which, under the direction of mind and will, the potentialities of the vital force in the Mūlādhāra may be forced to realization. The process of mental concentration on this centre is described as follows: "With mental Japa of the Mantra prescribed and acquisition thereby of Mantra-Śakti, Jīvātmā (individual Consciousness), which is thought of as being in the shape of the tapering flame of a lamp, is brought from the region of the heart to the Mūlādhāra. Jīvātmā here spoken of is the Ātmā of the subtle body—that is, the Antahkaraṇa or mind as Buddhi (including therein Ahaṁkāra) and Manas, the faculties of sense (Indriya) or mind operating to receive impression through the sense organs, and Prāṇa;[1] the constituents of the second, third, and fourth, bodily sheaths. Following such concentration and impact of the retained Vāyu on this centre, the Vāyu is again raised with the Bīja "Yaṁ". A revolution from left to right is given to the "air of Kāma" or Kandarpa (Kāmavāyu)[2]. This is a form of Icchā-Śakti. This, the pressure of the Prāṇa and Apāna held in Kuṁbhaka, the natural heat arising therefrom, and the Vahni-Bīja (Fire Mantra) "Raṁ," kindle the fire of Kāma (Kāmāgni). The fire encircles and arouses the slumbering serpent Kuṇḍalinī, who is then, in the language of the Śāstra, seized with the passion of "desire" for Her Spouse, the Para-haṁsah or Paramaśiva. Śakti thus rendered

[1] According to the Vedāntik definition; or the five Tanmātras, according to Sāṁkhya. The Citta (mind) therefore enters Suṣumnā along with Prāṇa (Yoga-tattva-Upaniṣad and Dhyāna-bindu Up).

[2] A form of Apāna-Vāyu.

active is drawn to Śiva, as in the case of ordinary positive and negative electric charges, which are themselves but other manifestations of the universal polarity which affects the manifested world.

The Yogakuṇḍalī-Upaniṣad [1] states the following methods and others mentioned: When Prāṇa is passing through Iḍā, assume Padmāsana and lengthen the Ākāśa of 12 points by 4—that is, as in exhalation Prāṇa goes out in 16 measures, and in inhalation comes in 12, inhale for 16 and thus gain power. Then, holding the sides by each hand, stir up Kuṇḍalinī with all one's strength from right to left fearlessly for 48 minutes. Draw the body up a little to let Kuṇḍalī enter Suṣumnā. The Yogī does a drawing-up-movement in which the shoulders are raised and dropped. Prāṇa enters of itself with Her. Compressing above and expanding below, and *vice versa*, Prāṇa rises.

In the commentary [2] on verse 32 of the Ānandalaharī it is said: "The sun and the moon, as they move always in Deva-yāna and Pitṛ-yāna (northern and southern orbs) in the Macrocosm, are travelling (incessantly in the Microcosm) by Iḍā and Piṅgalā day and night. The moon, ever travelling by the left Nāḍī (Iḍā), bedews the whole system with her nectar. The sun, travelling by the right Nāḍī (Piṅgala), dries the system (thus moistened by nectar). When the sun and the moon meet at Mūlādhāra, that day is called Amāvasyā (new moon day) . . . . The Kuṇḍalī also sleeps in Ādhārakuṇḍa . . . . When a Yogī whose mind is under control is able to confine the moon in her own place, as also the sun, then the moon and sun become confined, and consequently the moon cannot shed its nectar nor the sun dry it. Next, when the place of nectar becomes dried by the fire with the help of Vāyu, then the Kuṇḍalī wakes up for

[1] Ch. I.

[2] "Saundaryalahari," pp. 60, 61.

want of food and hisses like a serpent. Afterwards, breaking through the three knots, She runs to Sahasrāra and bites the Candra (moon), which is in the middle of the same. Then the nectar begins to flow, and wets the (other) Candra-Maṇḍala in Ājñā-Cakra. From the latter the whole body becomes bedewed with nectar. Afterwards the fifteen eternal Kalās (part) of Candra (moon) in Ājñā go to Viśuddhi and move thereon. The Candra-Maṇḍala in Sahasrāra is also called Baindava. One Kalā remains there always. That Kalā is nothing but Cit Itself, which is also called Ātman. We call Her Tripurasundarī. It is understood by this that, in order to rouse the Kuṇḍali, one should practise in the lunar fortnight alone, and not in the solar one."

Kuṇḍalinī is led upwards "as a rider guides a trained mare by the reins," through the aperture hitherto closed by Her own coils, but now open, within the entrance of the Citrini Nāḍī. She then pierces, in that Nāḍī, each of the lotuses, which turn their heads upwards as She passes through them. As Kuṇḍalinī united with the subtle Jīvātmā passes through each of these lotuses, She absorbs into Herself the regnant Tattvas of each of these centres, and all that has been above described to be in them. As the ascent is made, each of the grosser Tattvas enters into the Laya state, and is replaced by the energy of Kuṇḍalinī, which after the passage of the Viśuddha-Cakra replaces them all. The senses which operate in association with these grosser Tattvas are merged in Her, who then absorbs into Herself the subtle Tattvas of the Ājñā. Kuṇḍalinī Herself takes on a different aspect as She ascends the three planes, and unites with each of the Liṅgas in that form of Hers which is appropriate to such union. For whereas in the Mūlādhāra She is the Śakti of all in their gross or physical manifested state (Virāt), at the stage of Ājñā, She is the Śakti of the mental and psychic or subtle body (Hiraṇya-garbha), and in the region of the Sahasrāra She is the Śakti of the "spiritual" plane (Īśvara), which, though itself in its Śiva aspect undifferentiated, contains in its Power-aspect all lower planes in a concealed potential state. The Māyā-Tantra (see v. 51, *post*) says that the four sound-producing Śaktis—namely, Parā, Paśyantī, Madhyamā, and Vaikharī—are Kuṇḍalī Herself (Kuṇḍalinya-bhedarūpā). Hence, when Kuṇḍalī starts to go to Sahasrāra, She in Her form as Vaikharī bewitches Svayaṁbhu-Liṅga; She then similarly bewitches Bāṇa-Liṅga in the heart as Madhyamā and Itara-Liṅga in the eyebrows as Paśyantī. Then, when She reaches the stage of Para-bindu, She attains the state of Parā (Parā-bhāva).

The upward movement is from the gross to the more subtle, and the order of dissolution of the Tattvas is as follows: Pṛthivī with the Indriyas (smell and feet), the latter of which have Pṛthivī (the earth as ground) as their support, is dissolved into Gandha-Tattva, or Tanmātra of smell, which is in the Mūlādhāra; Gandha-Tattva is then taken to the Svādhiṣṭhāna, and it, Ap, and its connected Indriyas (taste and hands), are dissolved in Rasa (Taste) Tanmātra; the latter is taken to the Maṇipūra and there Rasa-Tattva, Tejas, and its connected Indriyas (sight and anus), are dissolved into Rūpa (sight) Tanmātra; then the latter is taken into the Anāhata, and it, Vāyu, and the connected Indriyas (touch and penis), are dissolved in Sparśa (Touch) Tanmātra; the latter is taken to the Viśuddha, and there it, Ākāśa, and associated Indriyas (hearing and mouth), are dissolved in the Śabda (sound) Tanmātra; the latter is then taken to the Ājñā, and, there and beyond it, Manas is dissolved in Mahat, Mahat in Sūkṣma-Prakṛti, and the latter is united with Para-bindu in the Sahasrāra. In the case of the latter merger there are various stages which are mentioned in the text (v. 52), as of Nāda into Nādānta, Nādānta into Vyāpikā, Vyāpikā into Samanī, Samanī into Unmanī, and the latter into Viṣṇu-vaktra or Puṁ-bindu, which is also Paramaśiva.[1] When all the letters have been thus dissolved, all the six Cakras are dissolved as the petals of the lotuses bear the letters.

On this upward movement, Brahmā, Sāvitrī, Ḍākinī, the Devas, Matṛkaś, and Vṛttis, of the Mūlādhāra, are absorbed in Kuṇḍalinī, as is also the Mahī-maṇḍala or Pṛthivī, and the Pṛthivī-Bīja "Laṁ" into which it passes. For these Bījas, or sound powers, express the subtle Mantra aspect of that which is dissolved in them. Thus "earth" springs from and is dissolved in its seed (Bīja), which is that particular aspect of the creative consciousness, which propelled it. The uttered Mantra (Vaikharī-Śabda) or "Laṁ" is the expression in gross sound of that.

When the Devī leaves the Mūlādhāra, that lotus, which by reason of the awakening of Kuṇḍalinī and the vivifying intensity of the Prāṇik current had opened and turned its flower upwards, again closes and hangs its head downwards. As Kuṇḍalinī reaches the Svādhiṣṭhāna, that lotus opens out and lifts its flower upwards. Upon Her entrance, Viṣṇu, Lakṣmī, Sarasvatī, Rākinī, Mātṛkās and Vṛtti, Vaikuṇṭha-dhāma, Goloka, and the Deva and Devī residing therein, are dissolved in the body of Kuṇḍalinī. The Pṛthivī or Earth Bīja "Laṁ" is dissolved in the Tattva water, and water converted into its Bīja "Vaṁ" remains the body of Kuṇḍalinī. When the Devī reaches the Maṇipūra Cakra or Brahma-granthi, all that is in that Cakra merges in Her. The Varuṇa-Bīja "Vaṁ" is dissolved in fire, which remains in Her body as the Bīja "Raṁ". The Śakti next reaches the Anāhata-Cakra, which is known as the Knot of Viṣṇu

[1] See as to all these Śaktis of the Praṇava, the "Garland of Letters".

(Viṣṇu-granthi), where also all which is therein is merged in Her. The Bīja of Fire "Raṁ" is sublimed in air, and air converted into its Bīja "Yaṁ" is absorbed in Kuṇḍalinī. She then ascends to the abode of Bhāratī or Sarasvatī, the Viṣuddha-Cakra. Upon Her entrance, Ardha-nārīśvara Śiva, Śākinī, the 16 vowels, Mantra, etc., are dissolved in Her. The Bīja of Air "Yaṁ" is dissolved in ether, which, itself being transformed into the Bīja "Haṁ," is merged in the body of Kuṇḍalinī. Piercing the concealed Lalanā-Cakra, the Devī reaches the Ājñā known as the "Knot of Rudra" (Rudra-granthi), where Paramaśiva, Siddha-Kālī, the Devas, and all else therein, are dissolved in Her. At length the Bīja of Vyoma (ether) or "Haṁ" is absorbed into the subtle Tattvas of the Ājñā, and then into the Devī. After passing through the Rudra-granthi, Kuṇḍalinī unites with Paramaśiva. As She proceeds upwards from the two-petalled lotus, the Nirālaṁba-purī Praṇava, Nāda, and so forth, are merged in the Devī. She has thus in Her progress upwards absorbed in Herself the twenty-three Tattvas, commencing with the gross elements, and then remaining Herself Śakti as Consciousness, the cause of all Śaktis, unites with Paramaśiva whose nature is one with Hers.

By this method of mental concentration, aided by the physical and other processes described, the gross is absorbed into the subtle, each dissolving into its immediate cause and all into Cidātmā or the Ātmā which is Cit. In language borrowed from the world of human passion, which is itself but a gross reflection on the physical plane of corresponding, though more subtle, supersensual activities and bliss, the Śakti-Kuṇḍalinī who has been seized by desire for Her Lord is said to make swift way to Him, and kissing the lotus mouth of Śiva, enjoys Him (See v. 51, *post*). By the term Sāmarasya is meant the sense of enjoyment arising from the union (Sāmarasya) of male and female.

This is the most intense form of physical delight representing on the worldly plane the Supreme Bliss arising from the union of Śiva and Śakti on the "spiritual" plane. So Dakṣa, the Dharma-śāstrakāra, says: "The Brahman is to be known by Itself alone, and to know It is as the bliss of knowing a virgin."[1] Similarly, the Sādhaka in Laya-siddhi-yoga, thinking of himself as Śakti and the Paramātmā as Puruṣa, feels himself in union (Saṅgama) with Śiva, and enjoys with him the bliss which is Śṛṅgāra-rasa, the first of the nine Rasas, or the love sentiment and bliss. This Ādirasa (Śṛṅgāra) which is aroused by Sattva-guṇa[2] is impartite (Akhaṇḍa), self-illuminating (Svaprakāśa), bliss (Ānanda) whose substance is Cit (Cinmaya).[3] It is so intense and all-exclusive as to render the lover unconscious of all other objects of knowledge (Vedyāntara-sparśa-śūnyah), and the own brother[4] of Brahma-bliss (Brahmāsvādasahodara).[5] But as the Brahma-bliss is known only to the Yogi, so, as the Alaṁkāra-Śāstra last cited observes, even the true love-bliss of the mortal-world "is known to a few knowers only" (Jñeyah kaiścit pramātṛbhih), such as poets and others. Sexual as well as other forms of love are reflections or fragments of the Brahman-bliss.

---

1 Svasaṁvedyaṁ etat brahma kumārī-strī-sukhaṁ yathā, cited in Commentary to v. 15 of Ch. I of the Haṭha-yoga-pradīpikā.

2 So all the eight Bhāvas commencing with Sveda, Staṁbha, including the well-known Romāncha or thrill in which the hair stands on end (Pulaka), the choking voice (Sara-bhaṅga), pallor (Vaivarṇaya), and so forth, are all Sāttvik. The objection of an Indian friend, that these Bhāvas could not be Sāttvik inasmuch as Sattva was "spiritual," is an apt instance of the disassociation from Indian thought effected by English education and the danger of rendering the terms of Saṁskrit into English.

3 It is not a Tāmasik thing such as dream or madness, etc.

4 Sahodara—that is, brothers born of the same mother. Sexual-bliss is the reflection (faint comparatively though it be) of formless Brahman-bliss of which it is a form.

5 Sāhitya-Darpaṇa, Ch. III.

This union of the Śakti-Kuṇḍalinī with Śiva in the body of the Sādhaka is that coition (Maithuna) of the Sāttvika Pañca-tattva which the Yoginī-Tantra says is "the best of all unions for those who have already controlled their passions," and are thus Yati.[1] Of this the Bṛhat-Śrīkrama (*vide* v. 51, *post*) says: "They with the eye of knowledge see the stainless Kalā united with Cidānanda on Nāda. He is the Mahādeva, white like a pure crystal, and is the effulgent Cause (Biṁba-rūpa-nidāna), and She is the lovely woman of beauteous limbs which are listless by reason of Her great passion." On their union nectar (Amṛta) flows, which in ambrosial stream runs from the Brahma-randhra, to the Mūlādhāra, flooding the Kṣudra-brahmāṇda, or microcosm, and satisfying the Devatās of its Cakras. It is then that the Sādhaka, forgetful of all in this world, is immersed in ineffable bliss. Refreshment, increased power and enjoyment, follows upon each visit to the Well of Life.

In the Cintāmaṇi-satva, attributed to Śrī-Śaṁkarācārya, it is said: "This family woman (*i. e.*, Kuṇḍalinī), entering the royal road (*i.e.*, Suṣumnā), taking rest at intervals in the sacred places (*i.e.*, Cakras), embraces the Supreme Husband (Para-śiva) and makes nectar to flow (*i.e.*, from the Sahasrāra)."

The Guru's instructions are to go above the Ājñā-Cakra, but no special directions are given; for after this Cakra has been pierced, the Sādhaka can, and indeed must, reach the Brahma-sthāṇa, or abode of Brahman, unaided by his own effort. Above the Ājñā the relationship of Guru and Śiṣya (Master and Disciple) ceases. Kuṇḍalinī having pierced the fourteen "Knots," (Granthis)—*viz.*, three Liṅgas, six Cakras,

---

[1] Ch. VI:

Sahasrāropari bindau kuṇḍalyā melanaṁ shive.
Maithunaṁ paramaṁ dravyaṁ yatīnāṁ parikīrtitaṁ

and the five Śivas which they contain, and then Herself drunk with the nectar which issues from Para-Śiva, returns along the path whence She came to Her own abode (Mūlādhāra).[1] As She returns She pours from Herself into the Cakras all that She had previously absorbed therefrom. In other words, as Her passage upwards was Laya-krama, causing all things in the Cakras to pass into the Laya state (dissolution), so Her return is Sṛṣṭi-krama, as She "recreates" or makes them manifest. In this manner She again reaches the Mūlādhāra, when all that has been already described to be in the Cakras appears in the positions which they occupied before Her awakening. In fact, the descending Jīvātmā makes for himself the idea of that separated multiple and individualized world which passed from him as he ascended to and became one with the Cause. She as Consciousness absorbs what She as conscious Power projected. In short, the return of Kuṇḍalinī is the setting again of the Jīvātmā in the phenomenal world of the lowest plane of being after he had been raised therefrom to a state of ecstasis, or Samādhi. The Yogī thus knows (because he experiences) the nature and state of Spirit and its pathway to and from the Māyik and embodied world. In this Yoga there is a gradual process of involution of the gross world with its elements into its Cause. Each gross element (Mahā-bhūta), together with the subtle element (Tanmātra) from which it proceeds and the connected organ of sense (Indriya), is dissolved into the next above it until the last element, ether, with the Tanmātra sound and Manas, are dissolved in Egoism (Ahaṁkāra), of which they are Vikṛtis. Ahaṁkāra is merged in Mahat, the first manifestation of creative ideation, and the latter into Bindu, which is the Supreme Being, Consciousness, and Bliss as the creative Brahman. Kuṇḍalī when aroused is felt as

[1] As to the Samaya practice, *v. post*, p. 246, *et seq.*

intense heat. As Kuṇḍalinī ascends, the lower limbs become as inert and cold as a corpse; so also does every part of the body when She has passed through and leaves it. This is due to the fact that She as the Power which supports the body as an organic whole is leaving Her centre. On the contrary, the upper part of the head becomes "lustrous," by which is not meant any external lustre (Prabhā), but brightness, warmth, and animation. When the Yoga is complete, the Yogī sits rigid in the posture selected, and the only trace of warmth to be found in the whole body is at the crown of the head, where the Śakti is united with Śiva. Those, therefore, who are sceptical can easily verify some of the facts should they be fortunate enough to find a successful Yogī who will let them see him at work. They may observe his ecstasis and the coldness of the body, which is not present in the case of what is called the Dhyāna-Yogī, or a Yogī operating by meditating only, and not rousing Kuṇḍalinī. This cold is an external and easily perceptible sign. Its progression may be seen, obviously denoting the passing away of something which supplied the previous heat. The body seems lifeless, indicating that its supporting power has (though not entirely) left it. The downward return of the Śakti thus moved is, on the other hand, indicated by the reappearance of warmth, vitality, and the normal consciousness. The return process is one of evolution from the highest state of attainment to the point of departure.

Though not dealt with in this work, reference may here be made to the Sādhana accompanying the return of Kuṇḍalinī to Her resting-place in the ritual practice called Bhūta-śuddhi, where the ascent and descent are imagined only.

The Sādhaka thinking of the Vāyu Bīja "Yaṁ" as being in the left nostril, inhales through Iḍā, making Japa of the Bīja sixteen times. Then, closing both nostrils, he makes Japa of the Bīja sixty-four times. He then thinks of the "black man of sin" (Pāpa-puruṣa)[1] in the left[2] cavity of the abdomen as being dried up (by the air), and so thinking he exhales through the right nostril Piṅgalā, making Japa of the Bīja thirty-two times. The Sādhaka then, meditating upon the red-coloured Bīja "Raṁ" in the Maṇipūra, inhales, making sixteen Japa of the Bīja, and then closes the nostrils, making sixty-four Japa. Whilst making Japa he thinks that the body of the "man of sin" is being burnt and reduced to ashes (by the fire). He then exhales through the right nostril with thirty-two Japa, and then meditates upon the white Candra-Bīja "Thaṁ". He next inhales through Iḍā, making Japa of the Bīja sixteen times, closes both nostrils with Japa done sixty-four times, and exhales through Piṅgalā with thirty-two Japa. During inhalation, holding of breath, and exhalation, he should consider that a new celestial body is being formed by the nectar (composed of all the Mātṛkā-varṇa, or sound-powers, embodied in their Vaikharī form as lettered sound) dropping from the "Moon". In a similar way with the Bīja of water "Vaṁ" the formation of the body is continued, and with Bīja "Laṁ" of the cohesive Pṛthivī-Tattva it is completed and strengthened. Lastly, with the Mantra "So'ham" ("He I am") the Sādhaka leads the Jīvātmā into its place in the heart. Some forms of meditation are given in v. 51.

Kuṇḍalī does not at first stay long in Sahasrāra. The length of stay depends on the strength of the Yogī's practice. There is then a natural tendency (Saṁskāra) on the part of Kuṇḍalī to return. The Yogī will use all effort at his disposal to retain Her above, for the longer this is done the nearer

---

[1] See Mahānirvāṇa-Tantra Ullāsa, Ch. V, vv. 98, 99, where the Bhūta-śuddhi process is shortly described. Also Devī-Bhāgavata, cited, *post*.

[2] The worse or weaker side.

approach is made to the time when She can be in a permanent manner retained there.[1] For it is to be observed that liberation is not gained by merely leading Kuṇḍalī to the Sahasrāra, and of course still less is it gained by stirring it up in the Mūlādhāra, or fixing it in any of the lower centres. Liberation is gained only when Kuṇḍalī takes up Her permanent abode in the Sahasrāra, so that She only returns by the will of the Sādhaka. It is said that after staying in Sahasrāra for a time, some Yogins lead the Kuṇḍalinī back to Hṛdaya (heart), and worship Her there. This is done by those who are unable to stay long in Sahasrāra. If they take the Kuṇḍalinī lower than Hṛdaya—*i.e.*, worship Her in the three Cakras below Anāhata they no longer, it is said, belong to the Samaya group.[2]

Thus, when by the preliminary Sādhana purity of physical and mental function is gained, the Sādhaka learns how to open the entrance of the Suṣumnā, which is ordinarily closed at the base. This is the meaning of the statement that the Serpent with its coil closes the gate of Brahmā. At the base of the Suṣumnā-Nāḍī and in the Ādhāra lotus the Śakti-Kuṇḍalinī lies slumbering coiled round the Liṅga, the Śiva or Puruṣa aspect in that centre of the Śabdabrahman, of which She is the Prakṛti aspect. Kuṇḍalī in the form of Her creative emanations as mind and matter is the whole moving body, but She Herself exists at the Mūlādhāra or earth centre as a gross aspect of Śakti in its sleeping form. This is the normal abode of the Śakti who is the Śabda-Brahman. For having so completely manifested Herself She rests or sleeps in what is her grossest and concluding manifestation. The "residual" vital force in this centre then exists in a latent and potential state. If its aid

[1] Great Power (Siddhi) is had by the man who can keep Kuṇḍalī Śakti in the Sahasrāra three days and three nights.

[2] Lakṣmīdhara, cited by Anantakṛṣṇa-Śāstrī, "Saundaryalahari," p. 62.

towards Yoga is sought, the first process must be that by which the Serpent is aroused from its slumber. In other words, this force is raised from its latent potential state to one of activity, and there reunited with Itself in its other aspect as the Static Light which shines[1] in the cerebral centre.

Kuṇḍalī-Śakti is Cit, or Consciousness, in its creative aspect as Power. As Śakti it is through Her activity that the world and all beings therein exist. Prakṛti-Śakti is in the Mūlādhāra in a state of sleep (Prasuptā)—that is latent activity looking *outwards* (Bahirmukhī). It is because She is in this state of latent activity that through Her all the outer material world functions of life are being performed by man. And it is for this reason that man is engrossed in the world, and under the lure of Māyā takes his body and egoism to be the real Self, and thus goes round the wheel of life in its unending cycle of births and deaths. When the Jīva thinks the world to be different from himself and the Brahman, it is through the influence of Kuṇḍalinī who dwells within him. Her sleep in the Mūlādhāra, is, therefore, for the bondage of the ignorant.[2] As long as She remains in the Mūlādhāra lotus—namely, in that state of Hers which is the concomitant of the cosmic appearance—so long must that appearance endure. In short, when She is asleep, man is in the waking state (Jāgrat). Hence it is said[3] that the Śakti of the initiate is awake, that of the Paśu asleep. She is therefore aroused from sleep, and when awake returns to Her Lord, who is but Herself in another aspect; Her return is, in fact, the withdrawal of that activity of Hers which produces the world of

---

[1] For this reason the Sahasrāra is also called Bhāloka (from the root *bhā*, "to shine").

[2] Śāṇḍilya Upaniṣad, Ch. I.

[3] Kulārṇava-Tantra, Ch. V. Maṇḍalabrāhmaṇa Up. Tamas is destroyed there.

appearances, and which with such withdrawal disappears. For on Her upward Path She absorbs into Herself all the Tattvas which had emanated from Her. The individual consciousness of the Yogī, the Jīvātmā, being united with the world-consciousness in Her, or Kuṇḍalī, then becomes the universal consciousness, or Paramātmā, from which it appeared to be different only by reason of the world-creating activity of Kuṇḍalī which is thus withdrawn. The establishment through Her of the pure state of Being-Consciousness-Bliss is Samādhi.

In short, Kuṇḍalī is the individual bodily representative of the great Cosmic Power (Śakti) which creates and sustains the universe. When this individual Śakti manifesting as the individual consciousness (Jīva) is merged in the consciousness of the Supreme Śiva, the world is for such Jīva dissolved, and Liberation (Mukti) is obtained. Under, however, the influence of the Cosmic Śakti, the universe continues for those who are liberated until the Great Dissolution (Mahā-pralaya), at the close of which the universe again evolves into those Jīvas whose Karma has not been exhausted, and who have therefore not been liberated. The rousing and stirring up of Kuṇḍalī-Yoga is thus a form of that merger of the individual into the universal consciousness or union of the two which is the end of every system of Indian Yoga.

Paṇḍit R. Anantakṛṣṇa Śāstrī says [1]: "The Samaya method of worshipping Śakti, called the Samayācāra,[2] is dealt with in five treatises whose reputed authors are the great sages Sanaka, Sananda, Sanatkumāra, Vaśiṣṭha, and Śuka.

---

[1] "Saundaryalahari," pp. 5-10.

[2] This term is apparently of varying significance. It seems to be used here in a sense opposed to, some forms at least of, Kulācāra, and is yet used in the Kaula-Śāstras, to denote their worship with the Pañcatattva.

The following is a summary of the teachings contained in these Samaya-Āgamas, each of which goes after the name of its author:

" The Śakti or energy, the development of which is the subject of these treatises, is called the Kuṇḍalinī. The place where it resides is called the Mūlādhāra (original abode). By a successful development and working of this Śakti, the liberation of the soul is attained. In the ordinary condition Kuṇḍalinī sleeps quietly at the Mūlādhāra. The first purpose of the practitioners is to awaken this sleeping snake, and this is effected in two ways:

" (1) By Tapas. Here Tapas refers to the process of Prāṇāyāma, which means the regulation of the breath and holding it for stated periods of time. This is also the course advocated by the Yoga-Śāstras.

" (2) By Mantras. The pupil is initiated in the chanting of certain Mantras which he has to repeat a fixed number of times at particular hours of the day, all the while having before his mind's eye the figure of the Mūrti or God connoted by the Mantra he chants. The most important of these Mantras is said to be the Pañcadaśī.

" When it is thus roused up, the Kuṇḍalinī ascends from (1) Mūlādhāra, where it was sleeping, to the next higher centre, called the (2) Svādhiṣṭhāna (own place). Thence with great effort this Śakti is carried to the following centres in regular ascending order; (3) Maṇipūra (full of rays); (4) Anāhata (sound, not emanating from the collision of bodies)—the Śakti here is transformed into sound; (5) Viśuddhi (place of purity)—here it becomes a pure Sāttvic element; and (6) Ājñā (ā-jñā, a little knowledge). At this stage the practitioner may be said to have so far been successful in securing a command over this Śakti, which now appears to him, though only for a moment, in the form of a sharp flash of lightning.

"The passage of the Kuṇḍalinī from the Mūlādhāra through the above centres of energy up to Ājñā constitutes the first part of the ascent. The disciple who takes to this practice has to undergo a course of Upāsanā (contemplation and worship of the prescribed Deity) and Mantra-Japa (chanting of incantations),[1] into which he will be initiated by his Guru (teacher and guide). The six centres of energy above enumerated from Mūlādhāra to Ājñā, joined together by imaginary straight lines, form a double-faced triangle—a hexagon, the six-pointed star—which is called the Śrī-Cakra in Sanskrit. The Anāhata centre (the heart) is the critical point in the course of this ascent, and hence much is found written in the Āgamas about this centre.

"These centres in the body of man (Piṇḍāṇḍa) have their correspondence in the cosmic planes, and each of these has its own quality, or Guṇa, and a Presiding Deity. When the disciple ascends centre by centre, he passes through the corresponding Lokas, or cosmic planes. The following table give the correspondences, Guṇa, and Presiding Deity:

No.	Psychic Centre in Man's Body	Loka, or Cosmic Plane	Guna, or Quality	Presiding Deity
1	Mūlādhārā at the stage when Śakti is roused up	Bhuvarloka	Tamas	Agni (Fire)
2	Svādhiṣṭhāna	Svarloka		
3	Maṇipūra	Maharloka	Rajas	Sun
4	Anāhata	Janaloka		
5	Viśuddhī	Tapoloka	Sattva	Moon
6	Ājñā	Satyaloka		

[1] In this and other citations from the Paṇḍit the English equivalents of Sanskrit terms are unsuitable, as might be expected in one to whom English is not his own tongue.

"If one should die after attaining any of these stages, he is born again having all the advantages of the stages gained; thus, a man dies after leading the Śakti to the Anāhata; in his next birth he begins where he has last left, and leads the Śakti onwards from the Anāhata.

"This aspiration to unify one's soul with the Eternal One has been held by some to be an attempt of a Tāmasa origin to rid itself of all Tamas and Rajas in it. Therefore the aspirant in the first and second stages is said to have more Tamas than in the succeeding stages, and to be therefore in the Tāmasic stage, which is presided over by Agni. In the next two stages he is similarly said to be in the Rājasic stage, presided over by the Sun. In the next two he is in the Sāttvic stage, presided over by the Moon, the Deity which is assigned a higher plane than the Sun and Agni. But it is to be noticed that the aspirant does not get a pure Sattva until he passes on to the Sahasrāra, and that Tamas, Rajas, and Sattva, referred to in the above table, are but relative, and bear no comparison with their common acceptation.

"Kuṇḍalinī is the grossest form of the Cit, the twenty-fourth Tattva, which lives in the Mūlādhāra; later on we shall have to speak of it in detail in our treatment of the second part of the aspirant's ascent. This Kuṇḍalinī, as soon as it is awakened, is in the Kumārī (girl) stage. On reaching the Anāhata, it attains the Yoṣit stage (womanhood). Hence the indication that it is the most difficult and important step in the ascent. The next stage is in the Sahasrāra, of which we shall speak hereafter, and the Śakti in that stage is called Pativratā (devoted to husband). See Taittirīya-Āraṇyaka, I. 27. 12.

"The second part of the ascent of Kuṇḍalinī consists of only one step: the Śakti should be taken into the Sahasrāra from the Ājñā, where we left her. The Sahasrāra (lit., a thousand-petalled lotus) forms in itself a Śrī-cakra.

The description of this place in Sanskrit is too difficult to be rendered satisfactorily into English. In the Sahasrāra there is a certain place of lustre known as Candra-Loka (a world of nectar). In this place live in union the Sat (Sadāśiva) and the Cit, the twenty-fifth and the twenty-fourth Tattvas. The Cit, or Śuddha-Vidyā, is also called Ṣadākhyā, the 16th Kalā of the moon. These two Tattvas are always in union, and this union itself is taken to be the twenty-sixth Tattva. It is this union of Sat and Cit that is the goal of the aspirant. The Kuṇḍalinī which has been led all the way to the Sahasrāra should be merged into this union; this is the end of the aspirant's journey; he now enjoys beatitude itself (Paramānanda).

"But this Kuṇḍalinī does not stay in the Sahasrāra for a long time. It always tends to return, and does return to its original position. The process should again and again be repeated by the aspirant several times, until the Śakti makes a permanent stay with her Pati (husband)—namely, Sadāśiva, or until the union of Sadāśiva and Cit is complete, and becomes Pativratā, as already mentioned. The aspirant is then a Jīvan-mukta, or pure Sattva. He is not conscious of this material limitation of the soul. He is all joy, and is the Eternal itself. See vv. 9 and 10. So much of Samayācāra.

"Now to the other methods of Śākta worship; the Kaulas worship the Kuṇḍalinī without rousing her from her sleep[1] in the Mūlādhāra, which is called Kula; and hence Kaulas (Sans. Ku = earth, Pṛthivī; so Mūlādhāra). Beyond

[1] A statement by the same author at p. 75 is in apparent contradiction with this. He there says, citing Lakṣmīdhara: The Kaulas who worship Kuṇḍalinī in the Mūlādhāra have no other aim than *awakening* it from its sleep. When this is done, they think that they have attained their object, and there they stop. In their own words, the Kaulas have Nirvāṇa always near at hand.

the Mūlādhāra they do not rise; they follow the Vāmācāra or black magic,[1] and gain their temporal objects and enjoy; they are not liberated from birth and death; they do not go beyond this earth. Nay, more, the Kaulas are now so far degraded that they have left off altogether the worship of the Kuṇḍalinī in the Mūlādhāra, and have betaken themselves to practices most inhuman, which are far from being divine.[2] The Miśras are far above the Kaulas. They perform all Karmas, worship the Devī or Śakti in the elements, such as the sun, air, etc., and do Upāsanā with Yantras made of gold or other metals. They worship the Kuṇḍalinī, awake her, and attempt to lead her on. Some of the Miśra worshippers rise even as far as the Anāhata.

"We learn from the Commentators that this whole subject of Śakti-worship is treated of in detail in the 'Taittirīya-Āraṇyaka' (1st chapter). Some of them even quote from that 'Āraṇyaka' in support of their explanations. This subject is vast and a very difficult one. It is not possible for one to go into the intricacies of the subject unless one be a great Guru of vast learning and much personal experience;[3]

---

[1] Vāmācāra is not "black magic," the nearest Sanskrit equivalent for which is Abhicāra. There may have been, as the Mahākāla-Saṁhitā says (Ullāsa II), some Kaulas who, like the Vaidikas, sought enjoyment in this and the next world, and not Liberation (Aihikārthaṁ kāmayanti amṛte ratiṁ na kurvanti). But to state baldly that Kaulas as a whole do not rouse Kuṇḍalinī and lead her to the Sahasrāra is incorrect. Pūrṇānanda-Swāmī, the author of the text here translated, was himself a Kaula, and the whole object of the work is to secure Liberation (Mokṣa).

[2] The Paṇḍit here apparently adopts the opinion of Lakṣmīdhara, a follower of the so-called Samaya School, and an opponent of the Kaulas. If (as is probably the case) "inhuman" is the Paṇḍit's phraseology, it is inapt. But there have been different communities with very differing views and practice, *e.g.*, a Brahma-Kaula and a Kāpālika. See as to the rituals to which the Paṇḍit refers "Śakti and Śākta," (Secret Ritual).

[3] Here I wholeheartedly agree with my distinguished friend the Paṇḍit.

great works have been written on even single points in the ascent of the aspirant up the psychic centres.[1]

"The followers of the Samaya group are prohibited from worshipping Devī in the Macrocosm. They should worship Her in any of the Cakras in the human body, choosing that centre which their practice and ability permits them to reach. They should contemplate on Devī and Her Lord Śiva as (1) having the same abode (Adhiṣṭhāna-sāmya), (2) occupying the same position (Avaṣṭhāna-sāmya), (3) performing the same functions (Anuṣṭhāna-sāmya), (4) having the same form (Rūpa), and (5) as having the same name (Nāma). Thus, in worshipping Devī in the Ādhāra-Cakra, Śiva and Śakti (1) have Mūlādhāra for their seat, (2) both of them occupy the position of dancers, (3) both together perform the function of creating the universe, (4) both are red in colour, (5) Śiva is called Bhairava, and Śakti Bhairavī.

"Similarly for other Cakras mentioned in the preceding Ślokas. This is the way how beginners have to practise. Advanced students worship Devī in the Sahasrāra, and not in the lower centres. How is the worship to be carried on in Sahasrāra?

"The worshipper should fix his attention on Baindava, which is the locality where the ever-existing 26th Tattva—the union of Śiva and Śakti—resides. It lies above all the 25 Tattvas, and is situated in Candra-maṇḍala (the sphere of the moon) in Sahasrāra. He should contemplate on the said union and identify himself with it. This shows that those who carry on Bāhya-Pūja, or worship in the external world, do not belong to the Samaya School. As regards the identification of oneself with the union of Śiva and Śakti at Baindava just spoken of, there are two ways of realizing it; one is known as the fourfold path, and the

[1] See "Saundaryalahari," pp. 5-10.

other the sixfold path. These should be learnt from the Guru.

"A novitiate in the Samaya School has to go the following course:

"(1) He should cherish the utmost regard for and confidence in his Guru. (2) He should receive the Pañcadaśī-Mantra from his Guru, and chant (repeat) the same according to instructions, with a knowledge of its seer (Ṛṣi), metre (Chandas), and the Deity (Devatā).[1] (3) On the eighth day in the bright fortnight of Āśvayuja month, Mahā-navamī, he should at midnight prostrate himself at his Guru's feet, when the latter will be pleased to initiate him in some Mantra and the real nature of the six Cakras and of the sixfold path of identification.

"After he is thus qualified, Lord Mahādeva[2] gives him the knowledge or capacity to see his inner soul. . . . Then the Kundalinī awakes, and, going up suddenly to Maṇipūra, becomes visible to the devotee-practitioner. Thence he has to take Her slowly to the higher Cakras one after another, and there perform the prescribed worship, and She will appear to him more and more clearly. When the Ājñā-Cakra is crossed, the Kuṇḍalinī quickly darts away like a flash of lightning to Sahasrāra, and enters the Island of Gems surrounded by the Kalpa trees in the Ocean of Nectar, unites with Sadāśiva there, and enjoys with Him.

"The practitioner should now wait outside the veil[3] until Kuṇḍalinī returns to Her own place, and on Her return

[1] The Ṛṣi of the Mantra is he to whom it was first revealed; the metre is that in which it was first uttered by Śiva; and the Devatā is the Artha of the Mantra as Śabda. The Artha is fivefold as Devatā, Ādhi-devatā, Pratyādhi-devatā, Varṇādhi-devta and Mantrādhi-devatā.

[2] Śiva initiates him in the knowledge of Brahman. Thus, Śiva is considered the Teacher of the Spiritual Gurus (Ādinātha).

[3] This, as well as some other details of this description, I do not follow. Who is waiting outside the veil? The Jīva is, on the case stated, within, if there be a veil, and what is it?

continue the process until She is joined for ever with Sadāśiva in the Sahasrāra, and never returns.

"The process heretofore described and others of a similar nature are always kept secret; yet the commentator says he has, out of compassion towards his disciples, given here an outline of the method.

"Even in the mere expectation of the return of Kuṇḍalinī from Sahasrāra, the aspirant feels Brahmānanda (Brahma bliss). He who has once taken Kuṇḍalinī to Sahasrāra is led to desire nothing but Mokṣa (Liberation), if he has no other expectation. Even if any of the Samaya practitioners have some worldly expectations, they must still worship in the microcosm only.

"'Subhagodaya' and other famous works on Śrīvidyā say that the practitioner should concentrate his mind on Devī who resides in Sūrya-maṇḍala (the sun's disc), and so on. This statement is not at variance with the teaching contained in this book, for the Sūrya-maṇḍala referred to applies to the Piṇḍāṇḍa (microcosm), and not to Brahmāṇḍa (macrocosm). Similarly, all the verses advocating outer worship are to be applied to the corresponding objects in the Piṇḍāṇḍa." [1]

The last, highest and most difficult form of Yoga is Rāja-Yoga. By means of Mantra, Haṭha and Laya-Yoga the practitioner by gradual attainment of purity becomes fit for Savikalpa-Samādhi. It is through Rāja-Yoga alone that he can attain to Nirvikalpa-Samādhi. The former Samādhi or Ecstasy is one in which, unless it perfects into the second kind, there is a return to the world and its experience. This is not so in the Samādhi of Rāja-Yoga in which there is not the slightest seed of attachment to

[1] "Saundaryalahari," pp. 75-77, ending with: "For full particulars of these principles *vide* 'Śuka Saṁhitā,' one of the five Saṁhitās of the Samaya group."

the world and in which therefore there is no return thereto but eternal unity with Brahman. The first three kinds of Yoga prepare the way for the fourth.[1] In the Samādhi of Mantra-Yoga the state of Mahābhāva is attained marked by immobility and speechlessness. In the Samādhi of Haṭha-Yoga respiration ceases and to outward experience the Yogī is without sign of animation and like a corpse. In the Samādhi of Laya-Yoga described in this book the Yogī has no outer consciousness and is also immersed in the Ocean of Bliss. The Samādhi of Rāja-Yoga is complete (Cit-svarūpa-bhāva) and final (Nirvikalpa) Liberation.[2] There are, it is said, four states of detachment (Vairāgya) from the world[3] corresponding to the four Yogas, the mildest form of Vairāgya being the mark of the first or Mantra-Yoga and the greatest degree of detachment being the mark of the highest Yoga or Rāja-Yoga. Another mark of distinction is the prominence given to the mental side. All Yoga is concerned with mental practices but this is more specially so of Rāja Yoga which has been described[4] as the discrimination of the real from the unreal, that is the infinite and enduring from the finite and transient by reasoning with the help of the Upaniṣads and the recognized systems of Philosophy.

The English reader must not, however, identify it with mere philosophising. It is the exercise of Reason by the morally pure and intellectually great under the conditions and subject to the discipline above described with Vairāgya or Renunciation. In the man of Knowledge (Jñānī), Buddhi

---

[1] Rāja-Yoga, by Swāmī Dayānanda, published by Śrī-Bhārata Dharma-Mahāmaṇḍala, Banaras.

[2] *Ibid.*, 19, 20.

[3] Mṛdu (intermittent, vague and weak), Madhyama (middling), Adhimātra (high degree when worldly enjoyment even becomes a source of pain), Para (highest when the mind is turned completely from worldly objects and cannot be brought back to them under any circumstances).

[4] *Ibid.*, 5.

or Reason holds full sway. Rāja-Yoga comprises sixteen divisions. There are seven varieties of Vicāra (reasoning) in seven planes of knowledge (Bhūmika) called Jñānadā, Sannyāsadā, Yogadā, Līlonmukti, Satpadā, Ānandapadā and Parātparā.[1] By exercise therein the Rāja-Yogī gradually effectively practises the two kinds of Dhāraṇā,[2] *viz.*, Prakṛtyāśraya and Brahmāśraya dependent on Nature or Brahman respectively. There are three kinds of Dhyāna whereby the power of self-realization (Ātmapratyakṣa) is produced. There are four forms of Samādhi. There are three aspects of Brahman, *viz.*, Its gross aspect as immanent in the universe known as the Virāt-Puruṣa, its subtle aspect as the creator, preserver and dissolver of all this as the Lord (Īśvara) and the supreme aspect beyond that is Saccidānanda. Rāja-Yoga lays down different modes of Dhyāna for the three aspects.[3] Of the four Samādhis won by these exercises, in the two first or Savicāra, there is still a subtle connection with the conscious working or the power of Vicāra (reasoning, discernment), but the last two are without this or Nirvicāra. On reaching this fourth state the Rāja-Yogī attains Liberation even when living in the body (Jīvan-mukta) and is severed from the Karmāśraya.[4] In the general view it is only by Rāja-Yoga that this Nirvikalpa-Samādhi is attained.

[1] Similarly there are seven Bhūmikās or planes of Karma, *viz.*, Vividiṣā or Śubhecchā, Vicāranā, Tanumānasā, Sattāpatti Asamśakti, Padārthābhāvini, Turyagā and also seven planes of Worship (Upāsanā Bhūmikā), *viz.*, Nāmapara, Rūpapara, Vibhūtipara, Śaktipara, Guṇapara, Bhāvapara, Svarūpapara.

[2] See p. 207, *ante*.

[3] Rāja-Yoga, by Dayānanda Swāmī, 19.

[4] The mass of Karma Saṁskāras in their seed (Bīja) state.

VII

THEORETICAL BASES OF THIS YOGA

This Yoga has been widely affirmed. The following review does not profess to be exhaustive, for the literature relating to Kuṇḍalinī and Laya-Yoga is very great, but includes merely a short reference to some of the Upaniṣads and Purāṇas which have come under my notice, and of which I kept a note, whilst engaged in this work.[1] It will, however, clearly establish that this doctrine concerning the Cakras, or portions of it, is to be found in other Śāstras than the Tantras, though the references in some cases are so curt that it is not always possible to say whether they are dealing with the matter in the same Yoga-sense as the work here translated or as forms of worship (Upāsanā). It is to noted in this connection that Bhūta-śuddhi is a rite which is considered to be a necessary preliminary to the worship of a Deva.[2] It is obvious that if we understand the Bhūta-śuddhi to here mean the Yoga practice described, then, with the exception of the Yogī expert in this Yoga, no one would be competent for worship at all. For it is only the accomplished (Siddha) Yogī who can really take Kuṇḍalinī to the Sahasrāra. In this ordinary daily Bhūta-śuddhi, therefore, the process is purely a mental or imaginary one, and therefore forms part of worship or Upāsanā, and not Yoga. Further, as a form of worship the Sādhaka may,

[1] There are many others. Some references kindly supplied to me by Mahāmahopādhyāya Ādityarāma Bhattācārya have also been inserted.

[2] See Taranga I of the Mantramahodadhi: Devārcā-yogyatā-prāptyai bhūta-śuddhiṁ samācaret.

and does, adore his Iṣṭa-devatā in various parts of his body. This, again, is a part of Upāsanā. Some of the Śāstras however; next mentioned, clearly refer to the Yoga process, and others appear to do so.

In what are called the earliest Upaniṣads,[1] mention is made of certain matters which are more explicitly described in such as are said by Western orientalists to be of later date. Thus, we find reference to the four states of consciousness, waking, and so forth; the four sheaths; and to the cavity of the heart as a "soul" centre.

As already stated, in the Indian schools the heart was considered to be the seat of the waking consciousness. The heart expands during waking, and contracts in sleep. Into it, during dreaming sleep (Svapna), the external senses are withdrawn, though the representative faculty is awake; until in dreamless sleep (Suṣupti), it also is withdrawn. Reference is also made to the 72,000 Nāḍīs; the entry and exit of the Prāṇa through the Brahma-randhra (above the foramen of Monro and the middle commissure); and "upbreathing" through one of these Nāḍīs. These to some extent probably involve the acceptance of other elements of doctrine not expressly stated. Thus, the reference to the Brahma-randhra and the "one nerve" imply the cerebro-spinal axis with its Suṣumnā, through which alone the Prāṇa passes to the Brahma-randhra; for which reason, apparently, the Suṣumnā itself is referred to in the Śiva-saṁhītā as the Brahma-randhra. Liberation is finally effected by "knowledge," which, as the ancient Aitareya-Āraṇyaka says,[2] "is Brahman".

---

[1] For some references from the older Upaniṣads, see an article by Professor Rhys Davids in J.R.A.S., p. 71 (January, 1899) "Theory of Soul in Upaniṣads". See also my "Principles of Tantra," referring amongst others to Praśna Upaniṣad, III. 6, 7.

[2] P. 236 (edited by Arthur Barriedale Keith) of "Anecdoṭa Oxoniensia".

The Haṁsa Upaniṣad[1] opens with the statement that the knowledge therein contained should be communicated only to the Brahmacārī of peaceful mind (Śānta), self-controlled (Dānta) and devoted to the Guru (Guru-bhakta). Nārāyaṇa, the Commentator, who cites amongst other works the Tāntrik Compendium the Śāradā-Tilaka, describes himself as "one whose sole support is Śruti"[2] (Nārāyaṇena śrutimātropajīvinā). The Upaniṣad (§ 4) mentions by their names the six Cakras, as also the method of raising of Vāyu from the Mūlādhāra—that is, the Kuṇḍalinī-Yoga. The Haṁsa (that is, Jīva) is stated to be in the eight-petalled lotus below Anāhata[3] (§ 7) where the Iṣṭa-devatā is worshipped. There are eight petals, with which are associated certain Vṛttis. With the Eastern petal is associated virtuous inclination (Puṇye matiḥ); with the South-Eastern, sleep (Nidrā) and laziness (Ālasya); with the Southern, badness or cruelty (Krūra-mati); with the South-Western, sinful inclination (Pāpe manīṣā); with the Western, various inferior or bad qualities (Krīdā); with the North-Western, intention in movement or action (Gamanādau buddhiḥ); with the Northern, attachment and pleasurable contentment (Rati and Prīti); and with the North-Eastern petal, manual appropriation of things (Dravya-grahaṇa).[4] In the centre of this lotus is dispassion (Vairāgya). In the filaments is the waking state (Jāgrad-avasthā); in the pericarp the sleeping state (Svapna); in the stalk the state of

---

[1] Upaniṣadāṁ Samuccayaḥ: Ānandāśrama Series, Vol. XXX, p. 593.

[2] The Tantra, like every other Indian Śāstra, claims to be based on Veda.

[3] This lotus is commonly confused with the Anāhata. The latter is a Cakra in the spinal column; the eight-petalled lotus is in the region of the heart (Hṛd) in the body.

[4] Lit., "taking of things". The translation of this and some of the other Vṛttis is tentative. It is not easy in every case to understand the precise meaning or to find an English equivalent.

dreamless slumber (Suṣupti). Above the lotus is "the place without support" (Nirālaṁba-pradeśa), which is the Turīya state. The Commentator Nārāyaṇa says that the Vṛtti of the petals are given in the Adhyātma-viveka which assigns them to the various lotuses. In the passage cited from the Haṁsopaniṣad, they, or a number of these, appear to be collected in the centre of meditation upon the Iṣṭa-devatā. In § 9 ten kinds of sound (Nāda) are mentioned which have definite physical effects, such as perspiration, shaking, and the like, and by the practice of the tenth kind of Nāda the Brahmapada is said to be attained.

The Brahma-Upaniṣad[1] mentions in v. 2 the navel (Nābhi), heart (Hṛdaya), throat (Kaṇtha), and head (Mūrdhā), places (Sthāna) "where the four quarters of the Brahman shine". The Commentator Nārāyaṇa says that the Brahmopaniṣad, by the mention of these four, indicates that they are the centres from which the Brahman may (according to the method there prescribed) be attained.[2] Reference is made to the lotuses at these four places, and the mind is spoken of as the "tenth door" the other nine apertures being the eyes, ears, nostrils, and so forth.

The Dhyānabindu-Upaniṣad[3] refers to the hearing of the Anāhata sounds by the Yogī (v. 3). The Upaniṣad directs that with Pūraka meditation should be done in the navel on the Great Powerful One (Mahā-vīra) with four arms and of the colour of the hemp flower (*i.e.*, Viṣṇu); with Kuṁbhaka meditate in the heart on the red Brahmā seated on a lotus; and with Recaka think of the three-eyed one (Rudra) in the forehead. The lowest of these

---

[1] Ānandāśrama Series, Vol. XXIX, p. 325.

[2] It will be observed that the two lower Tāmasic centres are not here mentioned.

[3] *Ibid.*, p. 262.

lotuses has eight petals; the second has its head downwards; and the third, which is compounded of all the Devatas (Sarvadevamaya), is like a plantain flower (vv. 9-12). In v. 13, meditation is directed on a hundred lotuses with a hundred petals each, and then on Sun, Moon, and Fire. It is Ātmā which rouses the lotus, and, taking the Bīja from it, goes to Moon, Fire, and Sun.

The Amṛtanāda-Upaniṣad[1] refers to the five elements and above them Ardha-mātra—that is, Ājñā (vv. 30, 31). The elements here are those in the Cakras, for v. 26 speaks of the heart entrance as the aerial entrance (for the Vāyu-Tattva is here). Above this, it is said, is the gate of Liberation (Mokṣa-dvāra). It is stated in v. 25 that Prāṇa and Manas go along the way the Yogī sees (paśyati), which the Commentator says refers to the way Prāṇa enters (and departs from) Mūlādhāra, and so forth. He also gives some Haṭha processes.

The Kṣurikā-Upaniṣad[2] speaks of the 72,000 Nāḍīs, and of Iḍā, Piṅgalā and Suṣumnā (vv. 14, 15). All these, with the exception of Suṣumnā, can "be served by Dhyāna-Yoga" (*ib.*). Verse 8 directs the Sādhaka "to get into the white and very subtle Nāda (*Quaere* Nāḍī) and to drive Prāṇa-Vāyu through it"; and Pūraka, Recaka, Kuṁbhaka, and Haṭha processes are referred to. The Commentator Nārāyaṇa on v. 8, remarks that Kuṇḍalī should be heated by the internal fire and then placed inside the Brahma-nāḍī, for which purpose the Jālandhara-Bandha should be employed.

The Nṛsimha-pūrvatāpanīya Upaniṣad[3] in Ch. V, v. 2, speaks of the Sudarśana (which is apparently here the Mūlādhāra) changing into lotuses of six, eight, twelve,

---

[1] *Op. cit.*, 43. The Amṛta-bindu-Upaniṣad at p. 71 deals generally with Yoga.

[2] *Ibid.*, Vol. XXIX, p. 145.

[3] Ānandāśrama Edition, Vol. XXX, p. 61.

sixteen, and thirty-two petals respectively. This corresponds with the number of petals as given in this work except as to the second. For, taking this to be the Svādhiṣṭhāna, the second lotus should be one of ten petals. Apparently this divergence is due to the fact that this is the number of letters in the Mantra assigned to this lotus. For in the six-petalled lotus is the six-lettered Mantra of Sudarśana; in the eight-petalled lotus the eight-lettered Mantra of Nārāyaṇa; and in the twelve-petalled lotus the twelve-lettered Mantra of Vāsudeva. As is the case ordinarily, in the sixteen-petalled lotus are the sixteen Kalās (here vowels) sounded with Bindu or Anusvāra. The thirty-two-petalled lotus (Ājñā) is really two-petalled because there are two Mantras here (each of sixteen letters) of Nṛsimha and His Śakti.

The sixth chapter of the Maitrī-Upaniṣad[1] speaks of the Nāḍīs; and in particular of the Suṣumnā; the piercing of the Maṇḍalas Sun, Moon, and Fire (each of these being within the other, Sattva in Fire, and in Sattva Acyuta); and of Amanā, which is another name for Unmanī.

Both the Yoga-tattva-Upaniṣad,[2] and Yoga-śikhā Upaniṣad[3] refer to Haṭha-yoga, and the latter speaks of the closing of the "inner door," the opening of the gateway of Suṣumnā (that is, by Kuṇḍalinī entering the Brahma-dvāra), and the piercing of the Sun. The Rāma-tāpanīya-Upaniṣad[4] refers to various Yoga and Tāntrik processes, such as Āsana, Dvāra-pūja, Pīṭha-pūja, and expressly mentions Bhūta-śuddhi, which, as above explained, is the purification of the elements

[1] Vol. XXIX of same edition, p. 345; see pp. 441, 450, 451, 458 and 460.

[2] Same edition, Vol. XXIX, p. 477.

[3] *Ibid.*, p. 483; and as to the passage of Kuṇḍalinī through the Brahma-dvāra, see p. 485.

[4] Ānandāśrama Edition, Vol. XXIX, p. 520.

in the Cakras, either as an imaginative or real process, by the aid of Kuṇḍalinī.

I have already cited in the Notes numerous passages on this Yoga from the Śāṇḍilya-Upaniṣad of the Atharva-veda, the Varāha and Yoga-kuṇḍalinī-Upaniṣads of the Kṛṣṇa-Yajurveda, the Maṇḍala-Brāhmaṇa-Upaniṣad of the Śukla-Yajurveda, and the Nāda-bindu-Upaniṣad of the Ṛgveda.[1]

The great Devī-bhāgavata-Purāṇa (VII. 35, XI. 8) mentions in a full account the Six Cakras or Lotuses; the rousing of Kuṇḍalinī (who is called the Para-devatā) in the Mūlādhāra by the manner here described, uniting Jīva therewith by the Haṁsa-Mantra; Bhūta-śuddhi; the dissolution of the gross Tattvas into the subtle Tattvas, ending with Mahat in Prakṛti, Māyā in Ātmā. The Dharā-maṇḍala is mentioned, and it and the other Maṇḍalas are described in the manner here stated. The Bījas of Pṛthivī and other Tattvas are given. Allusion is also made to the destruction of the "man of sin" (Pāpa-puruṣa), in terms similar to those to be found in the Mahā-nirvāṇa and other Tantras. A remarkable Dhyāna of Prāṇa-Śakti is to be found in this chapter, which reads very much like another which is given in the Prapañcasāra-Tantra.[2]

Liṅga-Purāṇa, Part I, Ch. LXXV, mentions the Cakras with their different petals, the names of which are given by the Commentator. Śiva is Nirguṇa, it says, but for the benefit of men He resides in the body with Umā, and Yogīs meditate upon Him in the different lotuses.

Chapter XXIII of the Agni-Purāṇa, which is replete with Tāntrik rituals, magic, and Mantras, also refers to the Bhūta-śuddhi rite wherein, after meditation with the

---

[1] These Yoga-Upaniṣads have been recently translated as part of "Thirty Minor Upaniṣads," by K. Nārāyaṇasvāmi Aiyar (Theosophical Society of Madras, 1914).

[2] See Ch. XXXV, Vol. III of my "Tāntrik Texts".

respective Bīja-Mantras on the navel, heart, and Ājñā centres the body of the Sādhaka is refreshed by the flow of nectar.

Finally, an adverse critic of this Yoga whom I cite later invokes the authority of the great Śaṁkara, though in fact, if tradition be correct, it is against him. Śaṁkara, in whose Maths may be found the great Tāntrīk Yantra called the Śrī Cakra, says in his Commentary on vv. 9 and 10 of Ch. VIII of the Bhagavad-Gītā: "First the heart lotus (Anāhata) is brought under control. Then, by conquering Bhūmi (Mūlādhāra, etc.) and by the upward going Nāḍī (Suṣumnā), after having placed Prāṇa between the two eyebrows (see v. 38, Ṣaṭcakra-nirūpaṇa), the Yogī reaches the lustrous light-giving Puruṣa." On this the Tīkā of Ānandagirī runs: "By the Suṣumnā-Nāḍī between Idā and Piṅgalā. The throat is reached by the same way—the space between the eyebrows. By conquering earth (Bhūmi) is meant the process by which the five Bhūtas are controlled." Śrīdhara-Śvamī says: "By the power of Yoga (Yoga-bala) Prāṇa must be led along the Suṣumnā." And Madhusūdana-Sarasvatī says: "The upward-going Nāḍī is Suṣumnā, and the conquest of Bhūmi and the rest is done by following the path indicated by the Guru; and by the space between the eyebrows is meant the Ājñā Cakra. By placing Prāṇa there, it passes out by the Brahma-randhra, and the Jīva becomes one with the Puruṣa." The famous hymn called Ānanda-laharī ("Wave of Bliss"), which is ascribed to Śaṁkara, deals with this Yoga (Ṣaṭcakra-bheda); and in the thirteenth chapter of Vidyāraṇya's Śaṁkara-vijaya the six lotuses are mentioned, as also the fruit to be gained by worshipping the Devatā in each Cakra.[1]

---

[1] See also Ānandagirī's Śaṁkaravijaya and Madhava's Śaṁkara-vijaya (Ch. XI; see also *ib.*, where Śri-Cakra is mentioned).

Paṇḍit R. Anantakṛṣṇa-Śāstri says:[1]

"Many a great man has successfully worked the Kuṇḍalini to the Sahasrāra, and effected her union with the Sat and Cit. Of these stands foremost the great and far-famed Śaṁkarācārya, a humble pupil of one of the students of Gauḍapādācārya, the author of the well-known 'Subhagodaya' (52 ślokas). Having well acquainted himself with the principles contained in this work, Śrī Śaṁkārācārya received special instructions based upon the personal experience of his Guru. And adding his own personal experience to the above advantages, he composed his famous work on the Mantra-śāstra, consisting of 100 ślokas; the first forty-one of these forming the 'Ānanda-Laharī,' and the rest forming the 'Saundarya-Laharī'; the latter apostrophizes the Devī as a being who is beauteous from head to foot.

"'Ānanda-Laharī' may be said to contain the quintessence of the Samayācāra. The work is all the more valuable because the author teaches it from personal experience. Lengthy commentaries are written on almost every syllable of the text. The value attached to the work may be adequately understood by the following theory. Some hold that Śiva is the real author of 'Ānanda-Laharī,' and not Śaṁkarācārya, who was but a Mantra-draṣṭā or Ṛṣi —*i.e.*, one who realized the process and gave it to the world. No less than thirty-and-six commentaries on this work are now extant. Among them we find one written by our great Appaya-Dīkṣita. The commentaries are not entirely different, but each has its own peculiar views and theories.

"As for the text of 'Ānanda-Laharī,' it contains forty-and-one ślokas. According to some commentators, the ślokas are 35 in number; some recognize only 30, and

[1] "Saundaryalaharī," pp. 10-15.

according to Sudhā-vidyotinī and others only the following ślokas constitute the text of 'Ānanda-Laharī': 1-2, 8-9, 10-11, 14-21, 26-27, 31-41. In my opinion, also, the last statement seems to be correct, as the other ślokas treat only of Prayogas (applications of Mantras) for worldly purposes.[1] Only a few of these Prayogas are recognized by all the commentators; while the rest are passed over as being entirely Kārmic.

"As has been remarked already, 'Ānanda-Laharī' is but an enlargement of the work called Subhagodaya by Gauḍapāda, who is the Guru of the author's Guru. That work gives only the main points, without any of the characteristic admixture of illustrations, etc., above noticed.

"Of all the commentaries on 'Ānanda-Laharī' Lakṣmīdhara's seems to be the most recent; yet in spite of this it is the most popular, and with reason, too. Other commentaries advocate this or that aspect of the various philosophical schools; but Lakṣmīdhara collates some of the views of others, and records them side by side with his own. His commentary is in this way the most elaborate. He sides with no party;[2] his views are broad and liberal. All schools of philosophers are represented in his commentaries. Lakṣmīdhara has also commented on many other works on Mantra-Śāstra, and is consequently of much high repute. So his commentaries are as valuable to both 'Ānanda-Laharī' and 'Saundarya-Laharī' as Sāyaṇa's are to the Vedas.

"Lakṣmīdhara seems to have been an inhabitant of Southern India; the observances and customs he describes all point to this conclusion; the illustrations he adduces

[1] Thus, vv. 13, 18, 19 are said to treat of Madana-prayoga—that is, application for the third Puruṣārtha or Kāma (desire).

[2] He seems to be adverse to the Uttara or Northern Kaula School. —A.A.

smack invariably of the South, and even to this day his views are more followed in the South than in the North. He has also written an elaborate commentary on Gauḍapāda's Subhagodaya. The references to that in the commentary to this work, and the commentator's apology here and there for repeating what he has written on the former occasion, lead to the inference that the author had for his life-work the commentary on the original book.

"Acyutānanda's commentaries are in Bengali characters, and are followed as authority in Bengal even to this day.[1] Various commentaries are followed in various places but few have risen to be universally accepted.

"There are only three or four works treating of Prayoga (application); I have had access to all of them. But here I have followed only one of them, as being the most prominent and important. It comes from an ancient family in Conjeevaram. It contains 100 ślokas. The Yantras (figures) for the Mantras contained in the ślokas, the different postures of the worshipper, and similar prescriptions, are clearly described in it to the minutest detail.

"There seems to be some mystical connection between each śloka and its Bījākṣara.[2] But it is not intelligible, nor has any of the Prayoga Kartās [3] explained the same.

"The following is a list of commentaries written upon 'Ānanda-Laharī'; some of them include 'Saundarya-Laharī' also:

"I. 'Manoramā' a Commentary. 2. A commentary by 'Appaya-Dīkṣita (Tanjore Palace Library). 3. 'Viṣṇupakṣī.' Perhaps this may be the same as No. 14 given below. 4. By Kavirāja-śarman—about 3,000 granthas (Deccan- College Library). 5. 'Manju-bhāṣinī,' by Kṛṣṇācārya, the son

[1] I have followed this commentary also in my "Wave of Bliss".—A.A.

[2] Bīja or root-mantra.—A.A.

[3] Those writers who deal with the practical application.—A.A.

of Vallabhācārya—śloka about 1,700. He says in his Introduction that Śrī-Śaṁkarācārya praised the Brahma-Śakti called Kuṇḍalinī when he was meditating on the banks of the Ganges. He gives the purport of this work in his first śloka: 'I praise constantly the Kuṇḍalinī, who creates innumerable worlds continuously, though She is like a filament of the lotus, and who resides at the root of the tree (Mūlādhāra) to be roused and led (to Sahasrāra).' This is popular in the Bengal Presidency. 6. Another Commentary, called 'Saubhāgyavardhanī,' by Kaivalyāśrama. The Adyar Library has a copy of it. This is popular throughout India, so we can get as many MSS. of the same as we require from different places. It contains about 2,000 granthas. 7. By Keśava-bhatta. 8. 'Tattva-dīpikā,' by Gangāhari, a small Commentary based on Tantra-Śāstra. 9. By Gangādhara. 10. By Gopīramaṇatarkapravacaṇa—granthas about 1,400. Seems to be of recent origin. 11. Gaurī-kānta-sārvabhauma-bhattācārya—granthas about 1,300. Of recent origin. 12. By Jagadiśa. 13. By Jagannātha-Pañcānana. 14. By Nārasiṁha—granthas 1,500. The chief peculiarity of this commentary is that it explains the text in two different ways, each śloka being applicable to Devī and Viṣṇu at the same time. Though some commentators have given different meanings to some of the verses, yet all of them apply to the different aspects of Devī alone, and not to the different Devatās. 15. 'Bhāvārthadīpa,' by Brahmānanda[1]—granthas about 1,700. 16. By Malla-bhatta. 17. By Mahādeva-vidyā-vāgīśa. 18. By Mādhavavaidya (Deccan College Library). 19. By Rāmacandra—granthas about 3,000 (Deccan College Library). 20. By Rāmānanda-tīrtha. 21. Lakṣmīdhara's; which is

[1] This is the celebrated Bengali Parama-haṁsa guru of Pūrnānanda-Svāmī, author of the Ṣaṭcakra-nirupaṇa. Brahmānanda was the author of the celebrated Śāktānanda-taraṅgiṇī.—A.A.

well known to the public, and needs no comment. This has been brought out excellently in Deva Nāgara type by the Mysore Government lately. 22. By Viśvaṁbhara. 23. By Śrīkaṇtha-bhaṭṭa. 24. Rāma-Sūri. 25. By Diṇḍima (Adyar Library.) 26. By Rāmacandra-Miśra—granthas about 1,000 (Deccan College Library). 27. By Acyutānanda (printed in Bengali characters). 28. Sadāśiva (Government Oriental Library, Madras). 29. Another nameless Commentary (Government Oriental Library, Madras). 30. By Śrīraṅga-dāsa. 31. By Govinda-Tarkā-vāgīśa-Bhattācārya—granthas 600. He seems to give the Yantra also for each verse. Further, he says that the god Mahādeva specially incarnated as Śaṁkarācārya to promulgate the Science of Śrī-vidyā. 32. Sudhā-vidyotinī, by the son of Pravaraśena. This commentator says that the author of this famous hymn was his father, Pravaraśena, Prince of the Dramidas. He tells us a story in connection with Pravaraśena's birth which is very peculiar. As he was born in an inauspicious hour, Dramida, the father of Pravaraśena, in consultation with his wise minister, by name Suka, threw him out in the forest, lest he the (father) should lose his kingdom. . . . The child praised Devī by this hymn, and, pleased with it, the Devī fostered and took care of him in the forest. The story ends by saying that the boy returned to his father's dominion and became King. By his command, his son, the present commentator, wrote Sudhā-vidyotinī, after being fully initiated into this mystic Śāstra, Śrī-vidyā. The account, however, appears to be rather fantastic. This MS. I got from South Malabar with much difficulty. It gives the esoteric meaning of the verses in 'Ānanda-Laharī,' and seems to be a valuable relic of occult literature. 33. The book of Yantras with Prayoga. This is very rare and important.

"Besides the above commentaries, we do not know how many more commentaries there are upon this hymn."

The celebrity of "Ānanda-Laharī" and the great number of commentaries upon it are proof of the widespread and authoritative character of the Yoga here described.

To conclude with the words of the Commentator on the Triśatī: "It is *well known in Yoga-Śāstras* that nectar (Amṛta) is in the head of all breathing creatures (Prāṇī), and that on Kuṇḍalī going there by the Yoga-path which is moistened by the current of that nectar Yogins become like Īśvara." [1]

The Cakras, however, mentioned are not always those of the body above stated, as would appear from the following account, which, it will be observed, is peculiar, and which is taken from the Ṣaṭcakra Upaniṣad of the Atharvaveda.[2] Apparently reference is here made to cosmic centres in the worship of the Viṣṇu Avatāra called Nṛsiṁha.

"Om. The Devas, coming to Śatyaloka, thus spoke to Prajāpati, saying, 'Tell us of the Nārasiṁha [3] Cakra,' (to which he replied): There are six Nārasiṁha Cakras. The first and second have each four spokes; the third, five; the fourth, six; the fifth, seven; and the sixth, eight spokes. These six are the Nārasiṁha Cakras. Now, what are their names (that is what you ask). They are Ācakra,[4] Sucakra,[5] Mahācakra,[6] Sakalaloka-rakṣaṇa-cakra,[7] Dyucakra,[8] Asurāntaka-cakra.[9] These are their respective names. [1]

---

[1] Sarveṣām prāninām shirasi amṛtam asti iti yogamārgena kuṇḍalinīgamane tatratya tatpravāhāplutena yoginām Īśvarasāmyam jāyate iti yogaśāstreṣu prasiddham (Comm. v. 1).

[2] Bibliotheca Indica, ed. Asiatic Society (1871). The notes are from the Commentary of Nārāyaṇa.

[3] The man-lion incarnation of Viṣṇu.

[4] Ānandātmaka; in the self of Ānanda (bliss).

[5] Good, perfect.

[6] Lustrous (Tejomaya).

[7] The Cakra which by the Śaktis of Jñāna and Kriyā protects all regions (Loka).

[8] The Cakra of the path reached by Yoga.

[9] The Cakra which is the death of all Asuras, or liars.

"Now, what are the three circles (Valaya)? These are inner, middle and outer.[1] The first is Bīja;[2] the second, Nārasiṁha-gāyatri;[3] and the third, or outer, is Mantra. Now, what is the inner circle? There are six such (for each Cakra has one); these are the Nārasiṁha, Mahālākṣmya, Sārasvata, Kāmadeva, Praṇava, Krodha-daivata (Bījas), respectively.[4] These are the six interior circles of the six Nārasiṁha-Cakras. [2]

"Now, what is the middle circle? There are six such. To each of these belong Nārasiṁhāya, Vidmahe, Vajranakhāya, Dhīmahi, Tannah, Siṁhah pracodayāt, respectively.[5] These are the six circles of the six Nārasiṁha-Cakras. Now, what are the six outer circles? The first is Ānandātmā or Ācakra; the second is Priyātmā or Sucakra; the third is Jyotirātmā or Mahā-Cakra; the fourth is Māyātmā or Sakalaloka-rakṣaṇa-Cakra; the fifth is Yogātmā or Dyu-Cakra, and the sixth is Samāptātmā or Asurāntaka-Cakra. These are the six outer circles of the six Nārasiṁha-Cakras.[6] [3]

---

[1] That is, each Cakra has three divisions—inner, middle, and outer; or Bīja, Nārasiṁha-Gāyatrī, Mantra.

[2] The root Mantra, which in this case are those given in the next note but one.

[3] That is, the Mantra. Nārasiṁhāya vidmahe vajranakhāya dhīmahi, tannah siṁhah pracodayāt. (May we contemplate on Nārasiṁha, may we meditate on his Vajra-like claws. May that man-lion direct us.)

[4] That is, the following Bījas: Kṣauṁ (in Ācakra); Śrīṁ, His Śakti (in Sucakra); Aiṁ (in Mahā-Cakra); Klīṁ (in Sakalaloka-rakṣaṇa-Cakra); Oṁ (in Dyu-Cakra); and Hūṁ (in Asurāntaka-Cakra).

[5] That is, to each of them is assigned the several parts of the Nārasiṁha-gāyatrī above-mentioned.

[6] The Ātmā as bliss, love, light or energy, Māyā, Yoga, and the concluding Cakra which is the destruction of all Asuras.

"Now, where should these be placed?[1] Let the first be placed in the heart;[2] the second in the head;[3] the third at the site of the crown-lock[4] (Śikhāyām); the fourth all over the body;[5] the fifth in all the eyes[6] (Sarveṣu netreṣu) and the sixth in all the regions[7] (Sarveṣu deśeṣu). [4]

"He who does Nyāsa of these Nārasiṁha-Cakras on two limbs becomes skilled Anuṣṭubh,[8] attains the favour of Lord Nṛsiṁha, success in all regions and amongst all beings, and (at the end) Liberation (Kaivalya). Therefore should this Nyāsa be done. This Nyāsa purifies. By this one is made perfect in worship, is pious, and pleases Nārasiṁha. By the omission thereof, on the other hand, the favour of Nṛsiṁha is not gained nor is strength, worship, nor piety generated. [5]

"He who reads this becomes versed in all Vedas, gains capacity to officiate as priest at all sacrifices, becomes like one who has bathed in all places of pilgrimage, an adept in all Mantras, and pure both within and without. He becomes the destroyer of all Rākṣasas, Bhūtas, Piśācas, Śākinīs, Pretas, and Vetālas.[9] He becomes freed of all fear; therefore should it not be spoken of to an unbeliever."[10] [6]

---

[1] That is, how should Nyāsa be done? That is explained in the text and following notes where the Nyāsa is given.

[2] Kṣauṁ Nārasiṁhāya ācakrāya ānandātmane svāhā hṛdayāya namah.

[3] Śrīṁ vidmahe sucakrāya priyātmane svāhā sirase svāhā.

[4] Aiṁ vajra-nakhāya mahā-cakrāya jyotirātmane svāhā śikhāyai vaṣat.

[5] Klīṁ dhīmahi sakala-loka-rakṣaṇa-cakrāya māyātmane svāhā kavacāya huṁ.

[6] Oṁ tanno dyu-cakrāya yogātmane svāhā netra-trayāya vauṣat.

[7] Hauṁ nṛsiṁhah pracodayāt asurāntaka-cakrāya satyātmane svāhā astrāya phat.

[8] That is, he becomes capable of speech—a poet. He knows the beginning and end of all things and is able to explain all things.

[9] Various forms of terrifying and malignant spiritual influences.

[10] That is, not to one who is not competent (Adhikārī) to receive this knowledge. Here ends the Ātharvaṇīya Ṣaṭcakropaniṣad.

Notwithstanding the universal acceptance of this Yoga, it has not escaped some modern criticism. The following passage in inverted commas is a summary [1] of that passed by an English-educated [2] Guru from one of whose disciples I received it. It was elicited by the gift of the Sanskrit text of the works here translated:

"Yoga as a means to liberation is attained by entry through the doors of Jñāna (Knowledge) and Karma (Action). Yoga is doubtless bliss, for it is the union of the Jīvātmā with the Brahman who is Bliss (Ānanda). But there are various forms of Bliss. There is, for instance, physical bliss, gross or subtle as it may be. It is a mistake to suppose that because a method of Yoga procures bliss it therefore secures liberation. In order that we be liberated we must secure that particular Bliss which is the Brahman. Some centuries ago, however, a band of Atheists (*i.e.*, the Buddhists) discovered the doctrine of the Void (Śūnyavāda), and by a false display of a new kind of Nirvāṇa-Mukti locked up these two doors which gave entry to liberation. To-day these doors are secured by three padlocks. The first is the doctrine that by faith one attains Kṛṣṇa, but where there is argument (Tarka) He is far away. The second is the error of the Brahmos, who in Western fashion think that they can control the formless, changeless Brahman by shutting their eyes in church and repeating that He is the merciful, loving Father who is ever occupied with our good, and that if He be flattered He will be pleased; for worship (Upāsanā) is flattery. The third is the opinion of those to whom all religious acts are nothing but superstition; to whom self-interest

[1] If my summary, taken from the Bengalī, points the piteous acerbities of the original, the critic would, I am sure, not complain.

[2] It is always important to record such a fact, for it generally influences the outlook on things. In some cases the mind is so westernized that it is unable to appreciate correctly ancient Indian ideas.

is the only good, and whose pleasure it is to throw dust into the eyes of others and secure the praise of those whom they have thus blinded. Viṣṇu, in order to cause the disappearance of the Vedas in the Kali age, manifested as the atheist Buddha and allowed various false doctrines, such as that of the Arhatas, to be proclaimed. Rudra was affected by the sin of destroying the head of Brahmā. Then he began to dance, and a number of Ucchiṣta (or low malignant) Rudras whose deeds are never good, issued from His body. Viṣṇu and Śiva asked each other, 'Can we do these people any good?' Their partial manifestations then promulgated Śāstras opposed to the Vedas, fitted for the atheistic bent of their minds, that they might haply thereby rise through them to higher things. God fools the wicked with such Scriptures. We must now, however, discriminate between Śāstras. It is not because it is said in Sanskrit 'Śiva says' (Śiva uvāca) that we should accept all which follows this announcement. All that is opposed to Veda and Smṛti must be rejected. Of the enemies of the Vedas [1] for whom such Śāstras were designed, some became Vaiṣṇavas, and others Śaivas. One of such Scriptures was the Tantra with a materialistic Yoga system called Ṣaṭcakra-Sādhana, which is nothing but a trickery on the part of the professional Gurus, who have not hesitated also to promulgate forged scriptures. 'The very mention of Tāntrik Śāstra fills us with shame.' The Ṣaṭ-cakra-Sādhana is a mere obstruction to spiritual advancement. The Bliss which is said to be attained by leading Kuṇḍalī to the Sahasrāra is not denied, since it is affirmed by those who say they have experienced it. But this Bliss (Ānanda) is merely a momentary superior kind of physical

[1] This no Tāntrik would, I think, admit. He would say that it is ignorance (Avidyā) which sees any differences between Veda and Āgama. The critic re-echoes some Western criticisms.

Bliss which disappears with the body, and not the Bliss which is Brahman and liberation. Mokṣa is not to be got by entering the Sahasrāra, but in leaving it by piercing the Brahma-randhra and becoming bodiless.[1]

" The Tāntrik seeks to remain in the body, and thus to obtain liberation cheaply, just as the Brahmos and Members of the Ārya-Samāja have become Brahmajñānīs (knowers of the Brahman) at a cheap price. Nectar, too, is cheap with the Tāntriks. But what is cheap is always worthless, and this shows itself when one attempts to earn some fruit from one's endeavours. ' And yet all men are attracted when they hear of Ṣaṭcakra.' Many are so steeped in Tāntrik faith that they can find nothing wrong with its Śāstras. And the Hindu now-a-days has been put in such a maze by his Tāntrik Gurus that he does not know what he wants. For centuries he has been accustomed to the Tāntrik Dharma,[2] and his eyes are therefore not clear enough to see that it is as truly unacceptable to a Hindu as it is to a Mussalman. In fact, these persons (for whose benefit this Guru makes these remarks) are full of Mlecchatā,[3] though, after all, it must be admitted to be some advance for such a creature as a Mleccha to adhere even to Tāntrik doctrine. For bad as it is, it is better than nothing at all. All the same, the Gurus delude

---

[1] It is true that complete Mukti or Kaivalya is bodiless (Videha). But there is a Mukti in which the Yogī retains his body (Jīvanmukti). In truth, there is no " leaving," for Ātmā, as Śaṁkara says, does not come and go.

[2] This, at any rate, attests its wide pervasiveness.

[3] This is a contemptuous term which has descended from the days when the stranger was looked on as an object of enmity or contempt. Just as the Greeks and Chinese called anyone not a Greek or a Chinese a " barbarian," so Hindus of the Exoteric School call all non-Hindus, whether aboriginal tribes or cultivated foreigners, Mlecchas. Mlecchatā is the state of being a Mleccha. It is to the credit of the Śākta-Tantra that it does not encourage such narrow ideas.

them with their fascinating talk about Ṣaṭcakra. Like a lot of the present-day advertisers, they offer to show their so-called 'Lotuses' to those who will join them. Men are sent to collect people to bring them to a Dīkṣā-guru (initiator). In this respect the Tāntriks act just like coolie recruiters for the tea-gardens.[1] The Tāntrik says there are really 'Lotuses' there; but if the Lotuses are really there, why are we not told how we may see them?[2] And there also are supposed to be Devatās, Dākinīs, Yoginīs, 'all ready at every moment for inspection'.[3] And, then, how material it all is! They speak of a Para-Śiva above Śiva, as if there was more than one Brahman.[4] And, then, the nectar is said to be of the colour of lac. Well, if so, it is a gross (Sthūla) and perceptible thing; and as a doctor can then squeeze it out there is not need for a Guru.[5] In short, the Tāntrik Ṣaṭcakra is nothing but 'a sweet in the hands of a child'. A child who is wayward is given a sweet to keep him quiet. But if he has sense enough to know that the sweet is given to distract him, he throws it away, and finds the key to the locked doors of Yoga, called Karma and Jñāna. This process of Yoga was expelled from Hindu society centuries ago. For nearly 2,500 years ago Śaṁkara,[6] when destroying atheism, exterminated also

---

[1] These wander about India persuading the villagers to go and work on the tea-gardens, to which they are then conveyed by means which, to say the least, are not always admirable. Truth makes it necessary to state that the allegation that the Gurus employ agents to secure followers is baseless. The Gurus of the right type as a matter of fact are very particular about the competency of the would-be disciple.

[2] The books and the Gurus claim to do so.

[3] It is not a peep-show open to any. Only those are said to see who have mastered the great difficulties in this path.

[4] There is one Brahman with His aspects.

[5] This nectar is in the body. What is perceptible is not always such a gross thing as those with which medicine is concerned.

[6] This is the Indian tradition as to the philosopher's date.

Ṣaṭcakra-Yoga.[1] Śaṁkara then showed the worthlessness of the Tantras. They are again to-day attempting to enter Hindu society, and must be again destroyed."

The writer of the note thus summarized omitted to notice or perhaps was unaware that the Cakras are mentioned in the Upaniṣads, but endeavoured to meet the fact that they are also described in the Purāṇas by the allegation that the Paurānik Cakras are in conformity with the Vedas, whereas the Tāntrik Cakras are not. It is admitted that in the Śiva-Purāṇa there is an account of the six centres, but it is said that they are not there alleged to actually exist, nor is anything mentioned of any Sādhana in connection with them. They are, it is contended, to be imagined only for the purpose of worship. In external worship Devas and Devīs are worshipped in similar Lotuses. The Purāṇas, in fact, according to this view, convert what is external worship into internal worship. If, according to the Purāṇa, one worships an interior lotus, it is not to be supposed that there is anything there. One is worshipping merely a figment of one's imagination, though it is curious to note that it is said that this figment secures certain advantages to the worshipper and the latter must commence, according to this critic, with the Cakra which he is qualified to worship. It is not obvious how any question of such competency arises when each of the Cakras is imagined only. Attention is drawn to he fact that in the Liṅga-Purāṇa there is nothing about the rousing of Kuṇḍalī, the piercing of the six centres, the drinking of nectar, and so forth. The Purāṇa merely says, "Meditate on Śiva and Devī in the different lotuses." There is, it is

[1] When Śaṁkara disputed with the Kāpālika Krakaca, the latter invoked to his aid the fierce form of Śiva called Bhairava. But on Śaṁkara's worshipping the God, the latter said to Krakaca, "Thy time has come," and absorbed His devotee into Himself. See Mādhava's Śaṁkara-vijaya, Ch. XV.

thus contended, a radical difference between the two systems. "In the Paurānik description of the Cakras everything is stated clearly; but with the Tāntrik all is mystery, or else how indeed, except by such mystification, could they dishonestly carry on their profession as Gurus?"

Buddhists may dispute this critic's understanding of their Śūnyavāda, as Tāntriks will contest his account of the origin of their Śāstra. The Historian will call in question the statement that Śaṁkara[1] abolished the Tantra. For, according to the Śaṁkara-vijaya, his action was not to abolish any of the sects existing at his time, but to reform and establish bonds of unity between them, and to induce them all through their differing methods to follow a common ideal. Thus, even though Krakaca was absorbed into his God, the extreme Tāntrik sect of Kāpālikas which he represented is said to have continued to exist with Śaṁkara's approval, though possibly in a modified form, under its leader Vatukanātha. The Brahmos, Āryasamāja, Vaiṣṇavas, and Śaivas, may resent this critic's remarks so far as they touch themselves. I am not here concerned with this religious faction, but will limit the following observations in reply to the subject in hand:

The criticism, notwithstanding its "pious" acerbity against forms of doctrine of which the writer disapproved, contains some just observations. I am not, however, here concerned to establish the reality or value of this Yoga method, nor is proof on either of these points available except through actual experiment and experience. From a doctrinal and historical point of view, however, some reply may be made. It is true that Karma and Jñāna are means for the attainment of Mokṣa. These and Bhakti (devotion) which may partake of the character of the first or the second,

---

[1] See *ante*, p. 277.

according to the nature of its display,[1] are all contained in the eight processes of yoga. Thus, they include Tapas, a form of Karma-Yoga,[2] and Dhyāna, a process of Jñāna-Yoga. As has been pointed out, the "eight-limbed" Yoga (Aṣṭāṅga-Yoga) includes Haṭha processes, such as Āsana and Prāṇāyāma. What Haṭha-Yogīs have done is to develop the physical or Haṭha processes and aspect. The true view of Haṭha-vidyā recognizes that it is an *auxiliary* of Jñāna whereby Mokṣa is obtained. It is also obviously true that all Bliss is not Mokṣa. Ānanda (Bliss) of a kind may be secured through drink or drugs, but no one supposes that this is liberating Bliss. Similarly, Haṭha-Yoga processes may secure various forms of gross or subtle bodily Bliss which are not The Bliss. There is, however, a misunderstanding of the system here described when it is described as merely materialistic. It has, like other forms of Yoga, a material side or Haṭha aspect, since man is gross, subtle, and spiritual; but it has a Jñāna aspect also. In all Yoga there is mental exercise. As the Jīva is both material and spiritual, discipline and progress in both the aspects is needed. Kuṇḍalī is aroused by Mantra, which is a form of Consciousness (Caitanya). "It is he whose being is immersed in the Brahman," who arouses the Devī Kuṇḍalī by the Mantra Hūṁkāra (v. 50). The Devī is Herself Śuddha-Sattva [3] (v. 51). "The wise and excellent Yogī, wrapt in Samādhi and devoted to the Lotus Feet of his Guru, should lead Kula-kuṇḍalī along with Jīva to Her Lord the Para-Śiva in the

---

[1] Thus, the offering of flowers and the like to the Divinity partakes of the nature of Karma; whilst Bhakti in its transcendental aspect, in which by love of the Lord the devotee is merged in Him, is a form of Samādhi.

[2] When, however, we deal with what are called the three Kāṇḍas —*viz.*, Karma, Upāsanā, and Jñāna—Tapas and the like practices form part of Upāsanā-Kāṇḍa. The above definition is for the purposes of Yoga classification only.

[3] Sattva, Atisattva, Parama-sattva, Śuddha-sattva, and Viśuddha-sattva, are five different forms of Caitanya.

abode of Liberation within the pure Lotus, and meditate upon Her who grants all desires as the Caitanyarūpā Bhagavatī (that is, the Devī whose substance is Consciousness itself); and as he leads Kula-kuṇḍalī he should make all things absorb in Her." Meditation is made on every centre in which She operates. In the Ājñā centre Manas can only unite with and be absorbed into Kuṇḍalinī by becoming one with the Jñāna-Sakti which She is, for She is all Śaktis. The Laya-Yoga is therefore a combination of Karma and Jñāna. The former mediately and the latter directly achieves Mokṣa. In the Ājñā is Manas and Om, and on this the Sādhaka meditates (v. 33). The Sādhaka's Ātmā must be transformed into a meditation on this lotus (v. 34). His Ātmā is the Dhyāna of Om, which is the inner Ātmā of those whose Buddhi is pure. He realizes that he and the Brahman are one, and that Brahman is alone real (Sat) and all else unreal (Asat). He thus becomes an Advaitavādī or one who realizes the identity of the individual and universal Self (*ib.*). The mind (Cetas) by repeated practice (Abhyāsa) is here dissolved, and such practice is mental operation itself (v. 36). For the Yogī meditating on the Mantra whereby he realizes the unity of Prāṇa and Manas closes the "house which hangs without support". That is, he disengages the Manas from all contact with the objective world (v. 36), in order to attain the Unmani-Avasthā. Here is Parama-Śiva. The Tāntrik does not suppose that there are several Śivas in the sense of several distinct Deities. The Brahman is one. Rudra, Śiva, Parama-Śiva, and so forth, are but names for different manifestations of the One. When it is said that any Devatā is in any Cakra, it is meant, that that is the seat of the operation of the Brahman, which operation in its Daiva aspect is known as Devatā. As these operations vary, so do the Devatās. The Haṁsah of the Sahasrāra contains in Himself all Devatās (v. 44). It is here in the Ājñā that the Yogī places at the time of death his Prāṇa and enters the supreme Puruṣa, "who was before the three worlds, and who is known by the Vedānta" (v. 38). It is true that this action, like others, is accompanied by Haṭha processes. But these are associated with meditation. This meditation unites Kuṇḍalinī and Jīvātmā with the Bindu which is Śiva and Śakti (Śiva-Śaktimaya), and the Yogī after such union, piercing the Brahma-randra is freed from the body at death and becomes one with Brahman (*ib.*). The secondary causal body (Kāraṇāvāntara Śarīra) above Ājñā and below Sahasrāra is to be seen only through meditation (v. 39), when perfection has been obtained in Yoga practice. V. 40 refers to Samādhi-Yoga.

Passing to the Sahasrāra, it is said, "well concealed and attainable only by great effort, is that subtle 'Void' (Śūnya) which is the chief root of Liberation" (v. 42); in Parama-Śiva are united two forms of Bliss (v. 42)—namely, Rasa or Paramānanda-Rasa (that is, the bliss of Mokṣa) and Virasa (or the bliss which is the product of the union of Śiva and Śakti). It is from the latter union that there arise the universe and the nectar which floods the lesser world (Kṣudra-brahmāṇda), or the body. The ascetic (Yati) of pure mind is instructed in the knowledge by which he realizes the unity of the Jīvātmā and Paramātmā (v. 43). It is "that most excellent of men who has controlled his mind (Niyatanija-citta)—that is, concentrated the inner faculties (Antahkaraṇa) on the Sahasrāra, and has known it—who is freed from rebirth," and thus attains Mokṣa (v. 45). He becomes Jīvanmukta, remaining only so long in the body as is necessary to work out the Karma, the activity of which has already commenced—just as a revolving wheel will yet run a little time after the cause of its revolving has ceased. It is the Bhagavatī Nirvāṇa-Kalā who grants divine liberating knowledge—that is, Tattva-Jñāna, or knowledge of the Brahman (v. 47). Within Her is Nityānanda, which is "pure Consciousness itself" (v. 49), and "is attainable only by Yogīs through pure Jñāna" (*ib.*). It is this Jñāna which secures liberation (*ib.*). The Māyā-Tantra says: "Those who are learned in Yoga say that it is the unity of Jīva and Ātmā (in Samādhi). According to the experience of others, it is the knowledge (Jñāna) of the identity of Śiva and Ātmā. The Āgamavādīs say that knowledge (Jñāna) of Śakti is Yoga. Otherwise men say that the knowledge (Jñāna) of the Purāna-Puruṣa is Yoga; and others again, the Prakṛti-vādīs declare that the knowledge of the union of Śiva and Śakti is Yoga" (v. 57). "The Devī, by dissolving Kuṇḍalinī in the Para-bindu, effects the liberation of some Sādhakas through their meditation upon the identity of Śiva and Ātmā in the Bindu. She does so in the case of others by a similar process and by meditation (Cintana) on Śakti. In other cases this is done by concentration of thought on the Parama-puruṣa and in other cases by the meditation of the Sādhaka on the union of Śiva and Śakti" (*ib.*). In fact, the worshipper of any particular Devatā should realize that he is one with the object of his worship. In Praṇava worship, for instance, the worshipper realizes his identity with the Oṁkāra. In other forms of worship he realizes his identity with Kuṇḍalinī who is embodied by the different Mantras worshipped by different worshippers. In short, Jñāna is Kriyā-Jñāna and Svarūpa-Jñāna. The latter is direct spiritual experience. The former are the meditative processes leading to it. There is here Kriya-Jñāna, and when Kuṇḍalinī unites with Śiva She gives Jñāna (Svarūpa), for Her nature (Svarūpa), as also His, is that.

After union with Śiva, Kuṇḍalinī makes Her return journey. After She has repeatedly[1] gone to Him, She

[1] This is necessary in order that the aptitude be attained. By repetition the act becomes natural, and its result in the end becomes permanent.

makes a journey from which, at the will of the Yogī, there is no return. Then the Sādhaka is Jīvanmukta. His body is preserved until such time as the active Karma is exhausted, when he can achieve bodiless (Videha) or Kaivalya-Mukti (Supreme Liberation). "The revered Lord Preceptor"—that is, Śaṁkarācārya—in his celebrated Ānanda-Laharī thus hymns Her return (v. 10):

"Kuhariṇi, Thou sprinklest all things with the stream of nectar which flows from the tips of Thy two feet; and as Thou returneth to Thine own place, Thou vivifiest and makest visible all things that were aforetime invisible; and on reaching Thy abode Thou resumest Thy snake-like coil and sleepest." That is, as Her passage upward was Laya-krama (dissolution of the Tattvas), so Her return is Sṛiṣṭi-krama (re-creation of the Tattvas). V. 54 says that the Yogī who has practised Yama and Niyama and the like (that is, the other processes of Aṣṭāṅga-Yoga, including Dhyāna with its resulting Samādhi), and whose mind has been thus controlled, is never again reborn. Gladdened by the constant realization of the Brahman, he is at peace.

Whether the method above described be or be not effectual or desirable, it must be obvious upon a perusal of the text, which gives an explanation of it, that the Yoga which the author affirms to be the cause of Liberation is not merely material, but that it is the arousing of the Power (Jīva-Śakti) of the World-Consciousness (Jagacaitanya) which makes man what he is. The Yogī thus does claim to secure the bliss of Liberation by making entry thereto through the doors of Karma and Jñāna-Yoga.

A Brahmo Author[1] who is so little favourable to the Tantra as to describe the difference between it and the

---

[1] Gāyatrīmūlaka-Ṣaṭcakrer vyākhyāna o sādhanā (Mangala Ganga Mission Press).

Veda as being "as great as that which exists between the Netherworld (Pātāla) and Heaven (Svarga)"[1] does not deny the efficiency of the Tāntrik Ṣaṭcakra-Sādhana, but contrasts it with the Vaidika-Gāyatrī-Sādhana in an account of the two methods which I here summarize in inverted commas.

"The Cakras (the existence of which is not disputed) are placed where the nerves and muscles unite."[2] The Ājñā is the place of the Command. This manifests in the operation of Buddhi. If the command is followed, the Sādhaka becomes pure of disposition (Bhāva) and speech. Speech displays itself in the throat, the region of the Viśuddha. The next lower Cakra is called Anāhata because of its connection with Nāda, which is self-produced in the heart. The Vāyu in Anāhata is Prāṇa-Śakti. Here when free from sin one can see the Ātmā. Here the Yogī realizes 'I am He'. Fire is at the navel. The seat of desire is at the root of the Svādhiṣṭhāna. In the lowest lotus, the Mūlādhāra, are the three Śaktis of Jīva—namely, Icchā, Kriyā, and Jñāna—in an unconscious unenlivened state. The Sādhaka by the aid of

[1] The unorthodox author cited, quoting the saying that "to attain Siddhi (fruition) in Śruti (study and practice of ordinances of the Vedas) the Brāhmaṇa should follow the Tantra," asks, in conformity with his views on the latter Śāstra, "How can those who are divorced from Veda get Siddhi or Śruti?" This echoes a common reproach, that the Tantra is opposed to the Vedas which the Śāstra itself denies. The Kulārṇava-Tantra speaks of it, on the contrary, as Vedātmaka. Of course it is one question to claim to be based on Veda and another whether a particular Śāstra is in fact in accordance with it. On this the Indian schools dispute, just as the Christian sects differ as to the Bible which all claim as their basis.

[2] This definition is inaccurate. As explained later, the physical ganglia are merely gross correspondences of the subtle vital Cakras which inform them.

the Parātmā as fire (Agni) and air (Vāyu) [1] awakens these three forces (Śaktis) and ultimately by the grace of the Parātmā he is united, with the Turīya-Brahman."

" In days of old, Sādhana commenced at the Mūlādhāra Cakra; that is, those who were not Sādhakas of the Gāyatri-Mantra commenced from below at the lowest centre. There was a good reason for this, for thereby the senses (Indriya) were controlled. Without such control purity of disposition (Bhāva) cannot be attained. If such purity be not gained, then the mind (Citta) cannot find its place in the heart; and if the Citta be not in the heart there can be no union with the Parātmā. The first thing, therefore, which a Sādhaka has to do is to control the senses. Those who achieved this without fixing their minds on the Lord (Īśvara) [2] had to go through many difficult and painful practices (such as the Mudrās, Bandhas, etc., mentioned later) which were necessary for the control of the Indriyas and of the action of the Guṇas. All this is unnecessary in the Gāyatrī-Sādhana or method. It is true that the senses should be controlled in the three lower centres (Cakras)—this is, cupidity (Lobha) in the Mūlādhāra, lust (Kāma) in the Svādhiṣṭhāna at the root of the genitals, and anger (Krodha) at the navel. These three passions are the chief to set the senses in motion, and are the main doors to Hell. The way, however, in which control should be effected is to place the Citta (mind) on Sattā (existence) of Paramātmā in these Cakras. The Citta should be taken to each of these three lowest centres and controlled, whereby

---

[1] The Author here refers to the processes subsequently described, whereby air is indrawn and the internal fires are set ablaze to rouse the sleeping serpent. The Parātmā is the Supreme Ātmā.

[2] This observation suggests a line of thought which is of value. Some pursue the path of devotion (Bhakti), but what of those who have it not or in less degree?

these passions which have their respective places at those centres are controlled. Whenever, therefore, the senses (Indriya) get out of control fix the Citta (mind) on the Paramātmā in the particular Cakra."

[To give the above an English turn of thought: if, say, anger is to be controlled, carry the mind to the navel, and there meditate upon the existence of the Supreme One (Paramātmā) in this centre, not merely as the Supreme without the body and within the body, but as embodied in that particular part of it; for that is Its manifestation. The result is that the passionate activity of this centre is subdued; for its functioning is attuned to the state of the Ātmā which informs it, and both the body and mind attain the peace of the Ātmā on which the self is centred.[1]]

"Having thus controlled the senses, the Gāyatrī-Sādhana commences, not at the lowest, but at the highest, of the six centres—namely, the Ājñā between the eyebrows. There is no necessity for the difficult and painful process of piercing the Cakras from below.[2] Fix the mind on the Lord (Īśvara) in the highest centre. For the ether (Ākāśa) there is the being (Sattā) of the Supreme Ātmā. There and in the two lower centres (Viśuddha and Anāhata) enjoyment is had with Īśvara. The union between Jīva and Prakṛti is called Honey (Madhu) in the Upaniṣads. By Sādhana of the Ājñā centre (Cakra) purity of being (Bhāva-śuddhi) is attained, and purity of speech follows on the attainment of such Bhāva. Yoga with the Supreme Devatā who is all-knowing is had here. He who is freed from all disturbing conditions

[1] The paragraph in brackets is mine.—A.A.

[2] This observation appears to show a misunderstanding of the specific character of the Yoga. If it is desired to rouse Kuṇḍalī, the operation must, I am told, commence at the lowest centre. There are, however, other forms of Yoga in which Kuṇḍalī is not aroused.—A.A.

of body and mind reaches the state which is beyond the Guṇas (Guṇātīta), which is that of the Supreme Brahman."

We may conclude these two criticisms with the true Indian saying somewhat inconsistently quoted in the first: "To dispute the religion (Dharma) of another is the mark of a narrow mind. O Lord! O Great Magician! with whatsoever faith or feeling we call on Thee, Thou art pleased."

Whatsoever difference there has been, or may be, as to forms and methods, whether in Upāsanā or Yoga, yet all Indian worshippers of the ancient type seek a common end in unity with Light of Consciousness, which is beyond the regions of Sun, Moon, and Fire.

It will now be asked what are the general principles which underlie the Yoga practice above described? How is it that the rousing of Kuṇḍalinī-Śakti and Her union with Śiva effects the state of ecstatic union (Samādhi) and spiritual experience which is alleged? The reader who has understood the general principles recorded in the previous sections should, if he has not already divined it, readily appreciate the answer here given.

In the first place, the preceding section will have indicated that there are two lines of Yoga—namely, Dhyāna or Bhāvanā-Yoga, and Kuṇḍalinī-Yoga, the subject of this work—and that there is a difference between the two. The First class of Yoga is that in which ecstasy (Samādhi) is attained by intellective processes (Kriyā Jñāna) of meditation and the like with the aid, it may be, in the preliminary stage of auxiliary processes of Mantra or Haṭha-Yoga[1] (other than the rousing of Kuṇḍalinī-Śakti) and by detachment from the world; the second is that Yoga in which, though intellective processes are not neglected, the creative and

[1] Such as Prāṇāyāma, Āsana. See *ante*, p. 192.

sustaining Śakti of the whole body as Kuṇḍalinī is actually and truly united with the Lord Consciousness so as to procure for the Yogī a result which the Jñāna-Yogī directly gains for himself. The Yogī makes Her introduce Him to Her Lord, and enjoys the bliss of union through Her. Though it is He who arouses Her, it is She who gives Jñāna, for She is Herself that. The Dhyāna-Yogī gains what acquaintance with the supreme state his own meditative powers can give him, and knows not the enjoyment of union with Śiva in and through his fundamental body-power. The two forms of Yoga differ both as to method and result. The Haṭha-Yogī in search of Laya regards his Yoga and its fruit as the highest. The Jñāna-Yogī thinks similarly of his own. And in fact Rāja-Yoga is generally regarded as the highest form of Yoga. Kuṇḍalinī is so renowned that many seek to know Her. Having studied the theory of this Yoga, I have often been asked "whether one can get on without it". The answer of the Śāstra is: "It depends upon what you are looking for and on your powers." If you want to rouse Kuṇḍalinī-Śakti to enjoy the bliss of union of Śiva and Śakti through Her, which your capacities do not otherwise allow you to have or if you wish to gain the accompanying powers (Siddhi),[1] it is obvious that this end can only be achieved by the Yoga here described. But if liberation is sought and the Yogī has capacity to attain it without Kuṇḍalinī, then such Yoga is not necessary, for liberation may be obtained by pure Jñāna-Yoga through detachment, the exercise, and then the stilling, of the mind without any reference to the central bodily power at all. Indeed perfect Liberation (Nirvikalpa Samādhi) can only be obtained in this way by Rāja-Yoga of which Kuṇḍalinī-Yoga is a preliminary

---

[1] Thus, by raising Kuṇḍalinī-Śakti to the Maṇipūra centre, power may (it is said) be acquired over fire.

method.[1] Samādhi may also be attained on the path of devotion (Bhakti), as on that of knowledge. Indeed, the highest devotion (Para-bhakti) is not different from knowledge. Both are realization. A Dhyāna-Yogī should not neglect his body, knowing that, as he is both mind and matter, each reacts the one upon the other. Neglect or mere mortification of the body is more apt to produce disordered imagination than a true spiritual experience. He is not concerned, however, with the body in the sense that the Haṭha-Yogī is. It is possible to be a successful Dhyāna-Yogī and yet to be weak in body and health, sick, and short-lived. His body, and not he himself, determines when he shall die. He cannot die at will. The ecstasis, which he calls "Liberation while yet living" (Jīvanmukti), is (so it was said to me) not a state like that of real Liberation. He may be still subject to a suffering body, from which he escapes only at death, when he is liberated. His ecstasy is in the nature of a meditation which passes into the Void (Bhāvanā-Samādhi) effected through negation of thought (Citta-vṛtti) and detachment from the world—a process in which the act of raising the central power of the body takes no part. By his effort[2] the mind, which is a product of Kuṇḍalinī as Prakṛti Śakti, together with its worldly desires, is stilled, so that the veil produced by mental functioning is removed from Consciousness. In Laya-Yoga Kuṇḍalinī Herself, when roused by the Yogī (for such rousing is his act and part), achieves for him this illumination. But why, it may be asked, should one trouble over the body and its central

---

[1] Subject to Dharma, Yama, Niyama, etc. In any case where the end sought is purely "spiritual" there is Vairāgya or renunciation.

[2] This makes Rāja-Yoga the highest and most difficult of Yogas, for mind is made to conquer itself. In Laya-Yoga the conquest is achieved for the sādhaka by Kuṇḍalinī-Śakti. He arouses Her and She achieves for him Siddhi. It is easier to arouse Kuṇḍalinī than to win by one's thought alone Nirvikalpa-Samādhi.

power, the more particularly that there are unusual risks and difficulties involved? The answer has been already given alleged certainty and facility of realization through the agency of the power which is Knowledge itself (Jñāna-rūpā-śaktī); an intermediate acquisition of powers (Siddhi); and both intermediate and final enjoyment. This answer may, however, usefully be developed, as a fundamental principle of the Śākta-Tantra is involved.

The Śākta-Tantra claims to give both enjoyment[1] (Bhukti) in this and the next world, and Liberation (Mukti) from all worlds. This claim is based on a profoundly true principle.[2] If the ultimate Reality is one which exists in two aspects of quiescent enjoyment of the Self in Liberation from all form and of active enjoyment of objects—that is, as pure 'Spirit' and 'Spirit' in matter—then a complete union with reality demands such unity in both of its aspects. It must be known both "here" (Iha) and "there" (Amutra). When rightly apprehended and practised, there is truth in the doctrine which teaches that man should make the best of both worlds.[3] There is no real incompatibility between the two, provided action is taken in conformity with the universal law of manifestation. It is held to be false teaching that happiness

---

[1] As there are persons who always associate with the word "enjoyment" (Bhoga) "beer and skittles," it is necessary to say that that is not the necessary implication of the word Bhoga, nor the sense in which it is here used. Philosophically, Bhoga is the perception of objects upon which enjoyment, or it may be suffering, ensues. Here any form of sense or intellectual enjoyment is intended. All life in the world of form is enjoyment. Bhoga in fact includes suffering.

[2] Which it is possible to adopt without approval of any particular *application* to which it may be put. There are some (to say the least) dangerous practices which in the hands of inferior persons have led to results which have given the Śāstra in this respect its ill repute.

[3] "Worlds," because that is the English phrase. Here, however, the antithesis is between the world (whether as earth or heaven) and liberation from all worlds.

hereafter can only be had by neglect to seek it now, or in deliberately sought for suffering and mortification. It is the one Śiva who is the supreme blissful experience, and who appears in the form of man with a life of mingled pleasure and pain. Both happiness here and the bliss of liberation here and hereafter may be attained if the identity of these Śivas be realized in every human act. This will be achieved by making every human function, without exception, a religious act of sacrifice and worship (Yajña). In the ancient Vaidik ritual, enjoyment by way of food and drink was preceded and accompanied by ceremonial sacrifice and ritual. Such enjoyment was the fruit of the sacrifice and the gift of the Gods. At a higher stage in the life of a Sādhaka it is offered to the One from whom all gifts come and of whom the Devatās are inferior limited forms. But this offering also involves a dualism from which the highest Monistic (Advaita) Sādhana of the Śākta-Tantra is free. Here the individual life and the world-life are known as one. And so the Tāntrik Sādhaka, when eating or drinking,[1] or fulfilling any other of the natural functions of the body, does so, saying and believing, Śivohaṁ ("I am Śiva"), Bhairavohaṁ ("I am Bhairava").[2] Sā-ahaṁ ("I am She").[3] It is not merely the separate individual who thus acts and enjoys. It is Śiva who does so *in* and *through* him. Such a one recognizes, as has been well said,[4] that his life and the play of all its activities are not a thing apart, to be held and pursued egotistically for its and his own separate sake, as though

---

[1] Thus in the Śākta ritual the Sādhaka who takes the wine-cup pours the wine as a libation into the mouth of Kuṇḍalinī-Śakti, the Śakti appearing in the form of himself.

[2] A name of Śiva.

[3] That is, the Mother of all appearing in the form of Her worshipper.

[4] By Sj. Aurobindo Ghose in "Arya".

enjoyment was something to be seized from life by his own unaided strength and with a sense of separateness; but his life and all its activities are conceived as part of the divine action in nature (Śakti) manifesting and operating in the form of man. He realizes in the pulsing beat of his heart the rhythm which throbs through, and is the sign of, the universal life. To neglect or to deny the needs of the body, to think of it as something not divine, is to neglect and deny that greater life of which it is a part, and to falsify the great doctrine of the unity of all and of the ultimate identity of Matter and Spirit. Governed by such a concept, even the lowliest physical needs take on a cosmic significance. The body is Śakti. Its needs are Śakti's needs; when man enjoys, it is Śakti who enjoys through him. In all he sees and does it is the Mother who looks and acts. His eyes and hands are Hers. The whole body and all its functions are Her manifestation. To fully realize Her, as such, is to perfect this particular manifestation of Hers which is himself. Man, when seeking to be the master of himself, so seeks on all the planes, physical, mental and spiritual; nor can they be severed, for they are all related, being but differing aspects of the one all-pervading Consciousness. Who is the more divine, he who neglects and spurns the body or mind that he may attain some fancied spiritual superiority, or he who rightly cherishes both as forms of the one Spirit which they clothe? Realization is more speedily and truly attained by discerning Spirit in, and as, all being and its activities, than by fleeing from and casting these aside as being either unspiritual or illusory and impediments in the path.[1] If not rightly conceived, they *may* be impediments and the cause of fall, otherwise they

[1] The first is the Tāntrik method of applying Vedāntic truth; the second, the ascetic or Māyāvādin method, with a greatness of its own, but perhaps in less conformity, with the needs of the *mass* of men.

become instruments of attainments; and what others are there to hand? And so the Kulārṇava-Tantra says: "By what men fall, by that they rise." When acts are done in the right feeling and frame of mind (Bhāva), those acts give enjoyments (Bhukti); and the repeated and prolonged Bhāva produces at length that divine experience (Tattva-jñāna) which is liberation. When the Mother is seen *in* all things, She is at length realized as She is when *beyond* them all.

These general principles have their more frequent application in the life of the world before entrance on the path of Yoga proper. The Yoga here described, is, however, also an application of these same principles in so far as it is claimed that thereby both Bhukti and Mukti are attained. Ordinarily it is said that where there is Yoga there is no Bhoga (enjoyment), but in Kaula teaching Yoga is Bhoga and Bhoga is Yoga, and the world itself becomes the seat of liberation ("Yogo bhogāyate, mokṣāyate saṁsārah").[1]

In Kuṇḍalinī-Yoga enjoyment (Bhoga), and powers (Siddhi) may be had at each of the centres to which the Central Power is brought and by continuance of the practice upward the enjoyment which is Liberation may be had.

By the lower processes of Haṭha-Yoga it is sought to attain a perfect physical body which will also be a wholly fit instrument by which the mind may function. A perfect mind again approaches, and in Samādhi passes into, pure Consciousness itself. The Haṭha-Yogī thus seeks a body which shall be as strong as steel, healthy, free from suffering and therefore long-lived. Master of the body, he is master of both life and death. His lustrous form enjoys the vitality of youth. He lives as long as be has the will to live and

---

[1] Yogo bhogāyate sākṣāt duṣkṛtaṁ sukṛtāyate,
Mokṣāyate hi saṁsārah kauladharme kuleśvari.
(Kulārṇava-Tantra)

enjoy in the world of forms. His death is the "death at will," when making the great and wonderfully expressive gesture of dissolution[1] he grandly departs. But it may be said the Haṭha-Yogīs do get sick and die. In the first place, the full discipline is one of difficulty and risk, and can only be pursued under the guidance of a skilled Guru. As the Gorakṣa-Saṁhitā says, unaided and unsuccessful practice may lead not only to disease, but death. He who seeks to conquer the Lord of Death incurs the risk of failure of a more speedy conquest by Him. All who attempt this Yoga do not, of course, succeed, or meet with the same measure of success. Those who fail, not only incur the infirmities of ordinary men, but others brought on by practices which have been ill pursued, or for which they are not fit. Those, again, who do succeed, do so in varying degree. One may prolong his life to the sacred age of 84, others to 100, others yet further. In theory, at least, those who are perfected (Siddha) go from this plane when they will. All have not the same capacity or opportunity through want of will, bodily strength, or circumstance. All may not be willing or able to follow the strict rules necessary for success. Nor does modern life offer in general the opportunities for so complete a physical culture. All men may not desire such a life, or may think the attainment of it not worth the trouble involved. Some may wish to be rid of their body, and that as speedily as possible. It is therefore said that it is easier to gain liberation than deathlessness. The former may be had by unselfishness, detachment from the world, moral and mental discipline. But to conquer death is harder than this; for these qualities and acts will not alone avail. He who does so conquer holds life in the hollow of one hand, and if he be

[1] Saṁhāra-mudrā, the gesture which signifies dissolution, "Now I am about to die".

a successful (Siddha) Yogī, liberation in the other. He has Enjoyment and Liberation. He is the Emperor who is master of the world and the possessor of the bliss which is beyond all worlds. Therefore it is claimed by the Haṭha-Yogī that every Sādhana is inferior to Haṭha-Yoga.

The Haṭha-Yogī who rouses Kuṇḍalinī gains various occult powers (Siddhi) and enjoyment thereby. At every centre to which he leads Kuṇḍalinī he experiences a special form of bliss (Ānanda) and gains special powers (Siddhi). If he has Vairāgya or distaste for these he carries Her to the Śiva of his cerebral centre, and enjoys the Supreme Bliss, which in its nature is that of Liberation, and which, when established in permanence, is Liberation itself on the loosening of the spirit and body. She who "shines like a chain of lights"—a lightning-flash—in the centre of his body is the "Inner Woman" to whom reference was made when it was said, "What need have I of any outer woman? I have an Inner Woman within myself." The Vīra ("heroic")[1] Sādhaka, knowing himself as the embodiment of Śiva (Ṣivohaṁ), unites with woman as the embodiment of Śakti on the physical plane.[2] The Divya ("divine") Sādhaka or Yogī unites within himself his own principles, female and male which are the "Heart of the Lord" (Hṛdayaṁ parameśituh)[3] or Śakti, and Her Lord Consciousness or Śiva. It is their

[1] See my "Śakti and Śākta".

[2] The statement in the Tantras that this union is liberation (Mukti) is mere Stuti—that is, praise in the Indian fashion of the subject in hand, which goes beyond the actual fact. The European reader who takes such statements *au pied de la lettre* and ridicules them makes himself (to the knowing) ridiculous. What actually happens in such case is a fugitive bliss, which, like all bliss, emanates from the Great Bliss, but is a pale reflection of it which nowise, in itself, secures immunity from future rebirth. It is the bliss of this lower Sādhana, as the union of Kuṇḍalinī-Śakti with Śiva is that of the higher.

[3] As the Parāprāveśika beautifully calls Her. Yoginīhṛdaya-Tantra says, "She is the heart, for from Her all things issue."

union which is the mystic coition (Maithuna) of the Tantras.[1] There are two forms of Union (Sāmarasya)[2]—namely, the first, which is the gross (Sthūla), or the union of the physical embodiments of the Supreme Consciousness; and the second, which is the subtle (Sūkṣma), or the union of the quiescent and active principles in Consciousness itself. It is the Latter which is Liberation.

Lastly, what in a philosophical sense is the nature of the process here described? Shortly stated, energy (Śakti) polarizes itself into two forms—namely, static or potential and dynamic as Prāṇa, the working forces of the body. Behind all activity there is a static background. The *static centre* in the human body is the central Serpent Power in the Mūlādhāra (root support). It is the power which is the static support (Ādhāra) of the whole body, and all its moving Prāṇik forces. This centre (Kendra) of power is a gross form of Cit or Consciousness—that is, in itself (Svarūpa) it is Consciousness and by appearance it is a power which, as the highest form of force, is a manifestation of it. Just as there is a distinction (though identity at base) between the supreme quiescent Consciousness and its active power (Śakti), so when Consciousness manifests as energy (Śakti), it possesses the twin aspects of potential and kinetic energy. In Advaita-Vedānta there can be no partition, in fact, of Reality. To the perfect eye of its Siddha the process of becoming is an ascription (Adhyāsa) to the ultimate Real.[3] To the eye of the Sādhaka—that is, the aspirant for Siddhi

---

[1] This, as the Yoginī-Tantra says, is the coition (Maithuna) of those who are Yati (who have controlled their passions).

[2] This term indicates the enjoyment which arises from the union of male and female, which may be either of bodies or of their inner principles.

[3] To the eye of Siddhi, to the spirit who is Udāsīna (simple witness unmindful of the external world), becoming is Adhyāsa and nothing real (in the Indian sense of that term, as used by Śaṁkara). Creation (Sṛṣti) is Vivarta, or apparent and not real evolution (Pariṇāma). Adhyāsa is attributing to something that which it does not really possess.

(perfected accomplishment)—to the spirit which is still toiling through the lower planes and variously identifying itself with them, becoming is tending to appear, and appearance is real. The Śākta-Tantra is a rendering of Vedāntic truth from this practical point of view, and represents the world-process as a polarization in Consciousness itself. This polarity as it exists in, and as, the body, is destroyed by Yoga, which disturbs the equilibrium of bodily consciousness which is the result of the maintenance of these two poles. In the human body the potential pole of energy, which is the supreme power, is stirred to action, on which the moving forces (dynamic Śakti) supported by it are drawn thereto, and the whole dynamism [1] thus engendered moves upward to unite with the quiescent Consciousness in the highest Lotus.[2] This matter has been so well put by my friend and collaborator Professor Pramathanātha Mukhyopādhyaya that I cannot improve on his account,[3] and therefore cite it in lieu of giving a further description of my own:

"When you say that Kuṇḍalī-Śakti is the primordial Śakti *at rest*, I am led to think of an analogy (and it may be more than an analogy) in modern science. Cosmic energy in its physical aspect may be considered either as static or as dynamic, the former being a condition of equilibrium, the latter a condition of motion or change of relative position.

---

[1] The projecting power of consciousness withdraws its projections into the sensuous world, and the power of Consciousness remains as Power to Be.

[2] Why here, it may be asked, seeing that Consciousness is all pervading? True; but there the Tāmasik force of Māyā is at its lowest strength. Therefore Consciousness is reached there.

[3] In a letter to me, in reply to one of mine answering some inquiries made by him as regards this Yoga. He wrote that my letter had suggested certain ideas "on a subject of supreme interest philosophically and practically in the life of a Hindu," which I reproduce in the text. The bracketed translations of the Sanskrit words are mine.

Thus a material thing apparently at rest (there being no absolute rest except in pure Consciousness or Cit) should be regarded as energy or Śakti equilibrated, the various elements of it holding one another in check (or, as the mathematicians will say, the algebraic sum of the forces being zero). Of course, in any given case the equilibrium is relative rather than absolute. The important thing to note is this polarization of Śakti into two forms—static and dynamic.

"In the tissues of a living body, again, the operative energy (whatever the nature of that may be, whether we believe in a special 'vital force' or not) polarizes itself into two similar forms—anabolic and katabolic—one tending to change and the other to conserve the tissues, the actual condition of the tissues being simply the resultant of these two co-existent or concurrent activities.

"In the mind or experience also this polarization or polarity is patent to reflection. In my own writings[1] I have constantly urged this polarity between pure Cit and the stress which is involved in it: there is a stress or Śakti developing the mind through an infinity of forms and changes but all these forms and changes are known as involved in the pure and unbounded ether of awareness (Cidākāśa). This analysis therefore exhibits the primordial Śakti in the same two polar forms as before—static and dynamic—and here the polarity is most fundamental and approaches absoluteness.

"Lastly, let us consider for one moment the atom of modern science. The chemical atom has ceased to be an atom (indivisible unit of matter). We have instead the electron theory. According to this, the so-called atom is a miniature universe very much like our own solar system.

---

[1] "Approaches to Truth" and "The Patent Wonder," two valuable presentments in modern terms of the ancient Vedantic teaching.

At the centre of this atomic system we have a charge of positive electricity round which a cloud of negative charges (called electrons) is supposed to revolve, just as myriads of planets and smaller bodies revolve round the sun. The positive and the negative charges hold each other in check, so that the atom is a condition of equilibrated energy, and does not therefore ordinarily break up, though it may possibly break up and set free its equilibrated store of energy, as probably it does in the emanations of radium. What do we notice here? The same polarity of Śakti into a static and a dynamic partner—*viz.*, the positive charge at rest at the centre, and the negative charges in motion round about the centre: a most suggestive analogy or illustration, perhaps, of the cosmic facts. The illustration may be carried into other domains of science and philosophy, but I may as well forbear going into details. For the present we may, I think, draw this important conclusion:

" Śakti, as manifesting itself in the universe, divides itself into two polar aspects—static and dynamic—which implies that you cannot have it in a dynamic form without at the same time having it in a corresponding static form, much like the poles of a magnet. In any given sphere of activity of force we must have, according to this cosmic principle, a static background—Śakti at rest or 'coiled,' as the Tantras say.

" Before I proceed, let me point out what I conceive to be the fundamental significance of our Tāntric and Purānic Kālī. This figure or Mūrti is both real and symbolic, as indeed every Mūrti in the so-called Hindu mythology is. Now, the Divine Mother Kālī is a symbol of the cosmic truth just explained. Sadāśiva, on whose breast She dances, nude and dark, is the static background of pure Cit, white and inert (Śava-rūpa) because pure Cit is in itself Svaprakāśa (self-manifest) and Niṣkriya (actionless). At the same time, apart from and beyond Consciousness there can be nothing—no power or Śakti—hence the Divine Mother stands on the bosom of the Divine Father. The Mother Herself is all activity and Guṇamayī (in Her aspect as Prakṛti composed of the Guṇas). Her nakedness means that though She encompasses all, there is nothing to encompass Herself; Her darkness means that She is inscrutable—Avāṅ-manasa-gocarā (beyond the reach of thought and speech). Of course, this is no partition of reality into two (there lies the imperfection of the Sāṁkhya doctrine of Puruṣa and Prakṛti, which is otherwise all right), but merely polarization in our experience of an indivisible fact which is the primordial (Ādyā) Śakti itself. Thus Cit is also Śakti. Śiva is Śakti and Śakti is Śiva, as the Tantras say. It is Guṇāśraya (support of Guṇas) as well as Guṇamaya (whose substance is Guṇas); Nirguṇa (attributeless) as well as Saguṇa (with attribute), as said in a well-known passage of the Caṇḍi.

"Your suggestive hint [1] makes the nature of the Kuṇḍalinī-Śakti rather clear to me. You are quite right, perhaps, in saying that the cosmic Śakti is the Samaṣṭi (collectivity) in relation to which the Kuṇḍalinī in the bodies is only the Vyaṣṭi (individual): it is an illustration, a reproduction on a miniature scale, a microcosmic plan, of the whole. The law or principle of the whole—that of macrocosmic Śakti—should therefore be found in the Kuṇḍalinī. That law we have seen to be the law of polarization into static-dynamic or potential-kinetic aspects. In the living body, therefore, there must be such polarization. Now, the Kuṇḍalinī coiled three times and a half at the Mūlādhāra is the indispensable and unfailing static-background of the dynamic Śakti operative in the whole body, carrying on processes and working out changes. The body, therefore, may be compared to a magnet with two poles.

[1] That Kuṇḍalinī is the static Śakti.

The Mūlādhāra is the static pole in relation to the rest of the body, which is dynamic; the working, the body necessarily presupposes and finds such a static support, hence perhaps[1] the name Mūlādhāra, the fundamental support. In one sense, the static Śakti at the Mūlādhāra is necessarily co-existent with the creating and evolving Śakti of the body, because the dynamic aspect or pole can never be without its static counterpart. In another sense, it is the Śakti *left over* (you have yourself pointed this out, and the italics are yours) after the Pṛthivī—the last of the Bhūtas—has been created, a magazine of power to be drawn upon and utilized for further activity, if there should arise any need for such. Taking the two senses together (yours as well as mine), Śakti at the Mūlādhāra is both co-existent with every act of creation or manifestation and is the residual effect of such act—both cause and effect, in fact—an idea which, deeply looked into, shows no real contradiction. There is, in fact, what the physicist will describe as a cycle or circuit in action. Let us take the impregnated ovum—the earliest embryological stage of the living body. In it the Kuṇḍalinī-Śakti is already present in its two polar aspects: the ovum, which the mother-element represents, one pole (possibly the static), and the spermatazoon, which is the father-element, represents the other (possibly the dynamic).[2] From their fusion proceed those processes which the biologist calls differentiation and integration; but in all this process of creation the cycle can be fairly easily traced. Shakti flows out of the germinal cell (fertilized ovum), seizes upon foreign matter, and assimilates it, and thereby grows in bulk; divides and sub-divides itself, and then again co-ordinates all its divided parts into one

[1] Certainly.

[2] The process of fertilization is dealt with in the Mātṛkābheda-Tantra.

organic whole. Now in all this we have the cycle. Seizing upon foreign matter is an outwardly directed activity, assimilation is an inwardly directed activity or return current; cell division and multiplication is an outwardly directed operation, co-ordination is inwardly directed;[1] and so on. The force in the germ-cell is overflowing, but also continuously it is flowing back into itself, the two operations presupposing and sustaining each other, as in every circuit. The given stock of force in the germ-cell, which is static so long as the fusion of the male and female elements does not take place in the womb, is the necessary starting-point of all creative activity; it is the primordial cause, therefore, in relation to the body—primordial as well as constantly given unceasing. On the other hand, the reaction of every creative action, the return current or flowing back of every unfolding overflow, constantly renews this starting force, changes it without changing its general condition of relative equilibrium (and this is quite possible, as in the case of any material system); the force in the germ-cell may therefore be also regarded as a perpetual effect, something left over and set against the working forces of the body. Many apparently inconsistent ideas enter into this conception and they have to be reconciled.

"1. We start with a force in the germ-cell which is statical at first (though, like a dicotyledon seed, or even a modern atom, it involves within itself both a statical and a dynamical pole; otherwise, from pure rest, involving no possibility of motion, no motion could ever arise). Let this be the Kuṇḍalinī coiled.

"2. Then there is creative impulse arising out of it; this is motion out of rest. By this, the Kuṇḍalinī becomes partly static and partly dynamic, or ejects, so to say, a

[1] This outflow and inflow is a common Tāntrik notion.

dynamic pole out of it in order to evolve the body, but remaining a static pole or background itself all along. In no part of the process has the Kuṇḍalinī really uncoiled itself altogether, or even curtailed its three coils and half. Without this Mūlādhāra-Śakti remaining intact no evolution could be possible at all. It is the hinge upon which everything else turns.

"3. Each creative act again reacts on the Mūlādhāra-Śakti, so that such reaction, without disturbing the relative rest of the coiled Śakti, changes its volume or intensity, but does not curtail or add to the number of coils. For instance, every natural act of respiration reacts on the coiled Śakti at the Mūlādhāra, but it does not commonly make much difference. But Prāṇāyāma powerfully reacts on it, so much so that it awakes the dormant power and sends it piercing through the centres. Now, the common description that the Kuṇḍalinī uncoils Herself then and goes up the Suṣumnā, leaving the Mūlādhāra, should, I think, be admitted with caution. That static background can never be absolutely dispensed with. As you have yourself rightly observed, 'Śakti can never be depleted, but this is how to look at it.' Precisely, the Kuṇḍalī, when powerfully worked upon by Yoga, sends forth an emanation or ejection in the likeness of Her own self (like the 'ethereal double' of the Theosophists and Spiritualists)[1] which pierces through the various centres until it becomes blended, as you point out, with the Mahā-Kuṇḍalī of Śiva at the highest or seventh centre. Thus, while this 'ethereal double' or self-ejection of the coiled power at the Mūlādhāra ascends the Suṣumnā, the coiled power itself does not and need not stir from its place. It is like a spark given from an over-saturated[2] electro-magnetic machine; or, rather,

[1] Spiritists.

[2] Overcharged.

it is like the emanations of radium which do not sensibly detract from the energy contained in it. This last, perhaps, is the closest physical parallel of the case that we are trying to understand. As a well-known passage in the Upaniṣad has it, 'The whole (Pūrṇa) is subtracted from the whole, and yet the whole remains.' I think our present case comes very near to this. The Kuṇḍalinī at the Mūlādhāra is the whole primordial Śakti in monad or germ or latency: that is why it is coiled. The Kuṇḍalinī that mounts up the Nāḍī is also the whole Śakti in a specially dynamic form—an eject likeness of the Eternal Serpent. The result of the last fusion (there are successive fusions in the various centres also) in the Sahasrāra is also the Whole, or Pūrṇa. This is how I look at it. In this conception the permanent static background is not really depleted, much less is it dispensed with.

"4. When again I say that the volume or intensity of the coiled power can be affected (though not its configuration and relative equilibrium), I do not mean to throw up the principle of conservation of energy in relation to the Kuṇḍalinī, which is the embodiment of all energy. It is merely the conversion of static (potential), energy into dynamic (kinetic) energy in part, the sum remaining constant. As we have to deal with infinities here, an exact physical rendering of this principle is not to be expected. The Yogī therefore simply 'awakens,' and never creates Śakti. By the way, the germ-cell which evolves the body does not, according to modern biology, cease to be a germ-cell in any stage of the complicated process. The original germ-cell splits up into two: one half gradually develops itself into the body of a plant or animal—this is the somatic cell; the other half remains encased within the body practically unchanged, and is transmitted in the process of reproduction to the offspring—that is, the germ-plasm. Now, this germ-plasm is unbroken through the whole line of propagation. This is Weismann's doctrine of 'continuity of the germ plasm,' which has been widely accepted, though it is but an hypothesis."

In a subsequent postscript the Professor wrote:

"1. Śakti being either static or dynamic, every dynamic form necessarily presupposes a static background. A purely dynamic activity (which is motion in its physical aspect) is impossible without a static support or ground (Ādhāra). Hence the philosophical doctrine of absolute motion or change, as taught by old Heraclitus and the Buddhists and by modern Bergson, is wrong; it is based neither upon correct logic nor upon clear intuition. The constitution of an atom reveals the static-dynamic polarization of Śakti; other and more complex forms of existence also do the same. In the living body this necessary static background is Mūlādhāra, where Śakti is Kuṇḍalinī coiled. All the functional activity of the body, starting from the development of the germ-cell, is correlated to, and sustained by the Śakti concentrated at, the Mūlādhāra. Cosmic creation, too, ending with the evolution of Pṛthivī-Tattva (it is, however, an unending process in a different sense, and there perhaps Henri Bergson, who claims that the creative impulse is ever original and resourceful, is right), also presupposes a cosmic static background (over and above Cidākāśa—ether of Consciousness), which is the Mahā-kuṇḍali-Śakti in the Cinmaya-deha (body of Consciousness) of Parameśvara or Parameśvarī (the Supreme Lord in male and female aspect). In the earliest stage of creation, when the world arises in Divine Consciousness, it requires, as the principle or pole of Tat (That), the correlate principle or pole of Aham (I); in the development of the former, the latter serves as the static background. In our own experiences, too, 'apperception' or consciousness of self is the sustaining background—a string, so to say, which holds together all the loose beads of our elements of feeling. The sustaining ground or Ādhāra, as the seat of static force, therefore is found, in one form or other, in every phase and stage of creative evolution. The absolute or ultimate form is, of course, Cit-Śakti (Consciousness as Power) itself, the unfailing Light of awareness about which our Gāyatrī (Mantra) says: 'Which sustains and impels all the activities of Buddhi.' This fact is symbolized by the Kālī-mūrti: not a mere symbol, however.

"2. My remarks about the rising or awakening of the Serpent Power at the Mūlādhāra have been, perhaps almost of the nature of a paradox. The coiled power, though awakened, uncoiled and rising, never really stirs from its place; only a sort of 'ethereal double' or 'eject' is unloosed and sent up through the system of centres. Now, in plain language, this ethereal double or eject means the dynamic equivalent of the static power concentrated at the Mūla, or root. Whenever by Prāṇāyāma of Bīja-mantra, or any other suitable means, the Mūlādhāra becomes, like an electro-magnetic machine, over-saturated (though the Kuṇḍalī-Śakti at the Mūla is infinite and exhaustless, yet the capacity of a given finite organism to contain it in a static form is limited, and therefore there may be over-saturation), a dynamic or operative equivalent of the static power is set up, possibly by a law similar to Nature's law of induction, by which the static power itself is not depleted or rendered other than static. It is not that static energy at the Mūla wholly passes over into a dynamic form—the coiled Kuṇḍalinī leaving the Mūla, thus making it a void; that cannot be, and, were it so, all dynamic operation in the body would cease directly for want of a background. The coiled power remains coiled or static, and yet something apparently passes out of the Mūla—*viz.*, the dynamic equivalent. This paradox can perhaps be explained in two ways:

"(*a*) One explanation was suggested in my main letter. The potential Kuṇḍalī-Śakti becomes partly converted into kinetic Śakti, and yet, since Śakti, even as given in the Mūla-centre, is an infinitude, it is not depleted: the potential store always remains unexhausted. I referred to a passage in the Upaniṣad about Pūrṇa. In this case the dynamic equivalent is a partial conversion of one mode of energy into another. In Laya-Yoga (here described) it is ordinarily so. When, however the infinite potential becomes an infinite kinetic—when, that is to say, the coiled power of the Mūla becomes absolutely uncoiled—we have necessarily the dissolution of the three bodies (Sthūla, Liṅga, and Kāraṇa—gross, subtle, causal), and consequently Videha-mukti (bodiless liberation), because the static background in relation to a particular form of existence has now wholly given way, according to our hypothesis. But Maha-Kuṇḍalī remains; hence individual Mukti (liberation) need not mean dissolution of Samsāra (transmigrating worlds) itself. Commonly, however, as the Tantra says, 'Pītvā pītvā punah pītva,' etc.[1]

" (*b*) The other explanation is suggested by the law of induction. Take an electro-magnetic machine;[2] if a suitable substance be placed near it, it will induce in it an equivalent and opposite kind of electro-magnetism[2] without losing its own stock of energy. In conduction, energy flows over into another thing, so that the source loses and the other thing gains what it has lost, and its gain is similar in kind to the loss. Not so induction. There the source does not lose, and the induced energy is equivalent and opposite in kind to the inducing energy. Thus a positive charge will induce an equivalent negative charge in a neighbouring object. Now, shall we suppose that the Mūlādhāra, when it becomes

[1] "Having drunk, having drunk, having again drunk," a passage in the Kulārṇava-Tantra signifying not actual drinking (as some suppose), but repeated raising of Kuṇḍalinī.

[2] We may say "Take a magnet" and "magnetism".

over-saturated, induces in the neighbouring centre (say, Svādhiṣṭhāna) a dynamic (not static) equivalent?[1] Is this what the rise of the Serpent Power really means? The explanation, I am tempted to think, is not perhaps altogether fantastic."

In reply to this highly interesting and illustrative account of my friend, I wrote suggesting some difficulties in the way of the acceptance of his statement that Kuṇḍalinī-Śakti did not, in fact, Herself uncoil and ascend, but projected upwards an emanation in the likeness of Her own self. The difficulty I felt was this: In the first place, the Yoga books, to which full credence must be given in this matter, unequivocally affirm that Kuṇḍalinī Herself does, in fact, ascend. This is borne out by some inquiries made of a Tāntrik Pandit very familiar with this Śāstra[2] after the receipt of the letter quoted. As the body of the Yogī still lives, though in an inert corpse-like condition, when consciousness of it is lost, I asked him how the body was sustained when Kuṇḍalinī left Her central abode. His answer was that it was maintained by the nectar which flows from the union of Śiva and Śakti in the Sahasrāra. This nectar is an ejection of power generated by their union. If Kuṇḍalinī does not ascend, but a mere emanative spark of Her, how (he further asked) is it that the body becomes cold and corpse-like? Would this follow if the power still remained at its centre, and merely sent forth a dynamic equivalent of itself? There were further difficulties in the theory put forward by my friend, though it may be that there are also difficulties in the acceptance of the statement that the Mūlādhāra is entirely depleted of the great power. I suggested that Kuṇḍalī was the static centre of the whole body as a

[1] Here is the seat of the first moving, or Paśyantī Śabda.

[2] Though not practising himself, his brother, from whom he had learnt, was an adept in the Yoga. His statements I have always found of peculiar value. It must, however, be remembered that, however learned or practised a Pandit or Yogī may be, it is possible for him to be ignorant of the scientific implications of his doctrine and practice.

complete conscious organism, and that each of the parts of the body and their constituent cells must have their own static centres, which would uphold such parts and cells; and that the life of the body, as a collection of material particles (from which the general organic consciousness as a whole was withdrawn), was sustained by the nectar which flowed from Kuṇḍalinī-Śakti when in union with Śiva in the Sahasrāra. In reply, Professor P. Mukhyopādhyāya dealt with the matter as follows:

"According to my presentation of the case, something—*viz.*, a dynamic equivalent or 'operative double'—is certainly sent forth from the Mūlādhāra, but this basic centre or seat is not depleted or rendered void of static energy in consequence of that operation. The Mūla (root), as the seat of static or coiled power, can never be dispensed with. It is the *sine qua non* of all functions of the triple body (gross, subtle, causal). It is, so to say, the buffer or base against which any activity of the Jiva (embodied consciousness) must react or recoil, like a naval or any other kind of heavy gun against its base or emplacement. Thus while the dynamic or uncoiled Śakti ascends the axis, the static or coiled Śakti retains its place at the Mūla, and remains as the very possibility of the dynamic upheaval. The ascending power is simply the dynamic counterpart of the static ground. To say that Kuṇḍalinī leaves its place and ascends is only to say that it ceases to be Kuṇḍalī and becomes dynamic. The ascending power is therefore uncoiled or non-Kuṇḍalinī power; it is the dynamic expression of the Kuṇḍalinī power. So far all can agree. But the question is: Is the Mūla depleted or deprived of all power (especially coiled power) when that dynamical expression leaves it and ascends the axis? Is the dynamic expression wholly at the expense of the static ground? Should the latter cease in order that the former may commence?

"Here, I think, I must answer in the negative. It is a case of Power leaving as well as remaining—leaving as dynamic and remaining as static; it is the case of the Kuṇḍalī being uncoiled in one aspect or pole and remaining still coiled in another aspect or pole. A paradox, perhaps, but, like most paradoxes, it is likely to be true.

"Is scriptural authority, which, by-the-by, I hold in utmost reverence, really challenged by this interpretation? The nature of the dynamic equivalent and its relation to the static background have been indicated in the previous two communications, and I need not dilate on them. I have claimed throughout that the Mūlādhāra, as the seat of static (*i.e.*, coiled) power, can never be rendered a vacuum in relation to such power except in the circumstances of Videha-mukti (bodiless liberation), when the triple body (gross, subtle, causal), must dissolve. I think, also, that the point of view which you have taken can be reconciled with this interpretation of the matter. The Kuṇḍalinī Śakti is the static aspect of the life of the whole organized body, as you say rightly. The relation between the lives of the individual cells and that of the whole organism is not clearly understood in science. Is the common life a merely mechanical resultant of the lives of the individual cells, or are the lives of the individual cells only detailed manifestations of the common life? In other words, is the common life cause and the cell-lives effects or *vice-versa*? Science is not yet settled on this point. As a subscriber to the Śakti-vāda (doctrine of Śakti) I am inclined, however, to give primacy to the common life; in the germ-cell itself the common life is given in substance, and the whole development of the Jīva-deha (Jīva body) is only the detailed carrying out in particulars of what has been already given in substance, according to the principle of Adṛṣṭa (Karma). Nevertheless, I am quite willing to concede to the individual cells lives of semi-independence. 'Semi,' because they require to be sustained to a considerable degree by the life of the whole. Benefit or injury to the life of the whole reacts on the condition of the cells; the death of the whole life is followed by the death of the cells, and so on.

"Now, in every cell there is, of course, static-dynamic polarity; in the whole organism, also, there is such polarity or correlation. In the whole organism the static pole or correlate is the coiled power at the Mūlādhāra, and the dynamic correlate is the operative power (the five Prāṇas--*viz.*, Prāṇa, Apāna, Samāna, Udāna, and Vyāna), which actually carries on the various functions of the body. Ordinarily, therefore, this dynamic power is distributed over the whole body, vitalizing not merely the larger tissues, but the microscopic cells. Now, the devitalization (as you say) of the body in Kuṇḍalinī-Yoga or Ṣaṭ-cakra-bheda is due, I venture to think, not to the depletion or privation of the static power at the Mūlādhāra, but to the concentration or convergence of the dynamic power ordinarily diffused over the whole body, so that the dynamic equivalent which is set up against the static background or Kuṇḍalinī-Śakti is only the diffused fivefold Prāṇa gathered home—withdrawn from the other tissues of the body—and concentrated in a line along the axis. Thus ordinarily the dynamic equivalent is the Prāṇa diffused over all the tissues; in Yoga it is converged along the axis, the static equivalent or Kuṇḍalinī-Śakti enduring in both cases. Thus also the polarity or correlation is maintained: in the former case between Śakti at Mūlādhāra and the diffused Prāṇa; in the latter case between Śakti at Mūla and the converged Prāṇa along the axis. This will perhaps adequately explain coldness, increased inertia, insensibility, etc., of the rest of the body in Kuṇḍalinī-Yoga of which you write. Commonly in Yoga this withdrawal and convergence of Prāṇa is incomplete; the residual Prāṇa, together with the lives of the cells, keeps the body alive, though inert or corpse-like. In the case of complete withdrawal and focussing, the cells will die and the body disintegrate.

"On the other hand if the coiled power were simply and wholly uncoiled (*i.e.*, dynamized) in Kuṇḍalinī-Yoga, then there should be an excess rather than a defect of vitality all over the body; nothing would be subtracted from the already available dynamic energy of the body, but something would be added to it on account of the static power at the Mūla being rendered kinetic, and going up the axis and influencing neighbouring tissues.

"Hence I should venture to conclude that the static power at the base of the axis, without itself being depleted or rendered other than static, induces or produces a dynamic equivalent which is the diffused Prāṇa of the body gathered and converged along the axis. The states in the process may thus be summarily indicated:

"1. To begin with, there is coiled power at the base of the axis and its necessary correlate, the dynamic Prāṇa, diffused all over the body in the five forms.

"2. In Kuṇḍalinī-Yoga some part of the already available dynamic Prāṇa is made to act at the base of the axis in a suitable manner, by which means the base—or particularly the four-petalled Padma (lotus) which represents this centre—becomes over-saturated, and reacts on the whole diffused dynamic power (or Prāṇa) of the body by withdrawing it from the tissues and converging it along the line of the axis. In this way the diffused dynamic equivalent becomes the converged dynamic equivalent along the axis. This is what the rising of the serpent perhaps means.

"(*a*) In thus reacting, the coiled power has not lost its general equilibrium or static condition.

"(*b*) The *modus operandi* of this reaction is difficult to indicate, but it is probably (as suggested in my previous communications) either (i) a partial conversion of the infinite coiled power into the sort of influence that can thus gather the diffused Prāṇa, and converge it in its own resultant line along the axis, or (ii) an inductive action, analogous to electro-magnetic action, by which the Prāṇas are collected and converged. In this latter case there is no need for conversion of the static energy. We shall have perhaps to choose between, or rather co-ordinate, these two explanations in understanding the *modus operandi*. In mathematical language, the diffused Prāṇa is a scalar quantity (having magnitude, but no direction), while the converged Prāṇa is a vector quantity (having both magnitude and definite direction).

"Suppose, lastly, we are witnessing with a Divya-cakṣus (inner eye) the progress of Kuṇḍalinī-Yoga. There something like condensed lightning (Taḍit) is rising from the Mūlādhāra, and gathering momentum in going up from Cakra to Cakra, till the consummation is reached at the Paramaśivasthāna) (abode of the Supreme Śiva). But look back, and behold the Kula-Kuṇḍalinī is also there at the Mūla coiled three times and a half round the Svayaṁbhū-Liṅga. She has left and yet remained or stayed, and is again coming back to Herself. Is not this vision supported by scriptural authority and the experience of the Yogī?"

Putting aside detail, the main principle appears to be that, when "wakened," Kuṇḍalinī-Śakti either Herself (or as my friend suggests in Her eject) ceases to be a static power which sustains the world-consciousness, the content of which is held only so long as She "sleeps," and, when once set in movement, is drawn to that other static centre in the thousand-petalled lotus (Sahasrāra), which is Herself in union with the Śiva-consciousness or the consciousness of ecstasy beyond the world of forms. When Kuṇḍalinī "sleeps" man is awake to this world. When She "awakes" he sleeps—that is, loses all consciousness of the world and enters his causal body. In Yoga he passes beyond to formless Consciousness.

I have only to add, without further discussion of the point, that practitioners of this Yoga claim that it is higher than any other;[1] and that the Samādhi (ecstasy) attained thereby is more perfect. The reason which they allege is this: In Dhyāna-Yoga ecstasy takes place through detachment from the world and mental concentration, leading to vacuity of mental operation (Vṛtti), or the uprising of pure Consciousness unhindered by the limitations of the mind.[2] The degree to which this unveiling of consciousness is effected depends upon the meditative powers (Jñāna-Śakti) of the Sādhaka and the extent of his detachment from the world. On the other hand Kuṇḍalinī, who is all Śaktis, and who is therefore Jñāna-Śakti itself, produces, when awakened by the Yogī, full Jñāna for him. Secondly, in the Samādhi of Dhyāna-Yoga there is no rousing and union of Kuṇḍalinī-Śakti, with the accompanying bliss and acquisition of special powers (Siddhi). Further, in Kuṇḍalinī-Yoga there is not merely a Samādhi through meditation, but through the central power of the Jīva, a power which carries with it the forces of both body and mind. The union in that sense is claimed to be more complete than that enacted through mental methods only. Though in both cases bodily consciousness is lost, in Kuṇḍalinī-Yoga not only the mind, but the body in so far as it is represented by its central power (or, maybe, its

[1] I do not say either that this is admitted or that it is a fact. Only he who has had all Yoga experiences can say. I merely here state the facts.

[2] What, I believe, the Christian Scientist calls the "mortal mind". In Indian doctrine, mind is a temporal and limited manifestation of the unlimited eternal Consciousness. As the states are different, two terms are better than one.

eject), is actually united with Śiva. This union produces an enjoyment (Bhukti) which the Dhyāna-Yogī does not possess. Whilst both the Divya-Yogī and the Vīra-Sādhaka have enjoyment (Bhukti), that of the former is infinitely more intense, being an experience of Bliss itself. The enjoyment of the Vīra-Sādhaka is but a reflection of it on the physical plane, a welling up of the true bliss through the deadening coverings and trammels of matter. Again, whilst it is said that both have liberation (Mukti), this word is used in Vīra Sādhana in a figurative sense only, indicating a bliss which is the nearest approach on the physical plane to that of Mukti, and a Bhāva or feeling of momentary union of Śiva and Śakti which ripens in the higher Yoga-Sādhana into the literal Liberation of the Yogī. He, in its fullest and literal sense, has both Enjoyment (Bhukti) and Liberation (Mukti). Hence its claim to be the Emperor of all Yogas.

However this may be, I leave at this point the subject, with the hope that others will continue the inquiry I have here initiated. It, and other matters in the Tantra Śāstra, seem to me (whatever be their inherent value) worthy of an investigation which they have not yet received.

A. A.

DESCRIPTION OF THE SIX CENTRES

ṢAṬ-CAKRA-NIRŪPAṆA

Preliminary Verse

Atha tantrānusāreṇa Ṣaṭ Cakradi kramodvataḥ
Ucyate paramānanda-nirvāha-prathamāṅkuraḥ

Now I speak of the first sprouting shoot (of the Yoga plant) of complete realization of the Brahman, which is to be achieved, according to the Tantras, by means of the six Cakras and so forth in their proper order."

Commentary

"He alone who has become acquainted with the wealth [1] of the six Lotuses [2] by Mahā-Yoga is able to explain the inner principles [3] thereof. Not even the most excellent among the wise, nor the oldest in experience, is able, without the mercy of the Guru,[4] to explain the inner principles relating to the six Lotuses, replete as they are with the greatness of Ṣa, Sa and Ha." [5]

---

[1] Paricita-ṣaḍaṁbhoja-vibhava.

[2] That is, the Ṣaṭ-cakra; six centres, which are: Mūlādhāra, Svādhiṣṭhāna, Maṇipūra. Anāhata, Viśuddha, and Ājñā.

[3] Antas-tattva—*i.e.*, relating to the ṣaṭ-cakra.

[4] Kṛpā-nātha, Lord of Mercy, *i.e.*, the Guru.

[5] Ṣa, Sa, Ha. Ṣa=Final Liberation, Sa=Knowledge. Ha=Supreme Spirit; also Brahmā, Viṣṇu and Śiva, respectively.

Now, the very merciful Pūrṇānanda-Svāmī, wishful to rescue the world sunk in the mire of misery, takes that task upon himself. He does so to guide Sādhakas;[1] to impart Tattva-jñāna,[2] which leads to liberation; and also with the desire of speaking of the union of Kuṇḍalinī[3] with the six Cakras.[4]

"*Now*" (Atha).—The force of this article is to show the connection of the book with the Author's work entitled Śrī-tattva-cintāmaṇi, the first five chapters of which deal with the rites and practices preliminary to Ṣaṭ-cakra-nirūpaṇa.[5] In this book he speaks of the first shoot of the realization of the Brahman.

Paramānanda (Supreme Bliss) means Brahman, who, says Śruti, is "Eternal (Nityaṁ) and Knowledge (Vijñānaṁ) and Bliss (Ānandaṁ)".

"*Following the Tantras*" (Tantrānusāreṇa)—*i.e.*, following the authority of the Tantras.[6]

"*First sprouting shoot*" (Prathamāṅkura)—*i.e.*, the first steps which lead to realization of the Brahman. The first cause of such realization is achieved by knowledge of the six Cakras, the Nāḍīs,[7] and so forth, which is the Tāntrika-Yoga-Sādhana.

"*Complete realization*" (Nirvāha)—The Sanskrit word means "accomplishment"; here it is the accomplishment of the immediate experimental realization of the Brahman.[8]

---

[1] Those who practise Sādhana, or spiritual discipline; here aspirants for Yoga.

[2] Tattva-jñāna=Brahma-knowledge or Brahman-knowledge.

[3] The Devī as Śabda Brahman (Śabda-brahma-rūpā Kuṇḍalinī, v. 2, *post*) in the world of the body (Piṇḍāṇda), or Kṣudra- brahmāṇda (microcosm). Verse 10 describes Her as She who maintains all beings in the world by inhalation and exhalation. Unmanifested "sound" assumes the form of Kuṇḍali in the animal body (vv. 10, 11).

[4] Mūlādhāra, etc.

[5] Ṣaṭ-cakra-nirūpaṇa. Nirūpaṇa=investigation, ascertainment into, and of the six Cakras. This forms the sixth chapter of Pūrṇānanda's Śrī-tattva-cintāmaṇi.

[6] In which is to be found a detailed description of the process here described, known as Ṣaṭ-cakra-bheda, or piercing of the six Cakras.

[7] The "nerves," or channels of energy (see v. 2). Nāḍī is derived from the root naḍ, "motion," and means a channel (Vivara).

[8] Brahma-sākṣātkāra-rūpa-niṣpattiḥ.

"*Achieved by means of the six Cakras, and other things*" (Ṣaṭ-cakrādi-kramodgata)—*i.e.*, attained by [1] meditating on the six Cakras, *viz.* : Mūlādhāra, Svādhiṣṭhāna, Maṇipūra, Anāhata, Viśuddha, and Ājñā and other things,[2] *viz*: on the Nāḍīs,[3] the Liṅgas,[4] the five Elements,[5] Śiva Śakti, etc., connected with the six Cakras, in their order.

The *order* (Krama) is, first, meditation on them, next awakening of Kuṇḍalinī, and Her passage to the Brahma lotus and then Her return therefrom; the union of Śiva and Śakti, and so forth.

"*Order*" (Krama) by which it is attained, and this is the same as Yoga practice.

The Author in substance says: "I speak of the first step (Aṅkura) of the practice which is the First Cause of the immediate or experimental realization [6] of the Brahman, brought about by a knowledge of the six Cakras, as is laid down in the Tantras."

---

[1] "Attained by". This is Udgata, which literally means "sprung out of" or "sprouted out of".

[2] According to Śaṁkara, by "other things" are meant the Sahasrāra, etc. This Śaṁkara here and hereafter referred to is a commentator on this work, and not the philosopher Śaṁkarācārya.

[3] See note 2, p. 5.

[4] In three of the Cakras—*viz.*, Svayaṁbhu, Bāṇa, and Itāra.

[5] Vyoma-pañcaka.

[6] Brahma-sākṣātkāra.

Verse 1

Merorbāhyapradeśe śaśi mihirasire savyadakṣe niṣaṇṇe
Madhye nāḍī suṣumnātritaya-guṇamayi Candrasūryagnirūpā.
Dhattūra-smera-puṣpagrathita-tamavapuḥ kandamadhyacchirahstā
Vajrākhyā meḍhradeśā cchirasi parigatā madyamessyā jvalanti.

In the space outside the Meru,[1] placed on the left and the right, are the two Sirās,[2] Śaśī[3] and Mihira.[4] The Nāḍī Suṣumnā, whose substance is the threefold Guṇas,[5] is in the middle. She is the form of Moon, Sun, and Fire;[6] Her body, a string of blooming Dhātūra[7] flowers, extends from the middle of the Kanda[8] to the Head, and the Vajrā inside Her extends, shining, from the Meḍhra[9] to the Head.

Commentary

Now, Yoga like that which is about to be spoken of cannot be achieved without a knowledge of the six Cakras and the Nāḍīs; the Author therefore describes the relative Nāḍis in this and the following two verses.

---

[1] The spinal column.

[2] *i.e.*, Nādīs.

[3] Moon—that is, the feminine, or Śakti-rūpā Nāḍī Iḍā, on the left.

[4] Sun, or the masculine Nāḍī Piṅgalā on the right.

[5] Meaning either (*v. post*) the Guṇas, Sattva, Rajas and the Tamas; or as "strings," the Nāḍī Suṣumnā with the Nāḍī Vajrā inside it, and the Nāḍī Citriṇī within the latter.

[6] That is, as Citriṇī, Vajriṇī and Suṣumnā.

[7] *Dhattūra fastuos.*

[8] The root of all the Nāḍīs (*v. post*). Kanda=Bulb.

[9] Penis.

"*In the space outside*" (Bāhya-pradeśe) the two Nāḍīs, *Śaśī* and *Mihira* (Śaśī-mihira-sire=the two Nāḍīs or Sirās, Śaktī and Mihira). Śaśī =Candra (Moon); Mihira=Sūrya (Sun). These two Nāḍīs, which are in the nature of the Moon and Sun,[1] are the Nāḍīs, Iḍa and Piṅgalā.

"*Meru.*"—This is the Meru-daṇḍa, the backbone or spinal column, extending from the Mūla (root) or Mūlādhāra to the neck. This will be explained later.

"*Placed on the left and the right*" (Savya-dakṣe niṣaṇṇe).

"*These two Nādīs.*"—"The Iḍā is placed on the left, and the Piṅgalā on the right of the Meru" says the Bhūta-śuddhi-Tantra. The Sammohana-Tantra[2] speaks of their likeness to the Sun and Moon as follows:

"The Iḍā Nādī on the left is pale, and is in the nature of the Moon[3] (Candra-svarūpiṇī). She is the Śakti-rūpā Devī,[4] and the very embodiment of nectar (Amṛta-vigrahā). On the right is the masculine Piṅgalā in the nature of the Sun. She, the great Devī, is Rudrātmikā,[5] and is lustrous red, like the filaments of the pomegranate flower."

These two Nāḍīs go upward singly from the Mūla (*i.e.*, Mūlādhāra), and, having reached the Ājñā-Cakra, proceed to the nostrils.

The Yāmala says: "On its (*i.e.*, the Meru's) left and right are Iḍā and Piṅgalā. These two go straight up, alternating from left to right and right to left, and, having thus gone round all the Lotuses, these auspicious ones proceed to the nostrils."

The above passage shows the twofold and differing positions of the two Nāḍīs. They go upward alternating from the left to right and right to left, and going round the Lotuses (Padma) they form a plait and go to the nostrils.

Elsewhere they are described as being placed like bows: "Know that the two Nāḍīs Iḍā and Piṅgalā are shaped like bows."

---

1 Candra-svarūpīṇī and Sūryarūpā.

2 Ch. iv, 5-6. The seventh verse, which is not quoted by the Commentator, runs: "Inside the Meru, she who extends from the Mūla to the place of Brahman is the fiery Suṣumṇā, the very self of all knowledge."

3 *Cf.* Rudra-yāmala, Ch. XXVII, v. 51.

4 Śakti-rūpā—the Devī as Śakti or "female".

5 Rudrātmikā—that is, of the nature of Rudra or "male".

Also[1]: "She who is connected with the left scrotum is united with the Suṣumnā, and, passing near by the right shoulder-joint, remains bent like a bow by the heart, and having reached the left shoulder-joint passes on to the nose. Similarly, She that comes from the right scrotum passes on to the left nostril."

These two Nāḍīs which come from the left and right scrotum, when they reach the space between the eyebrows, make with the Suṣumnā a plaited knot of three (Triveṇī) and proceed to the nostrils.

They are also thus described: "In the Iḍā is the Devī Yamunā, and in Piṅgalā is Sarasvatī, and in Suṣumnā dwells Gangā.[2] They form a threefold plait[3] united at the root of the Dhvaja,[4] they separate at the eyebrows, and hence it is called Triveṇī-Yoga, and bathing there[5] yields abundant fruit."

"*Whose substance is the threefold Guṇas*" (Tritaya-guṇa-mayī).—The compound word here used is capable of different interpretations. Reading Guṇa to mean "a string," it would mean "made up of three strings"—*viz.*, Suṣumna, Vajrā and Citriṇī.[6] These three form one, but considered separately they are distinct. If Guṇa be read to mean "quality," then it would mean "possessed of the qualities Sattva, Rajas and Tamas". Now, the substance of Citriṇī is Sattva (Sattvaguṇamayī), of Vajrā, Rajas, and of Suṣumnā, Tamas.

"*Is in the middle*" (Madhye)—*i.e.*, in the middle or inside the Meru.

"She who is inside the Meru from the Mūla to the region of the Brahma-randhra,"[7] etc.

---

[1] Passage is from Prapañcāsara (Vol. III, Tāntrik Texts), Ch. I, vv. 81, 82. There is a variant reading nādikā for nāsikā.

[2] Sammohana-Tantra, Ch. II, 13, thus: "In the Iḍā is the Devī Jāhnavī and Yamunā is in Piṅgalā, and Sarasvatī is in Suṣumnā"—all names of Indian sacred rivers.

[3] This is also interpreted to mean that the three Nāḍīs conjoin at the three Granthis—Brahma-granthi, Viṣṇu-granthi and Rudra-granthi.

[4] The penis.

[5] By "bathing there," etc., in the "rivers" is meant, when the mind is suffused with a full knowledge of this Cakra, great benefit is thereby attained.

[6] Suṣumnā is the outermost sheath, and Citriṇī the innermost, and within Citriṇī is Brahma-nāḍī, the channel along which Kuṇḍalī goes.

[7] Sammohana-Tantra, II, 7; also occurs in Ch. XXVII, v. 52, of Rudra-yāmala.

Tripurā-sāra-samuccaya says: "She who is within the hollow of the Daṇḍa, extending from the head to the Ādhāra" (*i.e.*, Mūlādhāra), and so forth.

Some persons rely on the following passage of the Tantra-cūḍāmaṇī, and urge that it shows that the Suṣuṁnā is outside the Meru: "O Śivā, on the left of Meru is placed the Nāḍī Iḍā, the Moon-nectar, and on its right the Sun-like Piṅgalā. Outside it (Tad-bāhye) [1] and between these two (Tayor madhye) is the fiery Suṣuṁnā."

But this is merely the opinion of these persons. Our Author speaks (in the following verse) of the Lotuses inside the Meru; and as the Suṣuṁnā supports these she must needs be within the Meru.

"*Form of Moon, Sun, and Fire*" (Candra-sūryāgni-rūpā.—Citriṇi is pale, and is the form of the Moon, Vajriṇī [2] is Sunlike, and hence has the lustre of the filaments of the pomegranate flower; Suṣuṁnā is fiery, and hence red. The Bhūta-śuddhi-Tantra, in describing the Suṣuṁnā, supports these three descriptions. Suṣuṁnā is the outermost and Citriṇī the innermost.

"Inside it, at a height of two finger's breadth, is Vajrā, and so is Citriṇī; hence it is that Suṣuṁnā is Tri-guṇā; she is tremulous like a passionate woman; she is the receptacle of the three Guṇas, Sattva, and others, and the very form of Moon, Sun and Fire."

"*From the middle of the Kanda to the Head*" (Kanda-madhyāt śirah-sthā).—Kanda is the root of all the Nāḍīs. It is spoken of as follows: "Two fingers above the anus and two fingers below the Meḍhra [3] is the Kanda-mūla, in shape like a bird's egg, and four fingers' breadth in extent. The Nāḍīs, 72,000 in number, emanate from it." The Nāḍīs come out of this Kanda.

Śirah-sthā (placed in the head): By this is to be understood that she ends in the middle of the Lotus of twelve petals which is near the pericarp of the Sahasrāra, hanging downwards in the head. See the opening verse of Pādukā-pañcaka: "I adore the twelve-petalled Lotus

[1] If Tad-bāhye be interpreted to mean outside these two, then this apparent contradiction is removed. Tad-bāhye is formed either by Tasya bāhye or Tayor bāhye: if the latter, then the meaning would be outside the two. Those who rely upon this passage read Tad-bāhye as equal to Tasya-bāhye.

[2] Vajriṇī=vajrā.

[3] Meḍhra=penis.

that is the crown of the Nāḍī along the channel (Randhra) [1] within which the Kuṇḍalī passes."

As the Citriṇī ends here, her Container, Suṣuṁnā, also ends here. If it be taken to mean that she exists above the Sahasrāra, then there will be a contradiction to the description in the fortieth verse, where the Sahasrāra is spoken of as "shining in vacant space" (Śūnya-deśe-prakāśaṁ). If Suṣuṁnā passes over it there can be no vacant space.

There are some who contend that all the three Nāḍīs—Iḍā, Piṅgalā, and Suṣuṁna—are inside the Meru, and quote the following as their authority from the Nigama-tattva-sāra: "The three Nāḍīs are said to be inside the Meru, in the middle of the back." But this cannot be; all the Tantras say that the Iḍā and Piṅgalā are outside the Meru, and on the authority of these our Author speaks of their being outside the Meru. Further, if they were inside the Meru they could not be bow-shaped and touch the hip and shoulder joints. The Nigama-tattva-sāra by the "three Nāḍīs" apparently means Suṣuṁnā, Vajrā and Citriṇī, and not Iḍā, Piṅgalā and Suṣuṁnā.

The position of the Suṣuṁnā from the Mūlādhāra to the head is thus described: "Suṣuṁnā goes forward, clinging like a Chavya-creeper [2] to the Meru, and reaching the end of the neck, O Beauteous One, she emerges and deflects, and, supporting herself on the stalk of the Śaṅkhinī,[3] goes towards the region of Brahman (Brahma-sadana).

Also *cf.*: "The other two are placed like bows. Suṣuṁnā is the embodiment of Praṇava; [4] emerging from the backbone, she goes to the forehead. Passing between the eyebrows and united with Kuṇḍalī,[5] she with her mouth [6] approaches the Brahma-randhra."

By this it becomes apparent that the backbone extends to the end of the back of the neck.

---

[1] This channel or passage within Citriṇī is Brama-nāḍ..

[2] *Tetranthera Apetala* (Colebrook's Amarakośa).

[3] Nāḍī of that name; *v. post.*

[4] Praṇavākṛti—the mantra Oṁ. This means that Praṇava manifests as the Suṣuṁnā.

[5] Devī Kuṇḍalinī; *v. ante.*

[6] Her mouth has neared the Brahma-randhra. The locative here is Sāmīpye saptamī—that is, locative in the sense of proximity. Suṣuṁnā does not actually reach Brahma-randhra, but goes near it, ending near the twelve-petalled lotus. *Cf.* v. I, Pādukā-Pañcaka.

"Supporting herself on the stalk of Śaṅkhinī," (Śaṅkhinī-nālamā laṁbya). Śaṅkhinī is thus described.

Īśvara said: "Sarasvatī and Kuhū are on either side of Suṣuṁnā; Gāndhārī and Hastijihvā again are on the right and left of Iḍā.

And again: "Between Gāndhārī and Sarasvatī is Śaṅkhinī. The Nāḍī named Śaṅkhinī goes to the left ear."

And also again: "Śaṅkhinī, emerging from the hollow of the throat, goes obliquely to the forehead, and then, O Aṁbikā,[1] united with and twisted round Citriṇī, she thereafter passes to the head."

Hence she (Śaṅkhinī) starts from Kanda-mūla, proceeds between Sarasvatī and Gāndhārī and reaches the throat, and then one of her branches proceeds obliquely to the left ear and the other goes to the top of the head.

"*Vajrā inside Her*" (Madhyame'syāḥ)—*i.e.*, inside Suṣuṁnā.

There are some who contend that the Meru-daṇḍa extends from the feet to the Brahma-randhra, and quote in support the following passage from Nigama-tattva-sāra: "The bony staff which goes from the feet[2] to the Brahma-randhra is called the Meru daṇḍa of the fourteen Lokas."

But the backbone is the spinal bone (Meru-daṇḍa). It extends from the Mūla-kanda to the end of the back of the neck. This is self-evident, and no authority can alter things which are patent. Moreover, it is impossible for one piece of bone to go to the end of the feet, for then the legs could not be bent or stretched. The Meru therefore does not go below the Mūla (Mūlādhāra). The meaning of the passage from the Nigama-tattva-sāra becomes clear if we read Pāda to mean "leg," and not "foot". "Beginning of the pāda" (Pādādhi) would then mean "where the legs begin". The sense would then be that the bone which controls the whole body from the feet right up to the head is the Meru-daṇḍa, which is like a stick, and begins from the penis, two fingers' breadth above the Mūla-kanda. The Bhūta-śuddhi-Tantra says: "Within it and two fingers' breadth above it are Vajrā and Citriṇī."

---

[1] "Mother," a title of the Devī.

[2] Pādādi, *lit.*, beginning of the pādā; *v. post.*

Verse 2

Tanmadhye citriṇī sā praṇavavilāsitā yogināṁ yogagamyā
lūtātantūpameyā sakalasarasijān merumadhyāntarasthān.
Bhittva dedīpyate tad-grathana-racanayā śuddha-bodha-svarūpā
tanamadhye brahmanāḍī haramukha-kuharadādi-devāntarātmā.

Inside her [1] is Citriṇī, who is lustrous with the lustre of the Praṇava [2] and attainable in Yoga by Yogīs. She (Citriṇī) is subtle as a spider's thread, and pierces all the Lotuses which are placed within the backbone, and is pure intelligence. [3] She (Citriṇī) is beautiful by reason of these (Lotuses) which are strung on her. Inside her (Citriṇī) is the Brahmanāḍī, [4] which extends from the orifice of the mouth of Hara [5] to the place beyond, where Ādi-deva [6] is.

Commentary

"*Inside Her*" (Tanmadhye)—*i.e.*, inside Vajrā.

"*Lustrous with the lustre of the Praṇava*" (Praṇava-vilāsitā).—She absorbs the luminous character of the Praṇava in Ājñā-cakra when she passes through it. *Cf. v.* 37, *post.*

---

[1] That is, inside Vajrā, which is, again, within Suṣumṇā.

[2] The mantra "Oṁ".

[3] Śuddha-bodha-svarūpā. From her is derived Jñāna by those who are pure (Śaṁkara).

[4] The Brahma-nāḍī is not a Nāḍī separate from Citriṇī, but the channel in the latter.

[5] Śiva; here the Svayaṁbhū-Liṅga.

[6] The Para-Bindu: *v. ib.* The Brahma-nādī reaches the proximity of, but not the Ādi-deva Himself.

"*Like a spider's thread*" (Lūtā-tantūpameyā).—She is fine like the spider's thread.

"*She pierces all the Lotuses,*" *etc.* (Sakala-sarasijān merumadhyāntara-sthān bhittvā dedīpyate).—She pierces the pericarp of the six Lotuses, and shines like a thread strung with gems.

There is a passage quoted as from the fourth Kāṇḍa of the Kalpa-Sūtra, and explained to mean: "In the hollow channel within Citriṇī are six Lotuses, and on the petals of these the Mahādevī Bhujaṅgī move about (viharanti)."

But this text, as it has given a plural verb to Bhujāṅgī [1] in the singular, seems to be incorrect. But if it be said that it is the word of Śiva, and that the plural is used as singular, it would then have to be understood that the locative in the phrase "In the channel within Citriṇī" is used as an instrumental, and the correct meaning of the passage would in that case be "that Bhujaṅgī goes along the channel within Citriṇī. And as She passes in her upward movement She pierces the Cakras, and moves about on the petals of the Cakras." Or it may also mean "that Bhujaṅgī, goes along the the hollow of the Citriṇī, and moves about on the petals of the six Lotuses within Suṣumṅā, and at length goes to Sahasrāra."

From the above authority it is not to be concluded that the six Lotuses are in the hollow of Citriṇī.[2]

"*Inside Her*" (Tan-madhye).—Within Citriṇī is Brahma-nāḍī. The word Nāḍi here means a channel (Vivara). It is derived from the root "Nada", (Nada gatau) motion. The word Brahma-nāḍī means the channel by which Kuṇḍalinī goes from the Mūlādhāra to the place of Parama-Śiva. Kuṇḍalini is a form of the Śabda-Brahman.[3] From this it is certain that the inside of Citriṇī is hollow, and there is no other Nāḍī inside her.

"*The orifice of the mouth of Hara*" (Hara-mukha-kuhara).—The orifice at the top of the Svayaṁbhū-Liṅga in the Mūlādhāra. Ādi-deva is the supreme Bindu in the pericarp of the thousand-petalled Lotus.

The rest of the verse requires no explanation.[4]

---

[1] *Lit.*, "Serpent," a name of Kuṇḍalini.

[2] Viśvanātha, quoting from Māyā-Tantra, says that all the six lotuses are attached to the Citriṇī (Citriṇī-grathitam).

[3] Śabda-Brahma-rūpā Kuṇḍalinī. The Śabda-brahman (see Introduction) is the Caitanya in all beings.

[4] Śaṁkara reads this verse in a slightly modified form, but the meaning is practically the same, the modifications being of a verbal character only.

Verse 3

Vidyanmālā-vilāsā munimanasilasat-tantu-rūpā susūkṣmā
śuddhajñanaprabodhā sakala-sukha-mayī śuddha-bodha-svabhāvā.
Brahma-dvāraṁ tadāsye pravilasati sudhādhāragamya-pradeśaṁ
granthi-sthānaṁ tadetat vadanamiti suṣuṁnākhya-nadyā lapanti.

She [1] is beautiful like a chain of lightning and fine like a (lotus) fibre, and shines in the minds of the sages. She is extremely subtle; the awakener of pure knowledge; the embodiment of all Bliss, whose true nature is pure Consciousness.[2] The Brahma-dvāra [3] shines in her mouth. This place in the entrance to the region sprinkled by ambrosia, and is called the Knot, as also the mouth of Suṣuṁnā.

Commentary

By this Śloka she is further described:

"*Fine like a* (*lotus*) *fibre and shines*" (Lasat-tantu-rūpā)—*i.e.*, She is luminous, albeit fine like the fibre in the lotus-stalk; she shines because of the presence of Kuṇḍalinī.

"*Embodiment of all bliss*" (Sakala-sukha-mayī).—Sukha is here used as the equivalent of Ānanda, which means Spiritual Bliss. She is the source of all Bliss.[4]

---

[1] That is, Citriṇī, the interior of which is called the Brahma-nāḍī.

[2] Śuddha-bodha-svabhāvā.

[3] See Commentary.

[4] Because, according to Viśvanātha, She drops nectar, and therefore contains all kinds of bliss. Śaṁkara says it is also capable of the interpretation "It is blissful to all".

"*Whose true nature is pure consciousness*" (Śuddha-bodha-svabhāvā).—Śuddha-bodha is Tattva-Jñāna, She whose Nature[1] is pure Consciousness.

"*Brahma-dvāraṁ*"[2] is the entrance and exit of Kuṇḍalinī in her passage to and from Śiva.

"*Her mouth*" (Tadāsye)—the mouth of Brahma-nāḍī, the orifice in the mouth of Hara.

"*This place*" (Tadetat)—*i.e.*, the place near the entrance.

"*The entrance to the region sprinkled by ambrosia*" (Sudhā-dhāra-gamya-pradeśaṁ).—The region which is sprinkled by the ambrosia (Sudhā) which flows from the union[3] of Parama-Śiva and Śakti, and which is attained by the help of Śiva and Śakti dwelling in the Mūlādhāra.

"*Knot*" (Granthi-sthānaṁ).—The place of the union of Suṣuṁnā and Kanda.[4]

"*Is called*"—that is, by those versed in the Āgamas.

---

[1] Sva-bhāvā is interpreted by Kālīcaraṇa to mean one's nature. Śaṁkara interprets the word to mean the Jñāna which is the Paramātmā, or, in other words, divine or spiritual Jñāna. According Śaṁkara, the reading is Śuddha-bhāva-svabhāvā.

[2] Door of Brahman.

[3] Sāmarasya, a term which is ordinarily applied to sexual union (Strīpuṁ-yogāt yat saukyaṁ tat sāmarasyaṁ)—here and elsewhere, of course, used symbolically.

[4] The root of all the Nāḍīs; see v. I, *ante*.

Verse 4

Athādhārapadmaṁ suṣumnākhya-lagnaṁ
dhvajādho gudordhvaṁ catuh-śoṇa-patraṁ.
Adhovaktramudyat-suvarṇābhavarṇaiḥ
vakarādisāntair yutaṁ veda-varṇaih.

Now we come to the Ādhāra Lotus.[1] It is attached to the mouth of the Suṣumnā, and is placed below the genitals and above the anus. It has four petals of crimson hue. Its head (mouth) hangs downwards. On its petals are the four letters from Va to Sa, of the shining colour of gold.

Commentary

After having described the Nāḍīs, the Author describes the Mūlādhāra-Cakra in detail in nine verses beginning with the present.

"*It is attached to the mouth of Suṣumnā*" (Suṣumnākhya-lagnaṁ).—The petals[2] are on four sides of the place where the Kanda[3] and Suṣumnā meet.

"*Below the genitals and above the anus*" (Dhvajādho-gudorddhvaṁ).—From below the root of the genitals to Suṣumnā.

"*Four petals of crimson hue*" (Catuh-śoṇa-patraṁ).—The four petals are red in colour. Śoṇa is the crimson colour of the red lotus.

"*On its petals are the four letters from Va to Sa*" (Vakārādisāntair-yutaṃ veda[4] varṇaih). The four letters are Va, Śa (palatal), Ṣa (cerebral),

---

[1] That is, Mūlādhāra-Cakra, so called from its being at the root of the six Cakras; see hence to v. 11, *post*.

[2] See Introduction.

[3] *V.* p. 7, *ante*.

[4] Veda-varṇa: Veda stands for "four". There are four Vedas, and the learned sometimes use the word Veda to mean four—*i.e.*, the number of the Vedas.

and Sa.[1] On each of the petals of the six Lotuses the letters of the alphabet are to be meditated upon, going round in a circle from the right (Dakṣināvartena). *Cf.* Viśvasāra-Tantra: "The petals of the Lotuses are known to contain the letters of the alphabet, and should be meditated upon as written in a circle from the right to the left."

[1] See Introduction.

Verse 5

Amuṣmin dharāyaś-catuṣkoṇa-cakraṁ
samudbhāsi śūlāṣṭakairāvṛtaṁ tat.
Lasat pītā-varṇaṁ taḍit-komalāṅgaṁ
tadante samāste dharāyāḥ svabījaṁ.

In this (Lotus) is the square region (Cakra) of Pṛthivī,[1] surrounded by eight shining spears.[2] It is of a shining yellow colour[3] and beautiful like lightning, as is also the Bīja of Dharā[4] which is within.

Commentary

In the pericarp of this Lotus is the square region Pṛthivī, which is described in detail. On the four sides and four angles of the square are eight shining spears. The region is of yellow colour.

Cf. "O Thou of dulcet speech, in the Mūlādhāra is the four-cornered region of Dharā, yellow in colour and surrounded by eight spears (Śūla) like Kulācalas."

---

[1] Earth element, which is that of this Cakra. The form of this tattva is a square.

[2] The Aṣṭa-śūla are directed towards the eight points of the compass.

[3] The colour of the earth element which presides in this Cakra. Each Tattva manifests the form, colour, and action, of its particular vibration.

[4] That is, the Bīja of Pṛthivī, the earth Tattva or "Laṁ". See Introduction.

Kulācala is by some interpreted to mean the breast of a woman. According to this view, the tips of these spears are shaped like a woman's breasts. Others understand by the expression the seven Kula Mountains.[1]

Cf. Nirvāṇa-Tantra: "O Devī, the seven Kula Mountains, *viz.*, Nīlācala, Mandara, Candra-śekhara, Himālaya, Suvela, Malaya, and Suparvata—dwell in the four corners." According to this notion, the eight spears are likened to the seven Kula Mountains on Earth.

"*Within it*" (Tad-ante).—Inside the region of Pṛthivī (Dharā maṇḍala) is the Bīja of Earth—*viz.*, "Laṁ". This Bīja is also of a yellow colour. The phrase "shining yellow colour" (Lasat-pīta-varṇaṁ) is descriptive of the Bīja also. So it has been said:

"Inside it is the Aindra-Bīja (Bīja of Indra), [2] of a yellow colour possessed of four arms, holding the thunder in one hand, mighty [3] and seated on the elephant Airāvata." [4]

---

[1] Mahendro Malayah Sahyah Śuktimān Ṛkṣaparvatah.
Vindhyaś ca Pariyātraś ca saptaite kulaparvatāh.

(quoted in Śabda-stoma-mahā-nidhi). Some read Pāriyātrah in place of Pāripātrah. Śaṁkara says that the spears are here because the Cakra is inhabited by Dākinī who is one of the great Bhairavīs.

[2] The Bīja of Indra and the Bīja of Earth are the same.

[3] Māhā-bāhu, "possessed of great long arms—sign of prowess. *Cf.* Ājānu-laṁbita-bāhu (arms reaching the knees).

[4] The elephant of Indra. This and other animals figured in the Cakras denote both qualities of the Tattva and the Vehicles (Vāhana) of the Devata therein. See Introduction.

Verse 6

Cuturbāhu-bhūṣaṁ gajendrādhi-rūḍhaṁ
tadaṅke navīnārka-tulya-prakāśaḥ.
Śiśuḥ sṛṣṭikārī lasadveda-bāhuḥ
mukhāṁbhojalakṣmiś-caturbhāgabhedaḥ.

Ornamented with four arms[1] and mounted on the King of Elephants,[2] He carries on His lap[3] the child Creator, resplendent like the young Sun, who has four lustrous arms, and the wealth of whose lotus-face is fourfold.[4]

Commentary

This is the Dhyāna of the Dharā-Bīja. The Bīja of Dharā or Pṛthivī is identical with that of Indra.

"*On his lap*" (Tad-aṅke)—*i.e.*, in the lap of Dharā-Bīja. The sense of this verse is that the Creator Brahmā dwells in the lap of Dharā-Bīja. By "aṅka" (lap) is to be understood the space within the Bindu or Dharā-Bīja. *Cf.* "In the Mūlādhāra is the Dharā-Bīja, and in its Bindu dwells Brahmā, the image of a Child, and King of the Immortals,[5] is mounted on an Elephant."

The above quoted passage, it is urged, means "the King of the Immortals is in the lap of Dharā-Bīja." But according to our view, as the Dharā-Bīja and the Indra-Bīja are the same, their identity is here spoken of; for it is also said, "the letters of the Mantra are the Devatā; the Devatā is in the form of Mantra (Mantra-rūpiṇī).

---

[1] These two adjectival phrases qualify Dharā-Bīja.

[2] Airāvata.

[3] That is, the Bindu of the Bīja (Dharā) or "Laṁ". This is explained, *post*.

[4] Brahmā is represented with four heads.

[5] *i.e.*, Indra-Deva.

Also *Cf.* Nirvāṇa-Tantra: "O beautiful one, the Indra Bīja is below the genitals. The very perfect and beautiful dwelling of Brahmā is above Nāda, and there dwells Brahmā the Creator,[1] the Lord of creatures[2]."

By "above Nāda" in this passage, we must understand that the abode of Brahmā is within the Bindu which is above Nāda. Some read "left of the genitals, and thus there is a difference of opinion. The Śāradā says that the Ādhāras are various according to different views.

"*Four lustrous arms*" (Lasad-veda[3]-bāhu).—Some interpret the Sanskrit compound word to mean "in whose arms shine the four Vedas, Sāma and others," thus thinking of Brahmā as being possessed of two arms only. But Brahmā is nowhere described as holding the Vedas in his hands, and that he should be meditated upon as having four arms is clear from the following passage in Bhūta-śuddhi-Tantra.

"Know, O Śivā, that in its lap is the four-armed, red-coloured child[4] Brahmā, who has four faces and is seated on the back of a swan."[5]

"*The wealth of whose lotus-face is fourfold*" (Mukhāṁbhojalakṣmīh catur-bhāga-bhedah).—By this is to be understood that Brahmā has four faces.

Some read the passage as "Catur-bhāgaveda"; thus read, the meaning practically is the same. If the Sanskrit text is read "Mukhāṁbhoja-lakṣmī-catur-bhāgaveda," the meaning would be," the four different Vedas enhance the beauty of his lotus-faces".[6]

As opposed to the opinion that Brahmā holds the four Vedas in his arms, the Viśva-sāra-Tantra in the Brāhmī-dhyāna says: "Meditate on Brāhmī (Śakti) as red in colour and garbed in the skin of the black antelope, and as holding the staff,[7] gourd,[8] the rosary of Rudrākṣa

---

[1] Sṛṣti-kartā.

[2] Prajā-pati.

[3] Veda is used to mean four, there being four Vedas.

[4] *i.e.*, Hiraṇya-garbha.

[5] Hamsa, or, as some say, goose or flamingo. See Woodroffe's "Garland of Letters", p. 155.

[6] The allusion is to the belief that the four Vedas came out of the four mouths of Brahmā.

[7] Daṇda.

[8] Kamaṇḍalu.

beads,[1] and making the gesture dispelling fear."[2] And in the Saptaśatī-Stotra[3] it has been said that Śiva and Śakti are to be meditated upon as having the same weapons.

Also *cf.* Yāmala: "The Ādi-Mūrti[4] should be meditated upon as making the gestures of dispelling fear and granting boons,[5] as also holding the Kuṇḍikā[6] and rosary of Rudrākṣa beads, and adorned with fine ornament."

This is how She should be meditated upon. The rest requires no explanation.

---

[1] Akṣa-sūtra.

[2] That is, the Abhaya-mudrā. The hand is uplifted, the palm being shown to the spectator. The four fingers are close together, and the thumb crosses the palm to the fourth finger.

[3] Mārkaṇḍeya-Caṇḍī.

[4] Brāhmī-Śakti.

[5] That is, the Varada-mudrā, the hand being held in the same position as in note 4 above, but with the palm held horizontally instead of vertically.

[6] Kamaṇḍalu: a vessel with a gourd-shaped body, and handle at the top, used for carrying water, generally by ascetics.

Verse 7

Vasedatra devī ca ḍākinyabhikhyā
lasadveda bā-hūjjvalā rakta-netrā
Samānoditāneka-sūrya-prakāśā
prakāśaṁ vahantī sadā śuddha-buddheḥ

Here dwells the Devī Dākinī[1] by name; her four arms shine with beauty, and her eyes are brilliant red. She is resplendent like the lustre of many Suns rising at one and the same time.[2] She is the carrier of the revelation of the ever-pure Intelligence.[3]

Commentary

In this Śloka the Author speaks of the presence of Dākinī-Śakti in the Ādhāra-Padma. The sense of this verse is that in this Lotus the Devī Dākinī dwells.

"*She is the Carrier of the revelation of the ever-pure Intelligence*"[4] (Prakāśam vahantī sadā śuddha-buddheḥ)—that is, she, Dākinī-Śakti, enables the Yogī to acquire knowledge of the Tattva (Tattva-Jñāna). By meditating on her, which is part of Yoga practice, one acquires Tattva-Jñāna. This Devī is the presiding Divinity of this region.

---

[1] Dākinī and other Śaktis of this class are in some Tantras called the Queens of the Cakras, and in others the doorrkeepers thereof.

[2] That is, according to Viśvanātha, she is very red.

[3] Śuddha-buddhi—*i.e.*, Tattva-Jñāna.

[4] If the word "sadā" is read separately from "śuddha-buddhi," it becomes an adverb qualifying "vahantī" and the passage would then mean that "she ever carries revelation of Divine Knowledge".

Cf. "The mouth[1] (the lotus) has the letters Va, Śa (palatal), Ṣa (lingual), and Sa, and is presided over by Dākinī."

"Dākinī, Rākinī, Kākinī, Lākinī, as also Śākinī and Hākinī, are the queens of the six respective Lotuses."[2] Elsewhere is given the Dhyāna of Dākinī thus: "Meditate on her, the red, the red-eyed Dākinī, in the Mūlādhāra, who strikes terror into the hearts of Paśus,[3] who holds in her two right hands the Spear[4] and the Khaṭvāṅga,[5] and in her two left hands the Sword[6] and a drinking-cup filled with wine. She is fierce of temper and shows her fierce teeth. She crushes the whole host of enemies. She is plump of body, and is fond of Pāyasānna.[7] It is thus that she should be meditated upon by those who desire immortality." Elsewhere she is described as "bright with a Tilaka[8] of vermilion, her eyes ornamented with collyrium, clad in black (antelope's skin) and decked with varied jewels," etc.

On the authority of the above passage, which occurs in a Dhyāna of Dākinī, she should be meditated upon as clad in black antelope skin.

The Devas Brahmā and others are to be meditated upon as having their faces down or up according to the frame of mind (Bhāva) of the Sādhaka.

The Śāktānanda-taraṅgiṇī[9] quotes the following from the Māyā-Tantra:

"Pārvatī asked: How can they be in the Lotuses which have their heads downward bent?

---

[1] Vaktra. This is possibly the transcriber's mistake for "Padma"= lotus.

[2] The Śāktānanda-taraṅgiṇī places them in a different order. See P. K. Śāstrī's edition, p. 75.

[3] The unillumined. See "Introduction to Tantra Śāstra".

[4] Śūla.

[5] A staff surmounted by a human skull.

[6] Khaḍga, a kind of sword used in the sacrifice of animals. Some read Kheta.

[7] A kind of milk pudding made of rice boiled in milk with ghee and sugar.

[8] Here the mark borne by a woman between the eyebrows showing that her husband is living—an auspicious mark. The Saubhāgyaratnākara says that Dākinī abides in Tvak-Dhātu.

[9] Fourth chapter; Prasanna Kumāra-Śāstrī's edition, pp. 78, 79. The passage in the text is incompletely quoted.

"Mahādeva said: The Lotuses, O Devī, have their heads in different directions. In the life of action [1] they should be thought of as having their heads downward, but in the path of renunciation [2] they are always meditated upon as having their heads upward turned."

The rest is clear.

[1] Pṛavrtti-mārga: the outgoing path as distinguished from the Nivṛtti-mārga, or the path of return to the Para-brahman.

[2] Nivṛtti-mārga.

Verse 8

Vajrākhyā viaktradeśe vlasati satataṁ karṇikā-madhyasaṁsṭhaṁ
koṇaṁ tat traipurākhyaṁ taḍidiva vilasat-komalaṁ kāmarūpam
Kandarpo nāma vayur nivasati satataṁ tasya madhye samantāt
jīveśo bandhu-jīva-prakaramabhí-hasan koṭisūrya-prakāṣaḥ

Near the mouth of the Nāḍī called Vajrā, and in the pericarp (of the Ādhāra Lotus), there constantly shines the beautifully luminous and soft, lightning-like triangle which is Kāmarūpa,[1] and known as Traipura.[2] There is always and everywhere the Vāyu called Kandarpa,[3] who is of a deeper red than the Bandhujīva flower,[4] and is the Lord of Beings and resplendent like ten million suns.

Commentary

In this Śloka is described the triangle in the pericarp of the Mūla-Cakra.

"*Near the mouth of the Nāḍī called Vajrā*" (Vajrākhyā-viaktradeśe).—The mouth of the Vajrā is two fingers above that of the Suṣuṁnā and below the base of the genitals.

"*The triangle known as Traipura*" (Trikoṇaṁ traipurākhyaṁ).—The triangle, is so called because of the presence of the Devī Tripurā

[1] See Commentary, *post*.

[2] This triangle, says Viśvanātha, citing Gautamīya-Tantra is Icchā-Jñāna-Kriyātmaka—that is, the powers of Will, Knowledge and Action. See Introduction.

[3] A Form of the Apāna-Vāyu. Kandarpa is a name of Kāma, the Deva of Love.

[4] *Pentapœles Phœnicea.*

within the Ka inside the triangle, and the letter Ka is the chief letter of the Kāma-bija.[1]

Cf. Śāktānanda-taraṅgiṇī [2]: "Inside dwells the Devi Sundarī,[3] the Paradevatā."

"*Soft*" (Komala)—*i.e.*, oily and smooth.

"*Kāma-rūpa*" [4]: that by which Kāma is caused to be felt—*i.e.*, it is Madanāgārātmaka.[5]

Cf. "The triangle should be known as the charming Śakti-pīṭha."

This triangle is above the Dharā-bīja. *Cf.* Sammohana-Tantra, speaking of Dharā-bīja: "Above it (Dharā-bīja) are three lines—Vāmā, Jyeṣṭā, and Raudrī."

"*Kandarpa*"—The presence in the Trikona of the Kandarpavāyu is here spoken of. It is *everywhere* (samantāt) that is, extended throughout the triangle.

"*Lord of Beings*" (Jīveśa).—So called because the continuance of life depends on Kāma or Kandarpa.

It is said that "In the Kanda (heart) region dwells Prāṇa; and Apāna dwells in the region of the anus." The air in the region of the anus is Apāna, and Kandarpa-Vāyu accordingly is a part of Apāna-Vāyu.[6] It is also said that [7] "Apāna draws Prāṇa, and Prāṇa draws Apāna—just as a falcon attached by a string is drawn back again when he flies away; these two by their disagreement prevent each other from leaving the body, but when in accord they leave it."

The two Vāyus, Prāṇa and Apāna, go different ways, pulling at one another; and neither of them, therefore, can leave the body, but

---

[1] That is, the Mantra "Klīṁ"; in Tantrarāja Śiva speaking to Devī says, "letter Ka is Thy form" The Nitya-pūjā-paddati, p. 80, mentions in this connection "Kaṁ," the Bīja of Kāminī.

[2] When dealing with the Kakāra-tattva, p. 165, Prasanna Kumāra-Śāstrī's edition.

[3] Sundari—*i.e.*, Tripura-sundarī, a name of the Devī. See Trantrarāja (Tāntrik Texts, VIII, Chs. 4-6).

[4] Śaṁkara defines this as "the embodiment of the devotee's desire" (Bhaktābhilāṣa-svarūpaṁ).

[5] Chamber of Madana (Deva of Love)—the Yoni.

[6] Vāyu here is a name for a manifestation of Prāna, the five most important of such manifestations being Prāna, Apāna Samāna, Vyāna, Udāna. See Introduction.

[7] This is an oft-repeated passage (Śāktānanda, p. 5).

when the two are in accord—that is, go in the same direction—they leave the body. Kandarpa-Vāyu, being a part of Apāna also pulls at Prāṇa-Vāyu, and prevents the latter from escaping from the body, hence Kandarpa-Vāyu is the Lord of Life.

In v. 10 the Author describes Kuṇḍalinī as " She who maintains all the beings of the world by Inspiration and Expiration." [1] He himself has thus said that Prāṇa and Apāna are the maintainers of animate being.

[1] The Inspired and Expired breath is Hamsaḥ.

Verse 9

Tanmadhye liṅgarūpī druta-kanaka-kalā-komalaḥ paścimāsyaḥ
jñāna dhyānaprakāśaḥ prathamakisalayākārarūpaḥ svayaṃbhuḥ
Vidyutpūrṇēṇdubiṁba-prakara-karacaya-snigdha-saṁtānahāsī
kāśīvāsí vilāsī vilasati saridāvartarūpaprakāraḥ

Inside it (the triangle) is Svayaṁbhu[1] in His Liṅga-form,[2] beautiful like molten gold, with His head downwards. He is revealed by Knowledge[3] and Meditation,[4] and is of the shape and colour of a new leaf. As the cool rays of lightning and of the full moon charm, so does His beauty. The Deva who resides happily here as in Kāśī is in forms like a whirlpool.[5]

Commentary

In this verse he speaks of the presence of the Svayaṁbhu-Liṅga in the triangle.

"*Svayaṁbhu in his Liṅga-form*" (Liṅga-rūpī svayaṁbhu)—*i.e.*, here dwells the Śiva-Liṅga whose name is Svayaṁbhu.

"*Beautiful like molten gold*" (Druta-kanaka-kalā-komala).—His body has the soft lustre of molten gold.

"*His head downwards*" (Paścimāsya).—*Cf.* Kālī-kulāmṛta: "There is placed the great Liṅga Svayaṁbhu, who is ever blissful, his head downward, active when moved by Kāma-Bīja."

---

[1] "Self-originated," "self-existent," the Śiva-Liṅga of that name.

[2] As the human phallus.

[3] Jñāna.

[4] Dhyāna.

[5] This refers to a depression on the top of the Liṅga.

"*Revealed by Knowledge and Meditation*" (Jñāna-dhyāna-prakāśa).—Whose existence is apprehended by us by Knowledge (Jñāna) and Meditation (Dhyāna). By Jñāna we realize the attributelessness and by Dhyāna the attributefulness (of the Brahman). Such is Svayaṁbhu.

"*The shape and colour of new leaves*" (Prathama-kisalayā-kāra-rūpa).—By this is conveyed the idea that the shape of the Svayaṁbhū-Liṅga is tapering like a new unopened leaf-bud. Like the pistil inside the Caṁpaka flower, it is broad at the bottom and tapers to a point at the end; this also shows that the Svayaṁbhu-Liṅga is of a blue-green colour (Śyāma).

Cf. Śāktānanda-taraṅginī: "O Maheśāni, meditate inside it (the triangle) upon the Svayṁbhu-Liṅga, who holds his head with an aperture therein downward—the beautiful and blue-green Śiva (Śivaṁ Śyāmala-sundaraṁ)."

In the Yāmala occurs the following passage: "Meditate upon the very beautiful celestial triangle (Trikoṇa) in the Mūlādhāra; within its three lines is Kuṇḍalī, charming like ten million lightning flashes in the dark blue [1] clouds."

This passage, which describes Kuṇḍalī as "lightning in the dark blue clouds," goes to show that the Svayammṁbhu-Liṅga is also blue; but Nīla (blue) and Śyāma (dark green) belong to the same category, and hence there is no contradiction.

As the cool rays of lightning and of the full moon charm, so does His beauty" (Vidyut-pūrṇēṇdu-biṁba-prakarakāra [2]-caya-snigdha-saṁtāna-hāsī).—As the strong light of the moon and of lightning emits no heat, so is the light which emanates from the Svayaṁbhu-Liṅga cool and pleasing bringing gladness into the hearts of men.

"*The Deva who resides happily here as in Kāśī*" [3] (Kāśī-vāsi-vilāsī). Kāśī is the place sacred to Śiva, His favourite abode. By these two adjectives it is implied that the Svayaṁbhu in the Ādhāra Lotus is happy as He is in His form of Viśveśvara in Kāśī, and He is as pleased to be here as at Kāśī. "Vilāsī" may also mean amorous because it has been

---

[1] Nīla.

[2] Viśvanātha for Kara (ray) reads Rasa—that is, the nectar flowing from the Moon.

[3] Benares or Vārāṇasī.

said above, "moved by Kāma-Bīja". Vilāsī is indicative of His Lordship of the Universe. [1]

"*Like a whirlpool*" (Sarid-āvarta-rūpa-prakāra).—The whirling water on its outer edge creates a depression in the middle and the centre thereof is raised like the shape of a conch. [2]

This Svayaṁbhu is placed on the Kāma-bīja. This has been said in Kālī-Kulāmṛta: "Surrounded by the filaments of the lotus, is the Śṛṅgāṭa [3] and over this is the beautiful Mahā-Liṅga Svayaṁbhu, with an opening on the top, ever happy, holding his head downwards, and active when moved by the Kāma-bījā."

Elsewhere the following occurs: "There, in the pericarp, is the above-mentioned Ḍākinī and thd triangle (Trikoṇa) within which is a small aperture and the red Kāma-bīja. There is also the Svayaṁbhu-Liṅga, his head downward and of a ruddy hue." This is, however, a different conception.

---

[1] The Universe is His Vilāsa or Līla.

[2] Śaṁkara says that he is so described because o his restless motion.

[3] The triangular pyramidical seat of Kāmā.

Verses 10 and 11 [1]

Tasyordhve bisatantu sodara-lasat sūkṣmā jaganmohinī
brahmavāramukhaṁ mukhena madhuraṁ saṁchadayantī svayaṁ
Śaṅkhāvarta nibhā navīna capalāmālā vilāsāspadā
suptā-sarpasamā śvopari lasāt sārdha-trivṛttākṛtiḥ

Kūjantī kulakuṇḍalī ca madhuraṁ mattalimālā-sphuṭaṁ
vācāṁ komalakāvya-bandharacanā bhedātibheda-kramaiḥ
Śvāsocchvāsa-vibhañjanena jagatāṁ jīvo yayā dhāryate
sā mūlāṁbuja gahvare vilasati proddāma-dīptāvaliḥ

Over it [2] shines the sleeping Kuṇḍalinī, fine as the fibre of the lotus-stalk. She is the world-bewilderer,[3] gently covering the mouth of Brahma-dvāra [4] by Her own. Like the spiral of the conch-shell, Her shining snake-like form goes three and a half times round Śiva,[5] and Her lustre is as that of a strong flash of young strong lightning. Her sweet murmur is like the indistinct hum of swarms of love-mad bees.[6] She produces

[1] Śaṁkara, unlike Kālīcaraṇa, has annotated the two verses separately.

[2] Svayaṁbhu-Liṅga—that is, round It with her body and over It with Her head.

[3] Kuṇḍalinī is the Śakti whereby the Māyik world exists, at rest. In the Kūrma-Purāṇa, Śiva says: "This Supreme Śakti is in me, and is Brahman Itself. This Māyā is dear to me, by which this world is bewildered." Hence the Devī in the Lalitā is called Sarvamohinī (all-bewildering).

[4] See Commentary.

[5] Śivopari.

[6] Viśvanātha says She makes this sound when awakened. According to Śaṁkara, this indicates the Vaikharī state of Kuṇḍalinī.

melodious poetry and Bandha[1] and all other compositions in prose or verse in sequence or otherwise[2] in Saṁskṛta, Prākṛta and other languages. It is She who maintains all the beings of the world by means of inspiration and expiration,[3] and shines in the cavity of the root (Mūla) Lotus like a chain of brilliant lights.

Commentary

In these two verses the author speaks of the presence of Kuṇḍalinī-Śakti in the Svayaṁbhu-Liṅga. It is the Devī Kuṇḍalinī who maintains the existence of individual beings (Jīva, Jīvātmā) by the functions of inspiration and expiration. She places them in individual bodies; She produces the humming sound resembling that of a swarm of bees, and is the source of Speech and She, as described below, dwells in the triangular hollow in the pericarp of the Mūlādhāra Lotus resting upon the Svayaṁbhu-Liṅga.

"*Shines fine as the fibres of the lotus stalk*" (Bisa-tantu-sodara-lasat-sūkṣmā)—*i.e.*, She is fine like the fibre of the lotus-stalk.

"*World-bewilderer*" (Jagan-mohinī)—*i.e.*, She is Māyā in this world.

"*Gently.*"[4]—Madhuraṁ.

"*The mouth of Brahma-dvāra*" (Brahma-dvāra-mukha)—the hollow on the head of Svayaṁbhu-Liṅga.

"*A strong flash of young lightning*" (Navīna-capalā-mālā-vilāsāspadā). —*Lit.*, "possessed of the wealth of a strong flash of young lightning." In youth every thing and person shows the characteristic qualities in a state of vigorous perfection. Hence a "young flash of lightning" means a strong flash.

"*She produces melodious poetry etc.*" (Komala-kāvya-banda-racana-bhedātibheda-krama).—This shows the mode in which words are produced.

---

[1] Is a class of literary composition in which the verse is arranged in the manner of a diagram or picture.

[2] Bheda-krama and Ati-bheda-krama.

[3] Viśvanātha quotes Dakṣiṇāmūrti as stating that during day and night man breathes in and out 21,600 times, taking both expiration and inspiration as the unit. See Introduction.

[4] Madhuraṁ: this is used as an adjective, according to Śaṁkara, and means sweet. He says She is drinking nectar by the Brahma-dvāra; as the nectar is coming through it, the Brahma-dvāra is sweet.

The soft music produced by a combination of soft and melodious words descriptive of beauty, virtue, etc., in all its modulations, resulting from perfecting of composition and regularity and irregularity in the disposition of words. By *Bandha* is here meant pictorial poetical composition in prose or verse arranged to look like a lotus (Padma-bandha), a horse (Aśva-bandha) and so on; and by *Ati-bheda* the author alludes to all the words in Saṁskṛta and Prākṛta. By using the word "order, sequence," the author emphasizes the fact that these compositions and words come out in the order laid down in the Śāstras. Kuṇḍalinī produces, both at random, and in set forms. Kuṇḍalinī produces words, Saṁskṛta and Prākṛta, distinct and indistinct. She is the source from which all sound emanates.

Cf. Śāradā [1]: "Upon the (bursting unfolding) of the supreme Bindu arose unmanifested Sound [2] (Avyakta-rava). It assumed the form of Kuṇḍalī in living bodies, and manifested itself in prose and verse by the aid of the letters of the Alphabet (*lit.*, the essence of the letters)."

By "Prose and Verse" all forms of speech are meant.

It has distinctly been said in Kādimata [3]: "By the action of the Icchā-Śakti of the Ātmā acting on Prāṇa-Vāyu there is produced in the Mūlādhāra the excellent Nāda (Sound) called Parā.[4] In its ascending movement it is thrown upward and opening out in the Svādhiṣṭhāna,[5] it receives the name of Paśyantī; and again gently led up as before

---

[1] Ch. I, second line of v. 11 and v. 14; the intermediate verses are omitted. These run as follows: "That sound is called, by those versed in the Āgamas, Śabda-brahman. Some teachers define Śabda-brahman to mean Śabdārtha, others (grammarians) define it to mean Śabda; but neither of them is correct, because both Śabda and Śabdārtha are Jaḍa (unconscious things). In my opinion, Śabda-brahman is the Caitanya of all beings." The Āgama in the text is Śruti; Rāghava quotes Śaṁkarācārya in Prapañcasāra, which speaks of men versed in Śruti. Caitanya is the Brahman considered as the essence of all beings—that is, Cit and Śakti, or Cit in manifestation.

[2] That is, the Principle or Cause of Sound.

[3] Tantrarāja (Vols. VIII and XII. Tāntrik Texts), Ch. XXVI, vv. 5-9.

[4] At pp. 120-122, Vol. II, Tāntrik Texts, Viśvanātha speaks of Parā, Paśyantī, and the other Śaktis. The form of Nāda, says the *Manoramā*, should be known from the Guru. This Icchā-Śakti is Kālamayī.

[5] Paśyantī is sometimes associated with Maṇi-pūra.

mentioned, it becomes united in the Anāhata with Buddhi-tattva, and is named Madhyamā. Going upward again, it reaches the Viśuddha in the throat, where it is called Vaikharī; and from there it goes on towards the head, (upper part of the throat, the palate, the lips, the teeth). It also spreads over the tongue from root to tip, and the tip of the nose; and remaining in the throat, the palate, and the lips, produces by the throat and the lips the letters of the Alphabet from A to Kṣa." [1]

It is needless to quote more.

Elsewhere has Kuṇḍalinī been thus described: "Meditate upon Devī Kuṇḍalinī, who surrounds the Svayaṁbhu-Liṅga, who is *Śyāmā* and subtle, who is Creation itself,[2] in whom are creation, existence, and dissolution,[3] who is beyond the universe,[4] and is consciousness [5] itself. Think of Her as the One who goes upwards." [6]

Also: "Meditate upon the Devī Kuṇḍalinī as your Iṣṭa-devatā,[7] as being ever in the form of a damsel of sixteen in the full bloom of her first youth, with large and beautifully formed breasts, decked with all the varied kinds of jewels, lustrous as the full moon, red in colour, with ever restless eyes." [8]

"Red (Raktā) as regards Sundarī," so says the Author of the Śāktānanda-taraṅgiṇī. Kuṇḍalinī, as a matter of fact, should always be meditated upon as red (Raktā) in colour.[9]

Sāmā (which ordinarily denotes "colour") is here meant to signify something different. In all Tantras and all Tāntrika collections

---

[1] The sense of this, says the *Manoramā*, is that Nāda which has four stages (Avasthā-catuṣṭyātmaka), after passing through the different centres mentioned in the Text, assumes the form of the 51 letters.

[2] Sṛṣṭi-rūpā.

[3] Sṛṣṭi-stithi-layātmikā.

[4] Viśvātītā. She is not only immanent, but transcends the universe.

[5] Jñāna-rūpā.

[6] Ūrddhva-vāhinī, for Kuṇḍalinī ascends to the Sahasrāra.

[7] Iṣṭa-deva-svarūpiṇī. The Iṣṭa-devatā is the particular Devatā of Sādhaka's worship.

[8] These in woman indicate a passionate nature.

[9] The Śāktānanda-taraṅgiṇī says: She is to be meditated upon as red only when the object of worship is Tripurā. The text may also be read as meaning that "red" is an attribute applicable to Śrī Sundarī —that is, the Devī Tripura-sundarī.

Kuṇḍalinī is described to be like lightning. "Śyāma is the name given to a woman who is warm in winter and cool in summer, and the lustre of molten gold."[1] This is what is meant here and colour is not intended. Thus the apparent discrepancy is removed.

The Kaṅkāla-mālinī-Tantra describes Kuṇḍalinī in the Brahma-dvāra, and before the piercing of the Cakras, thus: "She, the Brahman Itself, resplendent like millions of moons rising at the same time, has four arms and three eyes. Her hands make the gestures[2] of granting boons and dispelling fear, and hold a book and a Vīṇā.[3] She is seated on a lion, and as She passes to her own abode[4], the Awe-inspiring One (Bhīmā) assumes different forms."

---

[1] This is a quotation from the Alaṁkāra-Śāstra (Rhetoric).

[2] That, is the Mudrās Vara and Abhaya: *v. ante*, pp. 19, 20.

[3] The musical instrument of that name.

[4] The Mūlādhāra.

Verse 12

Tanmadhye paramā kalātikuśalā sūkṣmātisūkṣmā parā
nityānanda paramparātivigalat pīyūṣa-dhārādharā
Brahmāṇḍādī katāhameva sakalaṁ yadbhāsayā bhāsate
seyaṁ śrī parameśvarī vijayate nityaprabodhodayā

Within it [1] reigns dominant Parā,[2] the Śrī-Parameśvarī, the Awakener of eternal knowledge. She is the Omnipotent Kalā [3] who is wonderfully skilful to create, and is subtler than the subtlest. She is the receptacle of that continuous stream of ambrosia which flows from the Eternal Bliss. By Her radiance it is that the whole of this Universe and this Cauldron [4] is illumined.

Commentary

He is now speaking of the Staff-like Parā-Śakti, who is like a straight thread above Kuṇḍalinī, who is coiled round Svayaṁbhu-Liṅga. The Śrī-Parameśvarī, whose radiance illumines this Universe [5] and its cauldron, dwells in the Svayaṁbhu-Liṅga above where Kuṇḍalinī is coiled and holds supreme sway.

---

[1] Svayaṁbhu-Liṅga, round which Kuṇḍalī is coiled.

[2] According to Śaṁkara, Parā is in Kuṇḍalinī. She is called Brahmāṇī by Viśvanātha who quotes the Svacchanda-saṁgraha. In Kuṇḍalinī is the Parā state of Śabda.

[3] *Vide post.*

[4] Kaṭāha—that is, the lower half of the Brahmāṇḍa, and as such cauldron-shaped.

[5] Brahmāṇḍa—egg of Brahmā.

"*Omnipotent*" (Paramā).—She is the Māyā who is able to do that which is impossible.[1]

"*Kalā*" is a form of Nāda-Śakti (Kalā Nāda-śakti-rūpā); and is separate from Kuṇḍalinī.[2]

The Śāktānanda-taraṅgiṇī says: "Kalā is Kuṇḍalinī and She, Śiva has said, is Nāda-Śakti."[3]

And it has also been elsewhere said: "Above it, meditate in your mind on Cit-kalā united with Ī (Lakṣmī) who is tapering of shape like the flame of a lamp, and who is one with Kuṇḍalī."

Cf. Kālikā-Śruti: "Man becomes freed of all sins by meditating upon Kuṇḍalinī as within, above, and below the flame, as Brahmā, as Śiva, as Sūra,[4] and as Parameśvara Himself; as Viṣṇu, as Prāṇa, as Kālāgni,[5] and as Candra."[6]

By "within the flame" is meant the excellent Kāla (=Nāda-rūpā) above Kuṇḍalinī's threefold coil. This is what has been said by the author of the Lalitā-rahasya.

"*She (Parā) is wonderfully skilful to create*" (Ati-kuśala)—*i.e.*, She it is who possesses the wonderful skill and power of creation.

"*She is the receptacle of that continuous stream of ambrosia flowing from Eternal Bliss (Brahman)*" (Nityānanda-paraṁ-parātivigalat-pīyūṣa-dhārā-dharā).—By Eternal Bliss (Nityānanda) is meant the Nirguṇa or attributeless Brahman. *Paraṁpara* means "connected step by step". From Nityānanda, which is Nirguṇa-Brahman, there arises (in Its aspect as)

---

[1] So the Devī-Purāṇa (Ch. XLV), speaking of this power of the Supreme, says:

Vicitra-kāryakāraṇā cintitāti-phalapradā,
Svapnendrajālaval-loke māyā tena prakīrtitā.

Paramā may also mean Paraṁ mīyate anayā iti Paramā—*i.e.*, She by whom the Supreme "is measured," in the sense (for the Supreme is immeasurable) that she who is one with the Supreme, is formative activity. See Introduction. Viśvanātha, quoting an unnamed Tantra, says that this Māyā is within Kuṇḍalinī, and this Paramā is Paramātma-svarūpā.

[2] Kuṇḍalinyabheda-śarīriṇī.

[3] Nāda-Śakti = Sakti as Nāda.

[4] Sūra = Sūrya, or Sun.

[5] The fire which destroys all things at the time of dissolution (pralaya).

[6] Moon.

Saguṇa-Brahman; from Saguṇa-Brahman, Śakti; from Śakti, Nāda, from Nāda, Bindu; and from Bindu, Kuṇḍalinī.[1] Cit-kalā is another form of Kuṇḍalinī. It is thus that the ambrosia comes step by step to Parameśvarī, the Cit-kala. She is Nityānanda-paramparā—that is, She belongs to the chain of emanation from Nityānanda downwards; and She is Ativigalat-pīyūṣa-dhāradharā—that is, She is the receptacle of the stream of ambrosia which flows copiously from Nityānanda.[2]

This compound word may be interpreted to mean that She holds the copious flow of ambrosia caused by her union with the Brahman. From Nityānanda this nectar comes to Para-Bindu, and passes through the Ājñā-Cakra, Viśuddha-Cakra, etc., till it reaches the Mūlādhāra, and this nectar is that of which She is the receptacle. To interpret it to mean this, the entire word is read as one.

[1] See Introduction.

[2] That is, if the compound be read in two sections—*viz.*, Nityānanda-paramparā, and then separately, Ativigalatpīyūṣadhārā. The translation adopted in the text is that which is referred to in the paragraph which follows.

Verse 13

Dhyātvaitan-mūlacakrāntaravivaralasatkoṭisūryaprakāśāṁ
vācāmēśo narendrah sa bhavati sahasā sarvavidyāvinodī
Ārogyaṁ tasya nityaṁ niravadhi ca mahānandaittāntarātmā
Vākyaiḥ kāvyaprabandhaiḥ sakalasuragurūn sevate śuddhaśīlaḥ.

By meditating thus on Her who shines within the Mūla-Cakra, with the lustre of ten million Suns, a man becomes Lord of speech and King among men, and an Adept in all kinds of learning. He becomes ever free from all diseases, and his inmost Spirit becomes full of great gladness. Pure of disposition by his deep and musical words, he serves the foremost of the Devas.[1]

Commentary

In this verse the Author speaks of the benefit to be derived from meditating on Kuṇḍalinī. By *Mūla-Cakra* is meant the Mūlādhāra. "It is the root of the six Cakras—hence its name."

"*Within*" (Mūla-cakrāntara-vivara-lasat-koṭi-sūrya-prakāśāṁ).—She shines in the Mūlādhāra-Cakra like ten million suns shining at one and the same time.

"*His deep and musical words*" (Vākyaiḥ kāvya-prabandhaiḥ).—His speech is musical and full of meanings, as in a poetical composition.

"*He serves*" (Sevate).[2]—He uses his words in hymns of praise and for purposes of a like nature. He pleases them by words of adoration.

"*All the foremost of the Devas*" (Sakala-sura-gurūn).—The word Guru here means excellent, and the Author by Sura-gurūn means Brahmā, Viṣṇu, and Śiva, the principal Devas. Amara says that "adding the words Siṁha (lion), Śārdūla (tiger), Nāga (serpent), etc., to a male name implies excellence."

---

[1] That is, Brahmā, Viṣṇu, Śiva, etc.

[2] That is, by his mastery over words he becomes like Bṛhaspati, Guru of the Devas (Śaṁkara).

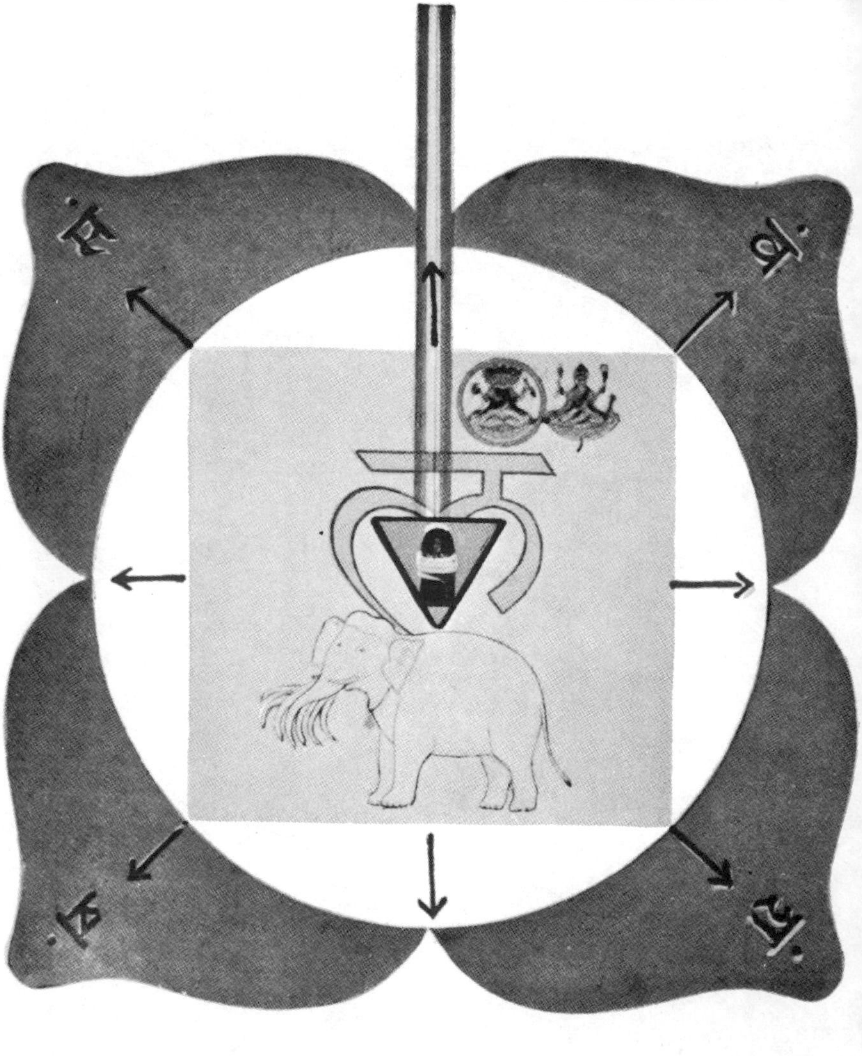

Plate II] Mūlādhāra-Cakra [To face Page 355

Summary

The Mūlādhāra is a Lotus of four petals. The petals are red, and have the letters Va, Śa (palatal), Ṣa (cerebral), Sa, in colours of gold. In the pericarp is the square Dharā-maṇḍala surrounded by eight spears, and within it and in the lower part is the Dharā-Bīja [1] who has four arms and is seated on the elephant Airāvata. He is of yellow colour, and holds the thunderbolt [2] in his hands. Inside the Bindu of the Dharā-Bīja is the Child Brahmā, who is red in colour, and has four hands with which he holds the staff,[3] the gourd,[4] the Rudrākṣa rosary, and makes the gesture which dispels fear.[5] He has four faces. In the pericarp there is a red lotus on which is the presiding Divinity of the Cakra (Cakrādhiṣṭhātrī), the Śakti Dākinī. She is red and has four arms, and in her hands are Śūla,[6] Khaṭvāṅga,[7] Khaḍga,[8] and Caṣaka.[9] In the pericarp there is also the lightning-like triangle, inside which are Kāma-Vāyu and Kāma-Bīja,[10] both of which are red. Above this is the Svayaṁbhu-Liṅga which is Śyāma-varṇa,[11] and above and round this Liṅga is Kuṇḍalinī coiled three and a half times, and above this last upstands, on the top of the Liṅga, Cit-kalā.[12]

(*This is the end of the first section.*) [13]

---

1 "Laṁ."

2 Vajra.

3 Daṇḍa.

4 Kamaṇḍalu.

5 Abhaya-mudrā.

6 Spear.

7 Skull-mounted staff.

8 Sword. Khaḍga is a heavy sacrificial sword.

9 Drinking-cup.

10 "Klīṁ."

11 Its colour.

12 Described in v. 12 as another from of Kuṇḍalinī.

13 Prakaraṇa. The commentator divides the text and his commentary into eight sections.

VERSE 14

Sindūra-pūraruciräruṇapadmamanyat
sauṣumṇamadhyaghaṭitaṁ dhvajamūladeśe
Aṅgacchadaiḥ parivṛtaṁ taḍidābhavarṇaiḥ
bādyaiḥ sabindu-lasitaiśca Puraṁdarāntaiḥ

THERE is another Lotus [1] placed inside the Suṣumṇā at the root of the genitals, of a beautiful vermilion colour. On its six petals are the letters from Ba to Puraṁdara,[2] with the Bindu [3] superposed, of the shining colour of lightning.

COMMENTARY

Having described the Mūlādhāra, he describes the Svādhiṣṭhāna-Cakra in five verses beginning with the present. This verse says that at the root of the genitals there is, distinct from the Mūlādhāra, another Lotus, of a beautiful vermilion colour.

"*Placed inside the Suṣumṇā*" (Sauṣumṇa [4]-madhya-ghaṭitaṁ).—The place of this Cakra or Padma is within Suṣumṇā.

"*At the root of gentials*" (Dhvaja-Mūladeśe).

"*Of a beautiful vermilion colour*" (Sindūra-pūra-rucirā-ruṇa).—This Lotus is of the charming red colour of vermilion.

"*On its six petals*" (Aṅga-chadaiḥ).—It is surrounded by its six petals which are the letters.[5]

---

[1] That is, the Svādhiṣṭhāna-Cakra. See Introduction.

[2] The letter La; *v. post.*

[3] The Anusvāra.

[4] Sausumṇa; Śaṁkara reads this word to mean the Brahma-nādī which is within Suṣumṇā, and says that the suffix "in" by which the change is effected is used in the sense of "relating to," and not "placed within".

[5] *V. ante*, Introduction.

"*The letters*" (Bādyaih sabindu-lasitaiḥ Puraṁdarāntaiḥ).—By Puraṁdara is meant the letter La, it being the Bīja of Puraṁdara or Indra. Each of these letters from Ba to La is on each petal of the lotus. They have the Bindu over them, and are of the shining colour of lightning. The above may also mean that the lustre of the letter is caused by their union with the Bindus placed over them.

VERSE 15

Tasyāntare pravilasadviśadaprakāśa-
mambhojamaṇḍalamatho varuṇasya tasya
Ardhendurūpalasitaṁ saradinduśubhraṁ
vaṁkārabījamamalaṁ makarādhirūḍhaṁ.

WITHIN it[1] is the white, shining, watery region of Varuṇa, of the shape of a half-moon,[2] and therein, seated on a Makara,[3] is the Bīja Vaṁ, stainless and white as the autumnal moon.

COMMENTARY

Here the Author speaks of the presence of the watery region of Varuṇa in the pericarp of the Svādhiṣṭhāna. This watery region (Aṁbhoja-maṇḍalaṁ) is in shape like the half-moon (Ardhendurūpa-lasitaṁ), and is luminously white (Viśadaprakāśaṁ).

The Śāradā says: "The region of water is lotus (shaped), that of earth is four-cornered[4] and has the thunderbolt (Vajra) and so forth." Rāghava-bhaṭṭa,[5] in describing it, says: "Draw a half-moon, and draw two Lotuses on its two sides." The Great Teacher[6] says that "the region of water is like the light of the Lotus-united Half-moon".

---

[1] Svādhiṣṭhāna.

[2] Water is the element of this Cakra, which is represented by the crescent.

[3] An animal of a legendary form, somewhat like an alligator. See Plate III.

[4] Ch. I, v. 24, Chaturasram; *sed qu*, for ordinarily the Maṇḍala is semi-circular.

[5] The famous commentator on the Śāradā-tilaka.

[6] Apparently Śaṁkarācārya, Prapañcasāra (Tāntrik Texts, Vol. III), i, 24.

Then he speaks of the Varuṇa-Bīja. This Bīja is also white, and is seated on a Makara, which is the Carrier [1] of Varuṇa. He has the noose in his hand.

Cf. " (Meditate) upon the white Bīja of Varuṇa (within the Lotus). Varuṇa is seated on a Makara, and carries the noose (Pāśa). And above him [2] (that is, in the Bindu) meditate on Hari [3] who is blue of colour (Śyāma) and four-armed."

The Va in Varuṇa-Bīja belongs to the Ya class—*i.e.*, to the group Ya, Ra, La, Va. This becomes clear from the arrangement of the letters in Kulākula-Cakra and in Bhūtalipi-Mantra.

The rest is clear.

---

[1] Vāhana.

[2] Tadūrddhvaṁ. See Comm. to next verse.

[3] Viṣṇu.

Verse 16

Tasyāṅkadeśakalito harireva pāyāt
nīlaprakāśarūciraśriyamādadhānaḥ
Pītāmbaraḥ prathamayauvanagarvadhārī
śrīvatsakaustubhadharo dhṛtavedabāhuḥ.

May Hari, who is within it,[1] who is in the pride of early youth, whose body is of a luminous blue beautiful to behold, who is dressed in yellow raiment, is four armed, and wears the Śrī-vatsa,[2] and the Kaustubha,[3] protect us!

Commentary

The Author here speaks of the presence of Viṣṇu in the Varuṇa-Bīja.

"*Within it*" (Aṅka-deśa-kalita)—*i.e.*, in the Bindu above Varuṇa-Bīja, in the same way as Brahmā is in the lap of Dharā-Bīja. The same explanation applies by analogy to the description of the other Lotuses.

"*Whose body, etc.*," (Nīla-prakāśa-rucira-śriyaṁ)—*Lit.*, He possesses the enchanting beauty of blue effulgence; *i.e.*, his body is of a luminous blue beautiful to behold.

"*Wears Śrī-vatsa and Kaustubha.*"—The following is his Dhyāna in the Gautamīya-Tantra: "On his heart is the gem Kaustubha, lustrous as

---

[1] *i.e.*, Viṣṇu is within "the lap" of the Bindu of Vāṁ.

[2] *Lit.*, Favourite of Śrī or Lakṣmī—an auspicious curl on the breast of Viṣṇu and His Avatāra; Kṛṣṇa. It is said to symbolically represent Prakṛti. See Ahirbuddhnya-Saṁhita, 52, 92, citing also the Astrabhūṣaṇa-Adhyāya of Viṣṇu-Purāṇa, I, 22.

[3] A great gem worn by Viṣṇu, which is said to symbolically signify the souls (see authorities in last note). These are said to be united with the Kaustubha of the Lord (Viṣṇutilaka, II, 100).

ten thousand Suns shining at the same time, and below it is the garland[1] with the lustre of ten thousand moons. Above Kaustubha is Śrī-vatsa, which also is luminous like ten thousand moons.

The Tantrāntara speaks of the weapons in the hands of Hari: "(Meditate on) Him who has the noose in His hand, and on Hari who is in His lap, and has four arms, and holds the Conch,[2] Discus,[3] Mace,[4] and Lotus,[5] is dark blue (Śyāma) and dressed in yellow raiment."

By "who has the noose in His hand" is meant Varuṇa as he has been described in the verse preceding the Text quoted.

Elsewhere he (Harī) is spoken of as "clad in yellow raiment, benign of aspect, and decked with a garland".[6]

We have seen that, in the Mūlādhāra, Brahmā is seated on the Haṁsa, and we should therefore think of Viṣṇu as seated on Garuḍa.[7]

---

[1] Vanamālā, the name for a large garland descending to the knee. It is defined as follows:

Ājānulambinī mālā sarvartu-kusumojjvalā.
Madhye sthūla-kadambādhyā vanamāleti kīrtitā.

(That is said to be Vanamālā which extends down to the knee, beauteous with flowers of all seasons with big Kadaṁba flowers in the middle.) This garland is celestial because in it the flowers of all the seasons are contained.

[2] Śaṅkha.

[3] Cakra.

[4] Gadā.

[5] Padma.

[6] The garland symbolizes the elements; the club, Mahat; the conch, Sāttvika-Ahaṁkāra; the bow, Tāmasika-Ahaṁkāra; the sword, knowledge; its sheath, ignorance; discus, the mind; and the arrows, the senses. See authorities cited at p. 43, *ante*.

[7] The Bird King, Vāhana of Viṣṇu.

Verse 17

Atraiva bhāti satataṁ khalu rākiṇī sā
nīlāṁbujodarasahodarakāntiśobhā
Nānāyudhodyatakarairlasitāṅgalakṣmīr-
divyāṁbarābharaṇabhūṣitamattacittā.

It is here that Rākiṇī always dwells.[1] She is of the colour of a blue lotus.[2] The beauty of Her body is enhanced by Her uplifted arms holding various weapons. She is dressed in celestial raiment and ornaments, and Her mind is exalted[3] with the drinking of ambrosia.

Commentary

In this Śloka the Author speaks of the presence of Rākiṇī in the Svādhiṣṭhāna.

Cf. Rākiṇī-dhyāna elsewhere: "Meditate on Rākiṇī, who is blue of colour (Śyāma). In Her hands are a spear,[4] a lotus, a drum[5] and a sharp battle-axe.[6] She is of furious aspect. Her three eyes are red, and Her teeth[7] show fiercely. She, the Shining Devī of Devas, is seated on a double

---

[1] Dwells (Bhāti): the Sanskrit word literally means "shines"—'here' that is, in the Svādhiṣṭhāna.

[2] Of the colour of a blue lotus (Nīlāmbujoddara-sahodarakānti-śobha); *lit.*, Her radiant beauty equals the interior of the blue lotus.

[3] Matta-cittā; for she drinks the nectar which drops from Sahasrāra. She is exalted with the divine energy which infuses Her.

[4] Śūla.

[5] Ḍamaru.

[6] Ṭaṅka.

[7] Daṁṣṭra—*i.e.*, She has long projecting teeth.

lotus, and from one of Her nostrils there flows a streak of blood.[1] She is fond of white rice,[2] and grants the wished-for boon."

As Rākiṇī is within another lotus[3] in this Lotus, therefore should the six Śaktis everywhere be understood to be in a red lotus as in the Mūlādhāra.

---

[1] Rakta-dhāraika-nāsāṁ. The Saubhāgyaratnākara has Rakta-dhātveka-nāthāṁ, that is, she who is the Lord of Raktadhātu.

[2] Śuklānna.

[3] There is another smaller Lotus in each of the main lotuses on which the Śakti sits.

Verse 18

Svādhiṣṭhānākhyametatsarasijamamalaṁ cintayedyomanuṣya-
stasyāhaṁkāradoṣādikasakalarepuḥ kṣīyate tatkṣaṇena
yogīśaḥsoऽpiṃohādbhutatimiracaye bhānutulyaprakāśo
gadyaih padyaiḥ prabandhairviracayati sudhāvākyasandoha
lakṣmīḥ.

He who meditates upon this stainless Lotus, which is named Svādhiṣṭhāna, is freed immediately from all his enemies,[1] such as the fault of Aha kāra [2] and so forth. He becomes a Lord among Yogīs, and is like the Sun illumining the dense darkness of ignorance.[3] The wealth of his nectar-like words flows in prose and verse in well-reasoned discourse.

Commentary

In this verse is described the benefit derived from the contemplation of the Svādhiṣṭhāna Lotus.

"*Svādhiṣṭhāna*".—"By *Sva* is meant the Para-Liṅga (Supreme Liṅga), and hence the Lotus is called Svādhiṣṭhāna." [4]

"*Fault of Ahaṁkāra and so forth*" (Ahaṁkāra-doṣādi).—By this is implied the six evil inclinations: Kāma (lust), Krodha (anger), etc. These six,[5] which are the six enemies of Man, are destroyed by contemplation on the Svādhiṣṭhāna Lotus. By contemplation upon it are also destroyed the darkness of Māyā, and Mohā,[6] and the Sun of knowledge (Jñāna) is acquired. The rest is clear.

---

[1] That is, his enemies the six passions.

[2] Egoism. See Introduction.

[3] Moha.

[4] This is from v. 58 of Ch. XXVII of the Rudra-yāmala.

[5] *Viz.*, Kāma (lust), Krodha (anger), Lobha (greed), Moha (delusion), Mada (pride), Mātsaryya (envy), which all arise from a sense of mineness (Ahaṁkāra).

[6] Ignorance, illusion, infatuation.

Plate III] **Svādhiṣṭhāna** [To face Page 365

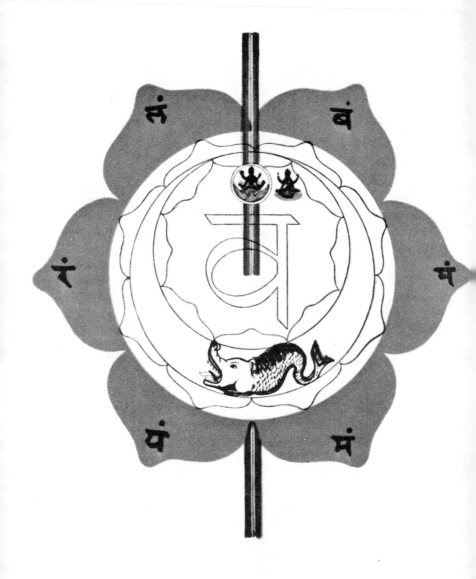

Summary of Verses 14 to 18

The Svādhiṣṭhāna-Cakra is of the colour of vermilion, and has six petals. On its six petals are the six letters Ba, Bha, Ma, Ya, Ra and La, with the Bindu placed thereon. They are of the colour of lightning. In the pericarp of this Lotus is the region of water in the form of an eight-petalled Lotus, with a half-moon in its centre. This region is white. Inside this latter is the Varuṇa-Bīja "Vaṁ," seated on a Makara, with a noose in his hand. In the lap of the latter (*i.e.*, in the hollow of the Bindu) is Viṣṇu seated on Garuḍa. He has four hands, and is carrying the Śaṅkha (conch shell), Cakra (discus), Gadā (mace), and Padma (lotus). He is dressed in yellow raiment, wears a long garland (Vanamālā) round his neck, the mark Śrī-vatsa and the gem Kaustubha on his breast, and is youthful in appearance. On a red lotus in the pericarp is the Śakti Rākiṇī. She is Śyāma-varṇā,[1] and in her four hands she holds the Śūla (spear or trident), Abja (lotus), Ḍamaru (drum) and Ṭaṅka (battle-axe). She is three-eyed and has fierce projecting fangs,[2] and is terrible to behold. She is fond of white rice,[3] and a stream of blood runs from her nostril.

(*Here ends the second section.*)

---

[1] See note to v. 11.

[2] Kuṭila-daṁṣṭrī.

[3] Śuklānna.

Verse 19

Tasyordhve nābhimūle daśadalalasite pūrṇameghaprakāśe
nīlāmbhojaprakāśairupahitajaṭhare ḍādipāntaiḥ sacandraiḥ
Dhāyedvaiśvānarasyāruṇamihirasamaṁ maṇḍalaṁ tat trikoṇaṁ
tadbāhye svastikāvyaistribhirabhilasitaṁ tatra vahneḥ svabījam.

Above it,[1] and at the root of the navel, is the shining Lotus of ten petals,[2] of the colour of heavy-laden rain-clouds. Within it are the letters Ḍa to Pha, of the colour of the blue lotus with the Nāda and Bindu above them. Meditate there on the region of Fire, triangular in form and shining like the rising sun. Outside it are three Svastika marks,[3] and within, the Bīja of Vahni himself.[4]

Commentary

The Maṇipūra-Cakra is described in this and the two following verses.

"*Shining lotus of ten petals*"[5] (Daśa-dala-lasite)—*i.e.*, the Lotus which shines by reason of its ten petals.

"*Of the colour of heavy rain-clouds*" (Pūrṇa-megha-prakāśe)—*i.e.*, of a dark hue.

---

[1] Svādhiṣṭhāna.

[2] The Maṇipūra-Cakra, the seat of the Element of Fire, the sign of which is a triangle. See Introduction.

[3] An auspicious mark; *v. post.*

[4] That is, "Raṁ," the Seed-mantra of Fire.

[5] Śaṁkara reads Daśa-dala-lalite—*i.e.*, the charming lotus of ten petals.

"*Within it are the letters, etc.*" (Nīlāṁbhoja-prakāśair upahita-jaṭhare ḍādi-phāntaiḥ sancandraiḥ).

The ten letters from Ḍa (cerebral) to Pha, with the Bindu placed above them, are of the colour of the blue lotus, and are each of them on the ten several petals. The letters are Ḍa, Ḍha, Ṇa, Ta, Tha, Da, Dha, Na, Pa, Pha. By Sacandraiḥ which qualifies Varṇaiḥ is meant that the letters have Bindu and Nāda over them, for these two go together.

"*Like the rising Sun*" (Aruṇa-mihira-samaṁ)—*i.e.*, like the young sun.

"*Svastika Marks*".[1]—These three marks or signs are on three sides of the triangle.

Rāghava-Bhaṭṭa says[2]: "A Svastika sign is made by the crossing of two straight lines going in four different directions." In this region of Fire is Raṁ, the Bīja of Fire.

---

[1] *i.e.*, like a cross 卐.

[2] In the note to v. 23 of Ch. I of the Śāradā-Tilaka.

Verse 20

Dhyāyenmeṣādhirūḍham navatapananibhaṁ vedabāhūjjvalāṅgaṁ
tatkroḍe rudramūrtirnivasati satataṁ suddhasindūrarāgaḥ
Bhasmāliptāṅgabhūṣābharaṇasitavapurvṛddhārūpī triṇetro
lokānāmiṣṭadātābhayalasitakaraḥ sṛṣṭisaṁhārakarī.

Meditate upon Him (Fire) seated on a ram, four-armed, radiant like the rising Sun. In His lap ever dwells Rudra, who is of a pure vermilion hue. He (Rudra) is white with the ashes with which He is smeared; of an ancient aspect and three-eyed, His hands are placed in the attitude of granting boons and of dispelling fear.[1] He is the destroyer of creation.

Commentary

Elsewhere the Dhyāna of Vahni is as follows: " Seated on a ram, a Rudrākṣa rosary in one hand, and the Śakti [2] in the other."

As there are no weapons placed in the other hands it is to be inferred that the other two hands are in the attitude of granting boons and of dispelling fear; that is how He is described to be in other Dhyānas of Him.

Rudra should here be meditated upon as seated on a bull.

"*He is white . . . smeared*" (Bhasmāliptāṅga-bhūṣābharaṇa-sita-vapuḥ).—The ashes with which his body is smeared and the ornaments he is wearing make him look white (though his hue is red).

---

[1] That is, making Vara and Abhaya-Mudrās.

[2] Vahni's or Fire's weapon. Bhāskararāya says it is the weapon which is called in Maharāṣtra Śāmti.

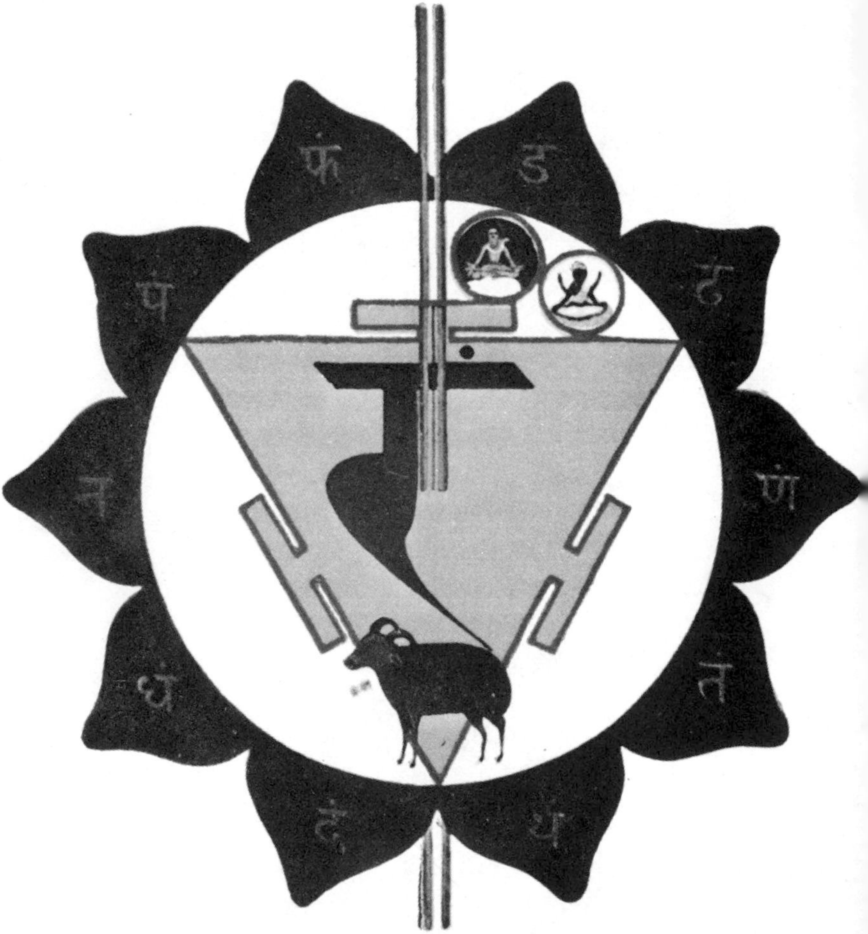

Plate IV] Maṇipūraka [To face Page 369

Verse 21

Atrāste lākinī sā sakalaśubhakarī vedabāhūjjvalāṅgī
śyāmā pītāmbarādyairvividhaviracanālaṁkṛtā mattacittā
Dhyātvaitannābhipadmaṁ prabhavati nitarāṁ saṁhṛtau pālane vā
vāṇī tasyānanābje nivasati satataṁ jñānasaṁdohalakṣmīḥ

Here abides Lākinī, the benefactress of all. She is four-armed, of radiant body, is dark[1] (of complexion), clothed in yellow raiment and decked with various ornaments, and exalted with the drinking of ambrosia.[2] By meditating on this[3] Navel Lotus[4] the power to destroy and create (the world) is acquired. Vāṇī[5] with all the wealth of knowledge ever abides in the lotus of His face.

Commentary

"*Decked with various ornaments*" (Vividha-viracanālaṃkṛtā).—She who is decorated with gems and pearls arranged in varied and beautiful designs.

Cf. Lākinī-dhyāna elsewhere: "Let the excellent worshipper meditate upon the Devī Lākinī, who is blue and has three faces, and three eyes (to each face), fierce of aspect, and with Her teeth protruding.[6] In Her right hand She holds the thunderbolt and the Śakti,[7] and in the left She

---

[1] Śyāma: see *ante*, p. 350.

[2] Matta-cittā; *vide ante*, p. 363, n. 3.

[3] Etat: a variant reading is evam, "in this manner".

[4] Nābhi-Padma.

[5] That is, the Devī of Speech, Sarasvatī.

[6] Viśvanātha quotes a Dhyāna in which She is described as hump-backed (Kubjinī) and as carrying a staff.

[7] The weapon of Vahni (Fire). See note 2, page 368.

makes the gestures [1] of dispelling fear and of granting boons. She is in the pericarp of the navel lotus, which has ten petals. She is fond of meat (Māmsāśī),[2] and her breast is ruddy with the blood and fat which drop from Her mouth."

The navel lotus is called Maṇi-pūra. The Gautamiya-Tantra says [3]: "This Lotus is called Maṇipūra because it is lustrous like a gem." [4]

Summary of Verses 19 to 21

The Nābhi-padma (Navel Lotus) is of the colour of the rain-cloud and has ten petals; on each of its petals are each of the ten letters, Ḍa, Ḍha, Ṇa, Ta, Tha, Da, Dha, Na, Pa, Pha, and of a lustrous blue colour, with the Bindu above each of them. In the pericarp of this Lotus is the red Region of Fire, which is triangular in shape, and outside it, on its three sides, are three Svastika signs. Within the triangle is the Bīja of Fire—"Raṁ". He (Bīja of Fire) is red in colour and is seated on a ram, is four-armed, and holds in his hands the Vajra (thunderbolt) and the Śakti weapon, and makes the signs of Vara and of Abhaya.[5] In the lap of Vahni-Bīja is Rudra, red of colour, seated on the bull, who, however, appears to be white on account of the ashes which He smears on His body. He is old in appearance. On a red lotus in the pericarp of this Lotus is the Śakti Lākinī. She is blue, has three faces with three eyes in each, is four-armed, and with Her hands holds the Vajra and the Śakti weapon, and makes the signs of dispelling fear and granting boons. She has fierce projecting teeth, and is fond of eating rice and dhal, cooked and mixed with meat and blood.[6]

(Here ends the third section)

---

[1] Mudrā.

[2] Some read "Māmsastāṁ"=She who abides in flesh.

[3] A Vaiṣṇava-Tantra of great authority. The quotation is from Ch. 34 of the same.

[4] Maṇi-vad bhinnaṁ. Bhinna here means "distinguished," for in the Maṇipūra is the Region of Fire. See also Rudra-yāmala, Ch. XXVII, v. 60.

[5] Vara and Abhaya—*i.e.*, the Mudrās granting boons and dispelling fear.

[6] Khecarānna—that is, meat mixed with rice and and dhal, such as Khicri, Pilau, etc.

VERSE 22

Tasyordhve hṛdi paṅkajaṁ sulalitaṁ bandhūkakāntyujjvalaṁ
kādyair dvādaśavarṇakairupahitaṁ sindūrarāgānvitaiḥ
Nāṁnānāhatasaṁjñakaṁ surataruṁ vāñchātiriktapradaṁ
vāyormaṇḍalamatra dhūmasadṛśaṁ ṣaṭkoṇaśobhānvitaṁ

ABOVE that, in the heart, is the charming Lotus,[1] of the shining colour of the Bandhūka flower,[2] with the twelve letters beginning with Ka, of the colour of vermilion, placed therein. It is known by its name of Anāhata, and is like the celestial wishing-tree,[3] bestowing even more than (the supplicant's) desire. The Region of Vāyu, beautiful and with six corners,[4] which is like unto the smoke in colour, is here.

COMMENTARY

The Anāhata Lotus is described in the six verses beginning with this.

This Lotus should be meditated upon in the heart; the verb *dhyāyet* is understood. The twelve letters beginning with Ka, that is, letters Ka to Tha are on the petals.

"*It is known by its name Anāhata*" (Nāmnāsnāhata-samjñakaṁ).—"It is so called by the Munis because it is here that the sound of Śabda

[1] The Anāhata, or heart Lotus, seat of the air element, the sign of which is described as hexagonal, is here. See Introduction.

[2] *Pentapoetes Phoenicea.*

[3] Kalpa-taru. Śaṁkara says the Kalpa-taru, one of the celestial trees in Indra's heaven, grants what is asked; but this gives more, since it leads him to Mokṣa.

[4] Ṣaṭ-koṇa—that is, interlacing triangles. See Plate V. See Introduction and Rudra-yāmala. Ch. XXVII, v. 64.

Brahman is heard, that Śabda or sound which issues without the striking of any two things together."[1]

"*Wishing-tree*"[2] is the tree in Heaven which grants all one asks; as it is like the Kalpa-taru so it bestows more than is desired.

"*Region of Vāyu*" (Vāyor maṇḍalaṁ).—In the pericarp of this Lotus is the Vāyu-maṇḍala.

---

[1] Viśvanātha quotes (p. 32, *post,* Verse 22, Ṣatcakranirūpaṇaṁ) the following: "Within it is Bāṇa-Liṅga, lustrous like ten thousand suns, also Sound which is Śabda-brahmamaya (whose substance is Brahman), and is produced by no cause (Ahetuka). Such is the lotus Anāhata wherein Puruṣa (that is, the Jīvātmā) dwells." As to Śabda-brahman see Rāghava Bhaṭṭa's Comm. on Śāradā, Ch. I, v. 12.

[2] Surataru=Kalpa-taru.

Verse 23

Tanmadhye pavanākṣaraṁ ca madhuraṁ dhūmāvalīdhūsaraṁ
dhyayolpāṇicatuṣṭayena lasitaṁ kṛṣṇādhiruḍhaṁ paraṁ
Tanmadhye karuṇānidhānamamalaṁ haṁsābhamīśabhidhaṁ
pāṇibhyāmabhayaṁ varaṁ ca vidadhallokatrayāṇāmapi

Meditate within it on the sweet and excellent Pavana Bīja,[1] grey as a mass of smoke,[2] with four arms, and seated on a black antelope. And within it also (meditate) upon the Abode of Mercy,[3] the Stainless Lord who is lustrous like the Sun,[4] and whose two hands [5] make the gestures which grant boons and dispel the fears of the three worlds.

Commentary

In this verse the Author speaks of the presence of the Vāyu-Bīja in the Anāhata-Cakra.

"*Pavana Bīja*" (Pavanākṣara)—*i.e.*, the Bīja Yaṁ.

"*Grey as a mass of smoke*" (Dhūmāvalī-dhūsara).—It has the greyish colour of smoke by reason of its being surrounded by masses of vapour.

---

[1] *i.e.*, Vāyu, whose Bīja is "Yaṁ".

[2] This smoke, Śaṁkara says, emanates from the Jīvātmā which is in the form of a flame.

[3] Śaṁkara reads "ocean of mercy" (Karuṇāvāridhi).

[4] Haṁsa, the Sun—a name also of the Supreme. *Cf.* "Hrīṁ the Supreme Haṁsa dwells in the brilliant heaven." See the Haṁsavatī Ṛk of Ṛgveda IV—40 quoted in Mahānirvāṇa-Tantra, vv. 196, 197, Ch. V. Haṁsa is from Haṁ=Gati, or motion. It is called Āditya because it is in perpetual motion (Sāyaṇa). Haṁsa is also the form of the Antarātmā, see v. 31, *post.* This Ṛk also runs in Yajurveda, X, 24, and XII, 14 and in some of the Upaniṣads.

[5] This shows that the Bīja has hands and feet (Śaṃkara).

"*A black antelope*," which is noted for its fleetness, is the Vāhana (carrier) of Vāyu. Vāyu carries his weapon, "Aṅkuśa,"[1] in the same way that Varuṇa carries his weapon, "Pāśa".[2]

He next speaks of the presence of Īśa in the Vāyu-Bīja. Everywhere Śiva is spoken of as having three eyes,[3] hence Īśa also has three eyes.

Elsewhere it is said: "Meditate upon him as wearing a jewelled necklet and a chain of gems round his neck, and bells on His toes, and also clad in silken raiment." In the same way of Him it has also been said: "The beautiful One possessed of the soft radiance of ten million moons, and shining with the radiance of his matted hair."

Īśa should therefore be thought of as clad in silken raiment, etc.

---

[1] Goad.

[2] Noose.

[3] The third eye, situate in the forehead in the region of the pineal gland, is the Eye of Wisdom (Jñānacakṣu).

VERSE 24

Atrāste khalu kākinī navataḍitpītā triṇetrā śubhā
sarvālaṁkaraṇānvitā hitakarī saṁyagjanānāṁ mudā
Hastaiḥ pāśakapālaśobhanavarān saṁbibhrati cābhayaṁ
mattā pūrṇasudhārasārdrahṛdayā kaṅkālamālādharā

HERE dwells Kākinī, who in colour is yellow like unto new lightning,[1] exhilarated and auspicious; three-eyed and the benefactress of all. She wears all kinds of ornaments, and in Her four hands She carries the noose and the skull, and makes the sign of blessing and the sign which dispels fear. Her heart is softened with the drinking of nectar.

COMMENTARY

In this verse the Author speaks of the presence of the Śakti Kākinī.

"*Exhilarated*"[2] (Mattā)—that is, She is not in an ordinary, but in a happy, excited mood.

"*With the drinking of nectar,*" *etc.* (Pūrṇa-sudhā-rasārdra-hṛdayā).—Her heart is softened to benevolence by the drinking of nectar; or it may be interpreted to mean that Her heart is softened by the supreme bliss caused by drinking the excellent nectar which drops from the Sahasrāra. Her heart expands with the supreme bliss. Kākinī should be thought of as wearing the skin of a black antelope.

Compare the following Dhyāna of Kākinī where She is so described: "If thou desirest that the practice of thy Mantra be crowned with success,

---

[1] Nava-taḍit-pītā—*i.e.*, where there is more thunder than rain, when the lightning shows itself very vividly. Pītā is yellow; Kākinī is of a shining yellow colour.

[2] Śaṁkara gives *unmattā* (maddened or exalted) as equivalent of Mattā.

meditate on the moon-faced, ever-existent[1] Śakti Kākinī, wearing the skin of a black antelope, adorned with all ornaments."[2]

[1] Nityāṁ. If this is not stutī, possibly the word is nityam, " always ".

[2] Viśvanātha, in his commentary on the Ṣaṭcakra, gives the following Dhyāna of Kākinī: " Meditate on Kākinī whose abode is in Fat (Meda-saṁsthāṁ), holding in Her hands Pāśa (noose), Śūla (trident), Kapāl (Skull), Ḍamaru (drum). She is yellow in colour, fond of eating curd and rice (Dadhyanna). Her beautiful body is in a slightly bending pose (Svavayava-namitā). Her heart is made joyous by the draught of rice-wine (Vāruṇī)." The Saubhāgya-ratnākara cites Seven Dhyānas of the Seven Śaktis or Yoginīs—Dākinī and others which show that each has Her abode in one of the seven Dhātus. The Seventh Śakti Yakṣiṇī is not mentioned in this book.

VERSE 25

Etannīrajakarṇikāntaralasacchaktistrikoṇābhidhā
vidyutkoṭisamānakomalavapuḥ sāste tadantargataḥ
Baṇākhyaḥ śivaliṅgakoʼpi kanakākārāṅgarāgojjvalo
maulau sūkṣmavibhedayuṅmaṇiriva prollāsalakṣmyālayaḥ

THE Śakti whose tender body is like ten million flashes of lightning is in the pericarp of this Lotus in the form of a triangle (Trikoṇa). Inside the triangle is the Śiva-Liṅga known by the name of Bāṇa. This Liṅga is like shining gold, and on his head is an orifice minute as that in a gem. He is the resplendent abode of Lakṣmī.

COMMENTARY

In this Śloka is described the triangle (Trikoṇa) which is in the pericarp of this Lotus.

"*Śakti in the form of a triangle*" (Trikoṇābhidha-Śaktīḥ).—By this we are to understand that the apex of the Triangle is downward.[1]

This Trikoṇa is below the Vāyu-Bīja, as has been said elsewhere. "In its lap is Īśa. Below it, within the Trikoṇa is Bāṇa-Liṅga."

"*On his head,*" *etc.* (Maulau sūkṣma-vibheda-yung maṇiḥ).—This is a description of Bāṇa-Liṅga. The orifice is the little space within the Bindu which is within the half-moon which is on the head of the Liṅga.

Elsewhere we find the following description: "The Bāṇa-Liṅga within the triangle, decked in jewels made of gold—the Deva with the half-moon on his head; in the middle is an excellent red lotus."

The red lotus in this quotation is one below the pericarp of the heart lotus; it has its head turned upwards, and has eight petals. It is in

[1] As it is a Trikoṇa-Śakti, it must have its apex downwards as in the case of the Yoni.

this lotus that mental worship (Mānasa-pūjā) should be made.[1] Compare the following: " Inside is the red eight-petalled lotus. There is also the Kalpa-tree and the seat of the Iṣṭa-deva under a beautiful awning (Candrātapa), surrounded by trees laden with flowers and fruits and sweet-voiced birds. There meditate on the Iṣṭa-deva according to the ritual [2] of the worshipper."

" *Orifice minute as*."—He here speaks of the Bindu which is the head of the Bāṇa-Liṅga. As a gem has a minute orifice in it (when pierced to be threaded), so has this Liṅga.[3] By this is meant that the Bindu is in the head of Śiva-Liṅga.

" *The resplendent abode of Lakṣmī*." [4]—By this one must know the great beauty of the Liṅga, due to a rush of desire.[5]

---

[1] This is not one of the six Cakras, but a lotus known as Ānanda-kanda, where the Iṣṭa-devatā is meditated upon. See Ch. V, v. 132, Mahānirvāṇa-Tantra.

[2] Kalpa. Tattat-kalpoktamārgatah. That is, in manner enjoined by the respective sampradāya of the sādhaka.

[3] The Liṅga itself is not pierced, but it carries the Bindu, which has an empty space (Śūnya) within its circle.

[4] That is, here, beauty.

[5] Kāmodgama.

VERSE 26

Dhyayedyo hṛdi paṅkajaṁ surataruṁ śarvasya pīṭhālayaṁ
devasyānila-hīna-dīpa-kalikā-haṁsena saṁ-śobhitaṁ
Bhānormaṇḍala-maṇḍitāntara-lasat kiñjalka-śobhādharaṁ
vācāmīśvara Īśvaro-pi jagatāṁ rakṣavināśe kṣamaḥ

HE who meditates on this Heart Lotus becomes (like) the Lord of Speech, and (like) Īśvara he is able to protect and destroy the worlds. This Lotus, is like the celestial wishing-tree,[1] the abode and seat of Śarva.[2] It is beautified by the Haṁsa,[3] which is like unto the steady tapering flame of a lamp in a windless place.[4] The filaments which surround and adorn its pericarp, illumined by the solar region, charm.

COMMENTARY

In this and the following verse he speaks of the good to be gained by meditating on the Heart Lotus.

"*He who meditates on this Lotus in the Heart becomes like the Lord of Speech*"—*i.e.*, Bṛhaspati, the Guru of the Devas—and able like Īśvara the Creator to protect and destroy the worlds. Briefly, he becomes the Creator, Protector and Destroyer of the Worlds.

He speaks of the presence of the Jīvātmā which is Haṁsa,[5] in the pericarp of this Lotus. The Jīvātmā is like the steady flame of a lamp in

---

[1] Sura-taru=Kalpa-taru.

[2] Mahā-deva, Śiva.

[3] Here the Jīvātmā.

[4] See Introduction.

[5] Viśvanātha quotes a verse in which this Haṁsa is spoken of as Puruṣa.

a windless place, and enhances the beauty of this Lotus (Anila-hīna-dīpa-kalikā-haṁsena sam-śobhitam). *Haṁsa* is the Jīvātmā. He also speaks of the presence of the Sūrya-maṇḍala in the pericarp of this Lotus.

" *The filaments which surround and adorn its pericarp, illumined by the solar region, charm* " (Bhānormaṇḍala-maṇḍitāntara-lasat kiñjalka-śobādharaṁ). —It is beautified by reason of the filaments which surround the pericarp being tinged by the rays of the Sun. The rays of the Sun beautify the filaments and not the space within the pericarp. The filaments of the other Lotuses are not so tinged, and it is the distinctive feature of this Lotus. By the expression " the Maṇḍala of Sūrya (Bhānu) " the reader is to understand that all the filaments in the pericarp are beauteous with the rays of the Sun, and not a portion of them.

All over the pericarp is spread the region of Vāyu. Above it is the region of Sūrya; and above these the Vāyu-Bīja and Trikoṇa, etc., should be meditated upon. This is quite consistent. In mental worship the *mantra* is " Maṁ—salutation to the region of Fire with his ten Kalās," [1] etc. From texts and Mantras like this we therefore see that the regions of Vahni (Fire), Arka (Sun), and Candra (Moon) are placed one above the other.

" *Īśvara* "—*i.e.*, Creator.

" *Able to protect and destroy the world* " (Rakṣā-vināśe-kṣamah)—*i.e.*, it is he who protects and destroys. The idea meant to be conveyed by these three attributes is that he becomes possessed of the power of creating, maintaining and destroying the Universe.[2]

---

[1] Kalā=Digits or portions of Śakti.

[2] By reason of his unification with the Brahma-substance.

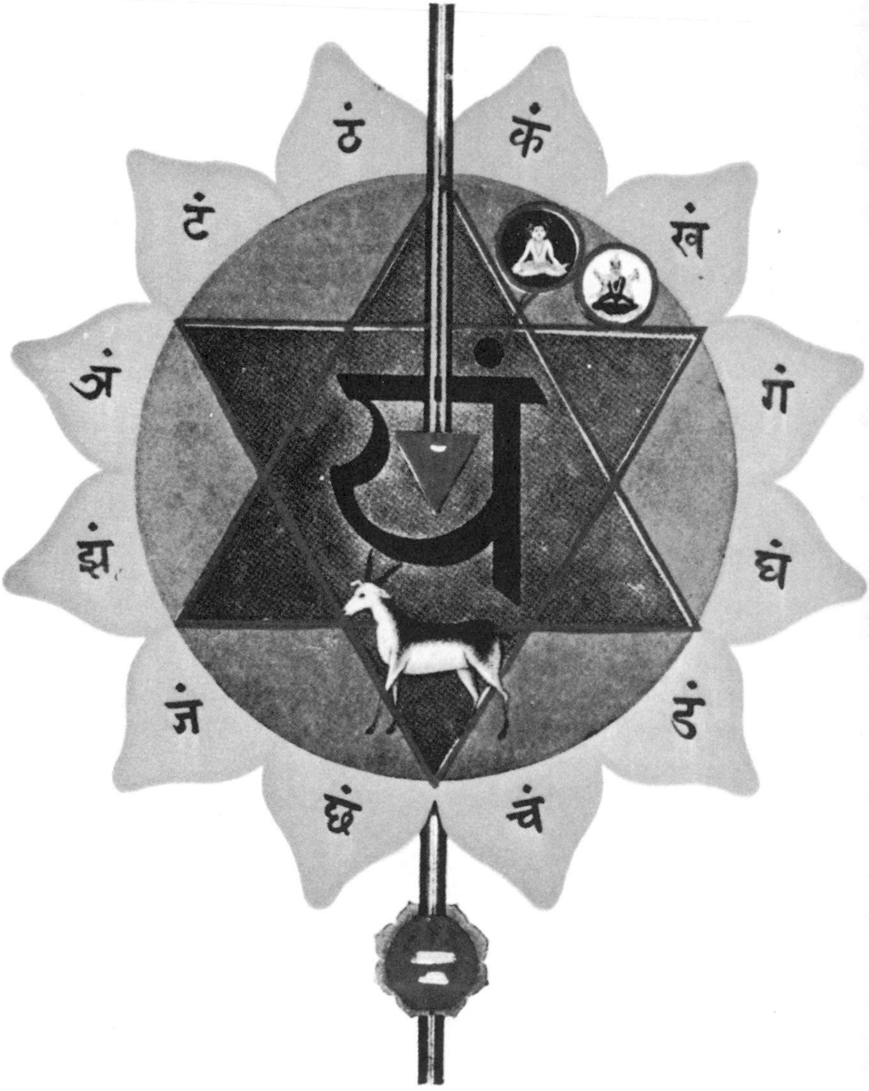

Plate V] Anāhata [To face Page 381

Verse 27

Yogīśo bhavati priyātpriyatamaḥ kāntākulasyāniśaṁ
jñānīśo'pi kṛtī jitendriyagaṇo dhyānāvadhānakṣamaḥ
Gadyaiḥ padyapadādibhiśca satataṁ kavyāmbudhārāvaho
lakṣmiraṅgaṇadaivataḥ parapure śaktaḥ praveṣṭuṁ kṣaṇāt.

Foremost among Yogīs, he ever is dearer than the dearest to women,[1] He is pre-eminently wise and full of noble deeds. His senses are completely under control. His mind in its intense concentration is engrossed in thoughts of the Brahman. His inspired speech flows like a stream of (clear) water. He is like the Devatā who is the beloved of Lakṣmī[2] and he is able at will to enter another's body.[3]

Commentary

"*Dearer than the dearest to women*" (Priyāt priyatamaḥ kāntākulasya) —*i.e.*, because he is skilful to please them.[4]

"*His senses are completely under control*" (Jitendriya-gaṇḥ)—*i.e.*, he is one who should be counted among those that have completely subjugated their senses.

"*His mind . . . . Brahman*" (Dhyānāvadhāna-kṣamaḥ).—Dhyāna is Brahma-cintana, and Avadhāna means steady and intense concentration of the mind. The Yogī is capable of both.

---

[1] Priyāt priyatamah—more beloved than those that are dear to them.

[2] According to Śaṁkara's reading, Lakṣmī becomes his family Devatā —that is, his family is always prosperous.

[3] Parapure; *v. post.*

[4] Karma-kuśalah—" dearer than their husbands " (Śaṁkara).

"*His inspired speech flows like a stream of (clear) water*" (Kāvyāṁbu-dhārā-vaha).—The flow of his speech is compared to an uninterrupted flow of water, and it is he from whom it flows.

"*He is like the Devatā who is the beloved of Lakṣmī*" (Lakṣmī-raṅgaṇa-daivataḥ).—He becomes like the Deva who is the beloved of Lakṣmī. Lakṣmī, the Devi of Prosperity, is the spouse of Viṣṇu. This compound word is capable of another meaning. It may mean: One who has enjoyed all prosperity (Lakṣmī) and all good fortune (Raṅgaṇa) in this world and who goes along the path of liberation. It has therefore been said:—"Having enjoyed in this world the best of pleasure, he in the end goes to the abode of Liberation."[1]

"*Another's body*" (Para-pure).—He is able at will to enter the enemy's fort or citadel (Durga), even though guarded and rendered difficult of access. And he gains power by which he may render himself invisible, fly across the sky, and other similar powers. It may also mean "another man's body".[2]

Summary of Verses 22 to 27

The Heart Lotus is of the colour of the Bandhūka[3] flower, and on its twelve petals are the letters Ka to Ṭha, with the Bindu above them, of the colour of vermilion. In its pericarp is the hexagonal[4] Vāyu-Maṇḍala, of a smoky colour, and above it Sūrya-Maṇḍala, with the Trikoṇa lustrous as ten million flashes of lightning within it. Above it the Vāyu-Bīja, of a smoky hue, is seated on a black antelope, four-armed and carrying the goad (Aṅkuśa). In his (Vāyu-Bīja's) lap is three-eyed Īśa. Like Haṁsa (Haṁsābha), His two arms extended in the gestures of granting boons and dispelling fear. In the pericarp of this Lotus, seated on a red lotus, is the Śakti Kākinī. She is four-armed, and carries the noose (Pāśa), the skull (Kapāla), and makes the boon (Vara) and fear-dispelling (Abhaya) signs. She is of a golden hue, is dressed in yellow raiment, and wears every variety

[1] *Iha bhuktvā varān bhogān ante mukti-padaṁ vrajet.*

[2] The Siddhi by which Yogīs transfer themselves into another's body, as Śaṁkarācārya is said to have done. The latter interpretation is preferable, for such an one will not have enemies, or if he have will not seek to overcome them.

[3] *Pentapœtes Phœnicea.*

[4] See Introduction.

of jewel and a garland of bones. Her heart is softened by nectar. In the middle of the Trikoṇa is Śiva in the form of a Bāṇa-Liṅga, with the crescent moon and Bindu on his head. He is of a golden colour.

He looks joyous with a rush of desire.[1] Below him is the Jīvātmā like Haṁsa. It is like the steady tapering flame of a lamp.[2] Below the pericarp of this Lotus is the red lotus of eight petals, with its head upturned. It is in this (red) lotus that there are the Kalpa Tree, the jewelled altar surmounted by an awning and decorated by flags and the like, which is the place of mental worship.[3]

(Here ends the fourth section)

---

[1] Kāmodgamollasita.

[2] See Introduction.

[3] See Mahānirvāṇa-Tantra, Ch. V. vv. 129, 130, where the Mantra is given.

Verses 28 and 29

Viśuddhākhyaṁ kaṇṭhe sarasijamamalaṁ dhūmadhūmrāvabhāsaṁ
svaraiḥ sarvaiḥ śoṇairdalaparilasitairdīpitaṁ dīptabuddheḥ
Samāste pūrnenduprathitatamanabhomaṇḍalaṁ vṛttarūpaṁ
himacchāyānōgopari lasitatanoḥ śuklavarṇāṁbarasya

Bhujaiḥ pāśābhītyaṅkuśavaralasitaiḥ śobhitāṅgasya tasya
manoraṅke nityaṁ nivasati girijābhinnadeho himābhaḥ
Triṇetraḥ pañcāsyo lalitadaśabhujo vyāghracarmāmbaraḍhyaḥ
sadāpūrvo devaḥ śiva iti ca samākhyānasiddhaḥ prasiddhaḥ

In the throat is the Lotus called Viśuddha, which is pure and of a smoky purple hue. All the (sixteen) shining vowels on its (sixteen) petals, of a crimson hue, are distinctly visible to him whose mind (Buddhi) is illumined. In the pericarp of this lotus there is the Ethereal Region, circular in shape, and white like the full Moon.[1] On an elephant white as snow is seated the Bīja[2] of Aṁbara,[3] who is white of colour.

Of His four arms, two hold the noose[4] and goad,[5] and the other two make the gestures[6] of granting boons and dispelling

[1] Ether is the element of this Cakra, the sign (Maṇḍala) of this Tattva being a circle (Vṛtta-rūpa). See Introduction.

[2] Manu=Mantra=(here) " Haṁ ".

[3] Aṁbara=the Ethereal Region; the word also means " apparel "—" Vyom-nivāṣasi " (*Amara-kośa*). On an elephant of the colour of snow is seated Aṁbara, white in colour in his Bīja form. The Saṁskṛt is capable of another meaning: " On an elephant is seated the Bīja whose raiment is white."

[4] Pāśa.

[5] Aṅkuśa.

[6] Mudrās.

fear. These add to His beauty. In His lap [1] there ever dwells the great snow-white Deva, three-eyed and five-faced, with ten beautiful arms, and clothed in a tiger's skin. His body is united with that of Girijā,[2] and He is known by what His name, Sadā-Śiva,[3] signifies.

Commentary

The Viśuddha Cakra is described in four verses beginning with these.

"Because by the sight of the Haṁsa the Jīva attains purity, this Padma (Lotus) is therefore called Viśuddha (pure), Ethereal, Great, and Excellent."

"*In the region of the throat is the Lotus called Viśuddha.*"—Pure (Amala, without impurity) by reason of its being *tejo-maya* [4] (its substance is *tejas*), and hence free from impurity.

"*All the vowels*" (Svaraiḥ sarvaiḥ)—*i.e.*, all the vowels, beginning with *A-kāra* and ending with Visarga—altogether sixteen in number.

"*Shining on the petals*" (Dala-parilasitaiḥ).—The vowels being sixteen in number, the number of petals which this lotus possesses is shown by implication to be sixteen also.

Elsewhere this has been clearly stated: "Above it (Anāhata) is the Lotus of sixteen petals, of a smoky purple colour; its petals bear the sixteen vowels, red in colour, with the Bindu above them. Its filaments are ruddy, and it is adorned by Vyoma-maṇḍala." [5]

"*Distinctly visible*" (Dīpitam).—These letters are lighted up, as it were, for the enlightened mind (Dīpta-buddhi).

"*Whose mind (buddhi) is illumined*" refers to the person whose *buddhi*, or intellect, has become free from the impurity of worldly pursuits as the result of the constant practice of Yoga.

---

[1] Of the Nabho-bīja or "Haṁ".

[2] "Mountain-born," a title of the Devī as the daughter of the Mountain King (Himavat—Himālaya). The reference is here to the Androgyne Śiva-Śakti form. See Commentary.

[3] Sadā=ever. Śiva=the Beneficent One. Beneficence.

[4] Fire purifies.

[5] The Ethereal Circle.

"*The Ethereal Region circular in shape, and white like the full Moon*" (Pūrṇendu-prathita-tama-nabhomaṇḍalaṁ vṛtta-rūpaṁ).—The Ethereal Region is circular in shape (Vṛttarūpa), and its roundness resembles that of the full Moon, and like the Moon it is also white. The Śāradā says: "The wise know that the Maṇḍalas participate in the lustre of their peculiar elements."[1] The Maṇḍalas are of the colour of their respective Devatās and elements: Ether is white, hence its Maṇḍala is also white.

"*In the pericarp of this lotus is the circular Ethereal Region*" (Nabhō-maṇḍalaṁ vṛtta-rūpaṁ).—In the lap of this white Aṁbara (or Ethereal Region) ever dwells Sadā-Śiva, who is spoken of in the second of these two verses.

"*On an elephant white as snow is seated*" (Hima-cchāyānāgopari lasita-tanu).—This qualifies Aṁbara.

Nāga here means an Elephant, and not a serpent. The Bhūta-śuddhi clearly says: "Inside it is the white Bīja of Vyoma on a snow-white elephant." Literally, "His body shows resplendent on an elephant," because He is seated thereon.

"*The Bīja of Aṁbara*" (Tasya manoh).—Tasya manoh means literally "His mantra" which is the Bīja of Ether or Haṁ.[2]

"*His four arms, (two of) which hold the Pāśa (noose), Aṅkuśa (goad) and (the other two) are in the gestures granting boons and dispelling fear, add to his beauty*" (Bhujaih pāśābhītyaṅkuśa-vara-lasitaih śobhitāṅgasya).—The meaning, in short, is that in His hands He is carrying the *pāśa* and *aṅkuśa*, and making the gestures of dispelling fear and granting boons.

"*In the lap of his Bīja*" (Tasya manor anke).—He is here in His Bīja form—in the form of Haṁ which is Ākāśa-Bīja. This shows the presence of the Bīja of Ether in the pericarp of this Lotus, and we are to meditate upon it as here described.

"*The snow-white Deva whose body is united with (or inseparable from) that of Giri-jā*" (Girijābhinna-deha).—By this is meant Arddhanārīśvara.[3] The Deva Arddhanārīśvara is of a golden colour on the left, and snow-white on the right. He dwells in the lap of Nabho-Bīja. He is described as "the Deva Sadā-Śiva garbed in white raiment. Half His body being inseparate from that of Girijā, He is both silvern and golden". He is

---

[1] That is, each Maṇḍala (*i.e.*, square, circle, triangle, etc.,) takes after the characteristics of its elements. (*Vide* Śāradā-tilaka, I, 24.)

[2] The Bīja of a thing is that thing in essence.

[3] Hara-Gaurī-mūrti (Śaṁkara).

also spoken of as " possessed of the down-turned digit (Kalā) of the Moon which constantly drops nectar ".[1]

The Nirvāṇa Tantra,[2] in dealing with the Viśuddha-Cakra, says: " Within the Yantra [3] is the Bull, and over it a lion-seat (Simhāsana). On this is the eternal Gaurī, and on Her right is Sadā-Śiva. He has five faces, and three eyes to each face. His body is smeared with ashes, and He is like a mountain of silver. The Deva is wearing the skin of a tiger, and garlands of snakes are His ornaments."

The Eternal Gaurī (Sadā Gaurī) is there as half of Śiva's body. She is in the same place spoken of as " the Gaurī, the Mother of the Universe, who is the other half of the body of Śiva ".

" *With ten beautiful arms* " (Lalita-daśa-bhuja).—The Author here has said nothing of what weapons the Deva has in His hands. In a Dhyāna elsewhere He is spoken of as carrying in His hands the Śūla (trident), the Ṭaṅka (battle-axe), the Kṛpāṇa (sword), the Vajra (thunderbolt), Dahana (fire), the Nāgendra (snake-king), the Ghaṇṭā (bell), the Aṅkuśa (goad), Pāśa (noose), and making the gesture dispelling fear (Abhītīkara).[4] In meditating on Him, therefore, He should be thought of as carrying these implements and substances and making these gestures in and by His ten arms. Great (Prasiddha, *lit.* known), here well-known for his greatness. The rest can be easily understood.

[1] This is the Amā-Kalā.

[2] Paṭala VIII. The text translated is incorrect. In Raśikamohana Chattopādhyāya's Edition it runs as: " Within the Yantra is the bull, half of whose body is that of a lion." This is consistent with the Arddha-nārīśvara, as the bull is the Vāhana (carrier) of Śiva, and the lion of the Devī.

[3] That is Ṣat-koṇa-yantra.

[4] This gesture is called also Astra or a weapon which is thrown, because it throws goodness on the Sādhaka.

Verse 30

Sudhāsindhoḥ śuddhā nivasati kamale sākinī pītavastrā
śaraṁ cāpaṁ pāśaṁ sṛṇimapi dadhatí hastapadmaiścaturbhiḥ·
Sudhāṁśoḥ saṁpūrṇaṁ śaśaparirahitaṁ maṇḍalaṁ karṇikāyāṁ
mahāmokṣadvāraṁ śriyamabhimataśīlasya śuddhendriyasya.

Purer than the Ocean of Nectar is the Śakti Sākinī who dwells in this Lotus. Her raiment is yellow, and in Her four lotus-hands She carries the bow, the arrow, the noose, and the goad. The whole region of the Moon without the mark of the hare [1] is in the pericarp of this Lotus. This (region) is the gateway of great Liberation for him who desires the wealth of Yoga and whose senses are pure and controlled.

Commentary

Here the Author speaks of the presence of Śākinī in the pericarp of the Viśuddha Lotus.

"*Purer than the Ocean of Nectar*" (Sudhā-sindhoḥ [2] Śuddhā).—The Ocean of Nectar is white and cool and makes immortal. Sākinī, who is the form of light itself (Jyotiḥ-svarūpā) is white and heatless.

In the following Dhyāna of Sākinī She is described in detail: "Let the excellent Sādhaka meditate in the throat lotus on the Devī Sākinī. She is light itself (Jyotiḥ-svarūpā): each of Her five beautiful faces is shining with three eyes. In Her lotus hands She carries the noose, the goad, the

---

[1] The "Man in the Moon".

[2] Sudhāsindhu, says Śaṁkara, is Candra (Moon). She is purer and whiter than the nectar in the moon. The translation here given is according to the construction of Śaṁkara and Viśvanātha, who read Sudhāsindhoh in the ablative. Kālīcaraṇa, however, reading it in the possessive case, gives the meaning "pure like the ocean of Nectar," which is the innermost ocean of the seven oceans, which surrounds the jeweled island (Maṇi-dvīpa).

sign of the book, and makes the Jñāna-mudrā.[1] She maddens (or distracts) all the mass of Paśus,[2] and She has her abode in the bone.[3] She is fond of milk food, and elated with the nectar which She has drunk."

By the expression "She is light itself" in the above Dhyāna, it is meant that She is white, whiteness being characteristic of light. The two Dhyānas differ as regards the weapons the Devī has in her hands. This is due to differences in the nature of the Sādhaka's aim.[4]

The Devī is in the lunar region (Candra-maṇḍala) within the pericarp. The Prema-yoga-Taraṅgiṇī says: "Here dwells the Śakti Sākinī in the auspicious region of the Moon."

"*In this Lotus*" (Kamale)—*i.e.*, in the pericarp of the Viśuddha-Cakra.

"*In this pericarp is the spotless region of the Moon, without the mark of a hare*" (Śaśa-pari-rahita), conveys the same meaning. The spots on the moon are called "the sign of the hare," "the stain on the moon". She is likened to the Stainless Moon.

"*The gateway of great liberation*" (Mahā-mokṣa-dvāra).—This is attributive of Maṇḍala, the lunar region, and is used in praise of the Maṇḍala. It is the gateway of Liberation, of Nirvāṇa-mukti, for those who have purified and conquered their senses, among other practices; by meditating on this in the path of Yoga they attain liberation (Mukti).

"*Who desires the wealth of Yoga*" (Śriyamabhimata-śīlasya)—By Śrī is meant "the wealth of Yoga". For him who by his very nature desires the wealth of Yoga, that is the gateway of Liberation. This clearly explains the meaning of Śuddhendriya, whose senses are pure and controlled.

In the pericarp of this Lotus is the Nabho-maṇḍala (ethereal region): inside the latter is the triangle (Trikoṇa); inside the triangle is the Candra-maṇḍala; and inside it is the Nabho-bīja[5]; and so forth. *Cf.* "Think of the full moon in the triangle within the pericarp; there think of the snowy Ākāśa seated on an elephant, and whose raiment is white. There is the Deva Sadā-Śiva." "Whose raiment is white" qualifies Ākāśa.

---

[1] Made by touching the thumb with the first finger of the right hand and placed over the heart.

[2] See *Introduction to Tantra-Śāstra*.

[3] *i.e.*, She is the Devata of the Asthi-Dhātu.

[4] The nature of the Dhyāna (meditation) varies with the aim which a Sādhaka wishes by his worship. See Tantrarāja. Tāntrik Texts, Vols. VIII and XII.

[5] The Bīja of Ether—Haṁ.

VERSE 31

Iha sthāne cittaṁ niravadhi vinidhāyātmasaṁpūrṇayogaḥ
kavirvāgmī jñānī sa bhavati nitarāṁ sādhakaḥ śāntacetāḥ
Trikālānāṁ darśī sakalahitakaro rogaśokapramuktaś-
ciraṁjīvī jīvī niravadhivipadāṁ dhvaṁsahaṁsaprakāśaḥ.

HE who has attained complete knowledge of the Ātmā (Brahman) becomes by constantly concentrating his mind (Citta) on this Lotus a great Sage,[1] eloquent and wise, and enjoys uninterrupted peace of mind.[2] He sees the three periods,[3] and becomes the benefactor of all, free from disease and sorrow and long-lived, and, like Haṁsa, the destroyer of endless dangers.

COMMENTARY

In this verse he speaks of the good gained by meditating on the Viśuddha-Cakra.

"*Who has attained, etc.*" (Ātma-saṁpūrṇa-yoga).[4]—He whose knowledge of the Ātman is complete by realisation of the fact that It is all-pervading. Ātman=Brahman.

According to another reading (Ātta-saṁpūrṇa-yoga), the meaning would be "one who has obtained perfection in Yoga". Hence the venerable Teacher [5] has said: "One who has attained complete knowledge of the Ātmā reposes like the still waters of the deep." The Sādhaka who fixes his Citta on this Lotus, and thereby acquires a full knowledge of the

---

[1] Kavi.

[2] Śanta-cetāh. Śama, says Śaṁkarācārya in his Ātmānātma-viveka, is Antarindriya-nigraha—*i.e.*, subjection of the inner sense.

[3] Past, present, and future.

[4] The word Yoga is here used as equivalent of Jñāna.

[5] Śrimadācārya, *i.e.*, Śaṁkarācārya.

Plate VI] Viśuddha [To face Page 391

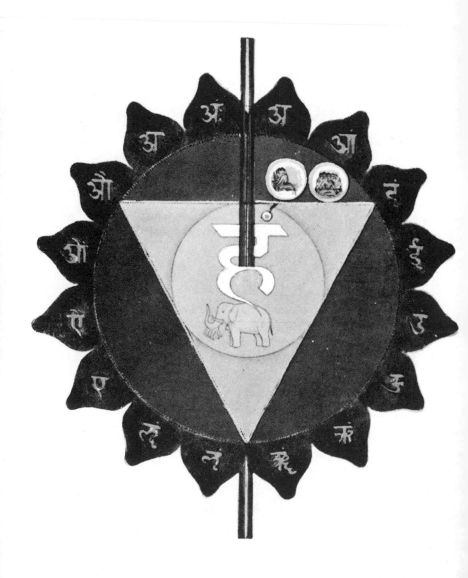

Brahman, becomes a knower (Jñānī) *i.e.*, becomes possessed of the knowledge of all the Śāstras without instruction therein. His Citta becomes peaceful; he becomes "merciful towards all, not looking for any return therefor. He is constant, gentle, steady, modest, courageous, forgiving, self-controlled, pure and the like, and free from greed, malice and pride." [1]

"*He sees the three periods*" (Tri-kāla-darśī)—*i.e.*, by the knowledge acquired by Yoga he sees everything in the past, present, and future. Some say that the meaning of this is that the Yogī has seen the Self (Ātmā), and, as all objects of knowledge are therein, they become visible to him.

"*Free from disease and sorrow*" (Roga-śoka-pramuktah) [2]—*i.e.*, by having attained Siddhi in his *mantra* he becomes free from diseases and long-lived, and by reason of his having freed himself from the bonds of Māyā he feels no sorrow.

"*Like Haṁsa, the destroyer of endless dangers*" (Niravadhi-vipadāṁ-dhvaṁsa-haṁsa-prakāśah).—From acts good and evil various dangers (Vipat) arise. The Sādhaka becomes like the Haṁsa which is the Antarātmā that dwells by the pericarp of the Sahasrāra,[3] for he can destroy all such dangers and in the result open the gate of Liberation (Mokṣa). Haṁsa is the form of the Antarātma. The rest is clear.

SUMMARY OF THE VIŚUDDHA CAKRA

At the base of the throat[4] is the Viśuddha Cakra, with sixteen petals of smoky purple hue. Its filaments are ruddy, and the sixteen vowels, which are red and have the Bindu above them, are on the petals. In its pericarp is the ethereal region (Nabho-maṇḍala), circular and white. Inside it is the Candra-maṇḍala, and above it is the Bīja Haṁ. This Bīja is white and garmented in white,[5] seated on an elephant, and is four-armed. In his four hands he holds the Pāśa (noose) and the Aṅkuśa (goad), and makes the Vara-mudrā and the Abhaya-mudrā. In his lap is Sadā-Śiva, seated on a great lion-seat which is placed on the back of a bull. He is in

---

[1] The portion within inverted commas is from the Bhagavad-Gītā, XVI, 2, 3.

[2] *Cf.* Sarva-roga-hara-cakra in Śrī-Yantra.

[3] That is, the Haṁsa is in the twelve-petalled Lotus below the Sahasrāra. Śaṁkara and Viśvanātha call Haṁsa the Sun.

[4] Kaṇṭha-mūle.

[5] That is, clothed in space.

his form of Arddha-nārīśvara, and as such half his body is the colour of snow, and the other half the colour of gold. He has five faces and ten arms, and in his hands he holds the Śūla (trident), the Ṭaṅka (battle-axe), the Khaḍga (sacrificial sword), the Vajra (thunderbolt), Dahana,[1] the Nāgendra (great snake), the Ghaṇta (bell) the Aṅkuśa (goad), the Pāśa (noose), and makes the Abhaya-mudrā. He wears a tiger's skin, his whole body is smeared with ashes, and he has a garland of snakes round his neck. The nectar dropping from the down-turned digit of the Moon is on his forehead. Within the pericarp, and in the Lunar Region and seated on bones, is the Śakti Sākinī, white in colour, four-armed, five-faced and three-eyed, clothed in yellow, and carrying in Her hand a bow, an arrow, a noose, and a goad.

---

[1] Agneya-astra.

VERSE 31A[1]

Iha sthāne cittaṁ niravadhi nidhāyāttapavano
yadi kruddho yogī calayati samastaṁ tribhuvanaṁ
Na ca brahmā viṣṇur na ca hariharo naiva khamaṇī-
stadīyaṁ sāmarthyaṁ śamayitumalaṁ nāpi gaṇapaḥ.

THE Yogī, his mind constantly fixed on this Lotus, his breath controlled by Kuṁbhaka,[2] is in his wrath [3] able to move all the three worlds. Neither Brahmā nor Viṣṇu, neither Hari-Hara [4] nor Sūrya [5] nor Gaṇapa [6] is able to control his power (resist him).

COMMENTARY

"*His breath controlled by Kuṁbhaka*" (Ātta-pavana).—Literally it means, who has taken the air in, which is done by Kuṁbhaka.

"*Hari-Hara*".—The Yugala (coupled) form, consisting of Viṣṇu and Śiva combined.

"*Surya*" (Kha-maṇi).—This word means the jewel of the sky, or Sūrya.

(Here ends the fifth section)

---

[1] This verse has not been taken into account either by Kālīcarṇa or Śaṁkara. It is given by Bala-deva in his text, and his Commentary is also here given. It is in Tripurā-sāra-samuccaya, Ch. v, 26.

[2] Retention of breath in Prāṇāyāma is Kuṁbhaka.

[3] This is praise (Stutivāda) of his great powers—that is, were he to get angry he could move the three worlds.

[4] See Commentary.

[5] Sun. See Commentary.

[6] Gaṇeśa.

Verse 32

Ājñānāmāṁbujaṁ taddhimakarasadṛśaṁ dhyānadhāmaprakāśaṁ
hakṣābhyāṁ vai kalābhyāṁ parilasitavapurnetrapatraṁ suśubhraṁ
Tanmadhye hākinī sā śaśisamadhavalā vaktraṣaṭkaṁ dadhānā
vidyāṁ mudrāṁ kapālaṁ ḍamarujapavaṭīṁ bibhratī śuddhacittā.

The Lotus named Ājñā [1] is like the moon, (beautifully white). On its two petals are the letters Ha and *Kṣa*, which are also white and enhance its beauty. It shines with the glory of Dhyāna.[2] Inside it is the Śakti Hākinī, whose six faces are like so many moons. She has six arms, in one of which She holds a book[3]; two others are lifted up in the gestures of dispelling fear and granting boons, and with the rest She holds a skull, a small drum,[4] and a rosary.[5] Her mind is pure (Śuddha-Cittā).

Commentary

The Author now describes the Ājñā-Cakra between the eyebrows in the seven verses beginning with this.

"*Lotus named Ājñā*" (Ājñā-nāma).—"Ājñā of the Guru is communicated here, hence it is called Ājñā." Here between the eyebrows is

---

[1] Ājñā—command. See Commentary. The Tantrāntara Tantra calls this Cakra the house of Śiva (Śiva-geha).

[2] The state of mind which is acquired by meditation (Dhyāna).

[3] Vidyāṁ mudrāṁ dadhānā, *i.e.*, she is making the gesture of Vidyā or Pustaka Mudrā and those of dispelling fear and granting boons. It is not that she is carrying a book in her hand. See *post.*

[4] Ḍamaru.

[5] Rosary with which "Recitation" (japa) of mantra is done.

the Ājñā (Command), which is communicated from above, hence it is called Ājñā. This Lotus which is well-known is here.[1]

This Lotus is between the eyebrows, as the following shows. "Going upwards after entering the throat and palate, the white and auspicious Lotus between the eyebrows is reached by Kuṇḍalī. It has two petals on which are the letters Ha and Kṣa, and it is the place of mind (Manas)."

The following are descriptions of the Lotus:

"*Like the Moon, beautifully white*" (Hima-kara-sadṛśaṁ). This comparison with Candra (Hima-kara) may also mean that this Lotus is cool like the moonbeams (the moon being the receptacle of Amṛta, or Nectar, whose characteristic is coolness), and that it is also beautifully white.

It has been said in "Īśvara-kārtikeya-samvāda":[2] "Ājñā-Cakra is above it; it is white and has two petals; the letters Ha and Kṣa, variegated in colour, also enhance its beauty. It is the seat of mind (Manas)."

"*Two petals*" (Netra-patra).—The petals of the lotus.

"*The letters Ha and Kṣa which are also white*" (Ha-kṣābhyāṁ kalābhyāṁ parilasitavapuh su-śubhraṁ).—These two letters are by their very nature white, and by their being on the white petals the whiteness thereof is made more charming by this very excess of whiteness.[3] The letters are called Kalās because they are Bījas of Kalās.[4]

"*It shines with the glory of Dhyāna*" (Dhyāna-dhāma-prakāśaṁ)—that is, its body shines like the glory of Dhyāna-Śakti.

"*Hākinī.*"—He next speaks of the presence of the Śaktī Hākinī here. The force of the pronoun Sā (She) in addition to Her name is that She is the well-known Hākinī.

"*The gestures of dispelling fear and granting boons*" (Mudrā).—This word stands for both Mudrās. There should be six weapons in Her hands, as She has six hands. There are some who read Vidyā and Mudrā as

---

[1] It is here that Ājñā of the Guru is communicated (Gautamīya-Tantra, cited by Viśvanātha). See Rudra-yāmala, Ch. XXVII, v. 68, which says that the Guru's Ājñā is communicated (Gurorājñeti).

[2] *i.e.*, the Saṁmohana-Tantra.

[3] Or the meaning may be that the Ājñā-Cakra has rays cool like the ambrosial rays of the Moon and like the Moon beautifully white.

[4] See Introduction, Prapañcasāra-Tantra, Vol. III, Tāntrik Texts, ed. A. Avalon.

one word, Vidyā-mudrā, and interpret it to mean Vyākhyā-mudrā—the gesture that conveys learning or knowledge—and speak of Her as possessed of four arms. Different manuscripts give different readings. Various manuscripts read these as two words. The wise reader should judge for himself.

In a Dhyāna in another place She is thus described: "Meditate upon Her, the divine Hākinī. She abides in the marrow [1] and is white. In Her hands are the Ḍamaru, the Rudrākṣa rosary, the skull, the Vidyā (the sign of the book), the Mudrā (gesture of granting boons and dispelling fear). She has six red-coloured faces with three eyes in each. She is fond of food cooked with Turminī, and is elated by drinking ambrosia. She is well seated on a white Lotus, and Her mind is exalted by the drink of the King of the Devas gathered from the Ocean."

The rest is clear.

[1] Majjasthā. According to another reading (cakrasthā) abides in the Cakra.

Verse 33

Etatpadmāntarāle nivasati ca manaḥ sūkṣmarūpaṁ prasiddhaṁ
yonau tatkarṇikāyāmitaraśivapadaṁ liṅgacihṇaprakāśaṁ
Vidyunmālāvilāsaṁ paramakulapadaṁ brahmasūtraprabodhaṁ
vedānāmādibījaṁ sthiratarahṛdayaścintayettatkrameṇa.

Within this Lotus dwells the subtle mind (Manas). It is well-known. Inside the Yoni in the pericarp is the Śiva called Itara,[1] in His phallic form. He here shines like a chain of lightning flashes. The first Bīja of the Vedas,[2] which is the abode of the most excellent Śakti and which by its lustre makes visible the Brahma-sūtra,[3] is also there. The Sādhaka with steady mind should meditate upon these according to the order (prescribed).

Commentary

He speaks of the presence of Manas in this Lotus.

"*Subtle*" (Sūkṣma-rūpa).—The Manas is beyond the scope of the senses; that being so, it may be asked, What is the proof of its existence? The answer is, It is well-known or universally accepted (Prasiddha) and handed down from Anādi-puruṣa, generation after generation as a thing realised, and is hence well-known. The evidence of the Śāstras, also, is that this Manas selects and rejects.[4] Here is the place of the Manas.

---

[1] Iṁ, Kālaṁ tarati iti Itarāh (Viśvanātha). "Itara" is that which enables one to cross Lāla. Iṁ—that is, the world of wandering.

[2] Oṁ.

[3] The Nādi-Citriṇī.

[4] Saṁkalpa-vikalpātmaka. This is the lower Manas, and not that referred to in the Commentary to v. 40, *post*. As to the mental faculties, see Introduction.

The presence of Manas is above the first Bīja of the Vedas as will appear from what is about to be spoken of.

"*Phallic form*" (Liṅga-cihṇa-prakāśaṁ).—He next speaks of the presence of the Śivalinga [1] in the Yoni which is within the pericarp. The Itara-Śiva who is there is in His phallic form, and within the Yoni. Within the triangle in the pericarp dwells Itara-Śivapada [2]—*i.e.*, the Śiva known by the name of Itara. This Liṅga is in the phallic form and white. As has been said in the Bhūta-śuddhi-Tantra: "Inside it is the Liṅga Itara, crystalline and with three eyes." Liṅga resembles continuous streaks of lightning flashes (Vidyun-mālā-vilāsaṁ).

"*First Bīja of the Vedas*" (Vedānāṁ-ādibījaṁ).—He then speaks of the presence of the Praṇava [3] in the pericarp of this Lotus. In the pericarp there is also the first Bīja—*i.e.*, Praṇava.[3]

"*Which is the abode of the most excellent Śakti*" (Paramakulapada).—Kula=Śakti which is here of a triangular form. Parama means most excellent, by reason of its resembling lightning and the like luminous substances; and *Pada* means place—*i.e.*, the triangular space. Hence this Bīja—namely, the Praṇava—we perceive is within the triangle. This is clearly stated in the following text:

"Within the pericarp, and placed in the triangle, is Ātmā in the form of the Praṇava, and above it, like the flame of a lamp, is the Charming Nāda, and Bindu which is Makāra,[4] and above it is the abode of Manas."

Now, if the Parama-kulapada [5] be the container (Ādhāra) of and therefore inseparate from the Praṇava, how is it that it is separately mentioned as one of the sixteen Ādhāras spoken of in the following passage? For it has been said that "the sixteen Ādhāras hard of attainment by the Yogī are Mūlādhāra, Svādhiṣṭhāna, Maṇipūra, Anāhata, Viśuddha, Ājñā-Cakra, Bindu, Kalāpada, Nibhodhikā, Arddhendu, Nāda, Nādānta, Unmanī, Viṣṇu-vaktra, Dhruvamaṇḍala,[6] and Śiva."

---

[1] Phallic emblem of Śiva.

[2] According to Viśvanātha, this is an Aṁśa (part) of the Nirguṇa Para-Śiva in the Sahasrāra.

[3] Oṁ.

[4] The letter Ma; that is, it is Makāra-rūpa or Ma before manifestation.

[5] Śaṁkara says that Paramakula=Mūladhāra-Padma, and Paramakulapada=He who has his abode in the Mūlādhāra.

[6] See Śāradā-Tilaka, Ch. V, 135, Ch. XII, v. 117 *et seq.*; Kulārṇava-Tantra, Ch. IV, and Introduction.

The answer is that the second Kulapada is not the one in the Ājña-Cakra, but is in the vacant space above Mahānāda which is spoken of later. This will become clear when dealing with the subject of Mahānāda.

" *Which makes manifest the Brahma-sūtra* " (Brahma-sūtra-prabodha). —Brahma-sūtra=Citriṇī-nāḍī. This Nāḍī is made visible by the lustre of the Praṇava. In v. 3 this Nāḍī has been described as " lustrous with the lustre of the Praṇava ".

The Sādhaka should with a steady mind meditate upon all these—*viz.*, Hākinī, Manas, Itara Liṅga and Praṇava—in the order prescribed. This is different from the order in which they are placed in the text by the author. But the arrangement of words according to their import is to be preferred to their positions in the text. The order as shown here should prevail. Thus, first Hākinī in the pericarp; in the triangle above her Itara-Liṅga; in the triangle above him the Praṇava; and last of all, above the Praṇava itself, Manas should be meditated upon.

Verse 34

Dhyānātmā sādhakendro bhavati parapure śīghragāmī munīndraḥ
sarvajñaḥ sarvadarśī sakalahitakaraḥ sarvaśāstrārthavetta
Advaitācāravādī vilasati paramāpūrvasiddhipraśiddho
dīrghāyuḥ so'pi kartā tribhuvanabhavane saṁhṛtau pālane ca.

The excellent Sādhaka, whose Ātmā is nothing but a meditation on this Lotus, is able quickly to enter another's body [1] at will, and becomes the most excellent among Munīs, and all-knowing and all-seeing. He becomes the benefactor of all, and versed in all the Śāstras. He realises his unity with the Brahman and acquires excellent and unknown powers.[2] Full of fame and long-lived, he ever becomes the Creator, Destroyer, and Preserver, of the three worlds.

Commentary

In this verse he speaks of the good to be gained by the Dhyāna of this Lotus.

"*Most excellent among Munīs*" (Munīndra).—A Munī is one who is accomplished in Dhyāna and Yoga [3] and other excellent acquirements. The suffix Indra means King or Chieftain, and is added to names to signify excellence.

"*Versed in all the Śāstras*" (Sarva-śāstrārthavettā).—Such an one becomes proficient in the Śāstras and in Divine knowledge, and thus he becomes all-seeing (Sarva-darśī)—*i.e.*, able to look at things from all points by reason of his being possessed of wisdom and knowledge which harmonises with Śāstras, manners, and customs.

---

[1] Para-pūra—may also mean another's house.

[2] Siddhi.

[3] Dhyāna-yogādi-saṁpannah.—The word may also mean one who is an adept in Dhyānayoga and other acquirements.

"*He realises,*" *etc.*, (Advaitācāra-vādī).—He knows that this Universe and all material existence is the Brahman, from such sayings of Śruti as, "The worlds are Its Pāda (that is Aṁśas)"; "All that exists is the Brahman";[1] and "I am the Deva, and no one else; I am the very Brahman, and sorrow is not my share."[2] He knows that the Brahman alone is the Real (Sat), and everything else is unreal (Asat), and that they all shine by the light of the Brahman.[3] The man who by such knowledge is able to realise the identity of the Individual with the Supreme Spirit[4] (Jīvātmā and Paramātmā), and preaches it, is an Advaitavādī.

"*Excellent and unknown powers*" (Paramāpūrva-siddhi)—that is, most exalted and excellent powers.

"*Full of fame*" (Prasiddha)—*i.e.*, famous by reason of his excellence.

"*He ever becomes,*" *etc.*, (So'pi kartā tribhuvana-bhavane samhṛtau pālane ca).—This is Praśaṁsā-vāda;[5] or it may mean that such Sādhaka becomes absorbed in the Supreme on the dissolution of the body, and thus becomes the source of Creation, Preservation, and Destruction.

---

[1] 'Pādo'sya viśvā bhūtānī Iti.' 'Tadidaṁ sarvaṁ Brahma.' The Chā. Up. reads (3. 12. 6), 'Pādo'sya sarvā bhūtānī' and (3. 14. 1), 'Sarvaṁ khalvidaṁ Brahma'—which mean the same thing.

[2] Ahaṁ devo na cānyo'smi Brahmaivāsmi na śokabhāk.

[3] Brahmaivaikaṁ sad-vastu tadanyad asat prapañca-samudāyastu Brahmābhāsatayā bhāsate.

[4] Jīvātma-paramātmanor aikyacintanaṁ.

[5] *i.e.*, Stuti-vāda, or praise; or, as we should say, compliment, which, while real in the sense of the presence of a desire to praise that which is in fact praiseworthy, is unreal so far as regards the actual words in which that desire is voiced.

VERSE 35

Tadantaścakreꝫsminnivasati satataṁ śuddhabuddhyantarātmā
pradīpābhajyotiḥ praṇavaviracanārūpavarṇaprakāśaḥ
Tadūrdhve candrārdhastadupari vilasadbindurūpī makāra-
stadūrdhve nādoꝫsau baladhavalasudhādhārasaṁtānahāsī.

WITHIN the triangle in this Cakra ever dwells the combination of letters [1] which form the Praṇava. It is the inner Ātmā as pure mind (Buddhi), and resembles a flame in its radiance. Above it is the half (crescent) moon, and above this, again, is Ma-kāra, [2] shining in its form of Bindu. Above this is Nāda, whose whiteness equals that of Balarāma [3] and diffuses the rays of the Moon. [3]

COMMENTARY

The author desires to speak of the presence of the Praṇava in the Ājñā-Cakra and says that in this Cakra, and within the triangle which has already been spoken of, ever dwells the combination of the letters A and U which by the rules of Sandhi make the thirteenth vowel O. This combination of letters is Śuddha-buddhyantarātmā—*i.e.*, the innermost Spirit manifesting as pure intelligence (Buddhi). The question may be asked if the thirteenth vowel (O) is that. To obviate this the author qualifies it by saying " above it is the half Moon, etc." It is by adding the half Moon (Nāda) and Bindu to O that the Praṇava is formed.

---

[1] That is, *a* and *u*, which by Saṁdhi becomes *O*, and with anusvāra (*m*) thus form the Praṇava, or mantra *Oṁ*.

[2] The letter M in its Bindu form in Candra-bindu.

[3] Śaṁkara reads it as Jala-dhavala, etc., and explains it by " white like water ". The last portion may also mean " smiling whiteness equals that of the Moon ".

He next gives its attributes:

"*Resembles a flame in its radiance*" (Pradīpābha-jyotiḥ).—But how can this thirteenth vowel by itself be Śuddha-buddhyantarātmā? He therefore says:

"*Above it is the crescent moon*" (Tadūrdhve candrārdhah).

"*And above this, again, is Ma-kāra, shining in its form of Bindu*" (Tadupari vilasad-bindu-rūpī Ma-Kāraḥ).—It is thus shown that by the placing of the crescent moon and the Bindu [1] over the thirteenth vowel the Praṇava is completely formed.

"*Above this is Nāda*" (Tadūrdhve nādo'sau)—*i.e.*, above the Praṇava is the Avāntara (final or second) Nāda, which challenges as it were the whiteness of Baladeva and the Moon (Bala-dhavala-sudhā-dhāra-saṁtāna-hāsī). By this he means to say that it is extremely white, excelling, in whiteness both Baladeva and the rays of the Moon.[2]

Some read Tadādye nādo'sau (in the place of Tadūrdhve nādo'sau) and interpret it as, "Below Bindu-rūpī Ma-kāra is Nāda". But that is incorrect. The text says: "Above this, again, is Ma-kāra, shining in its form of Bindu," and there is Nāda below it; that being so, it is useless to repeat that Nāda is below.

Besides, this Nāda is beyond the Nāda, which forms part of the Praṇava, and is part of the differentiating (Bhidyamāna) Para-bindu placed above the Praṇava. If, however, it be urged that it is necessary to state the details in describing the special Praṇava (Viśiṣṭa-Praṇava), and it is asked, "Why do you say a second Nāda is inappropriate?" then the reading Tadādye nādo'sau may be accepted.

But read thus it should be interpreted in the manner following: "This Nāda shown below the Bindu-rūpī Ma-kāra is Bala-dhavala-sudhā-dhāra-saṁthāna-hāsī (*v. ante*), and the Nāda first spoken of is also so described. Such repetition is free from blame on the authority of the maxim that "the great are subject to no limitations."

[1] That is, Anusvāra.

[2] Sudhādhārasaṁtāna, Viśvanātha says, means a multitude of moons.

VERSE 36

Iha sthāne līne susukhasadane cetasi puraṁ
nirālaṁbāṁ badhvā paramagurusevāsuviditāṁ
Tadabhyāsād yōgī pavanasuhṛdāṁ paśyati kaṇāṅ
tatastanmadhyāntaḥ pravilasitarūpānapi sadā.

WHEN the Yogī closes the house which hangs without support,[1] the knowledge whereof he has gained by the service of Parama-guru, and when the Cetas[2] by repeated practice becomes dissolved in this place which is the abode of uninterrupted bliss, he then sees within the middle of and in the space above (the triangle) sparks of fire distinctly shining.

COMMENTARY

Having described the Praṇava, he now speaks of its union (with Cetas), *i.e.*, Praṇava-yoga.

The Yogī should close the house (Puraṁ baddhvā)—*i.e.*, he should, with his mind set on the act, close the inner house; or, in other words, he should make Yoni-Mudrā[3] in the manner prescribed and thus effectually close the inner house. The use of the word *Pur* shows that the Yoni-Mudrā is meant. Then, when his Cetas by repeated practice (Abhyāsa) or meditation on the Praṇava becomes dissolved (Līna) in this place (the Ājñā-Cakra), he sees, within and in the space above the triangle wherein the Praṇava is, sparks of Fire[4] (Pavana-suhṛdāṁ kaṇān), or, to put it

---

[1] Nirālaṁba-purī. Nirālaṁba (*v. post*) means that which has no support—*viz.*, that by which the mind's connection with the world has been removed and realization of the infinite established. Ākāśamāṁsī= whose flesh or substance is Ākāśa (Rājanighantu Dict.)

[2] See next page and Introduction.

[3] *i.e.*, closes the avenues of the mind and concentrates it within itself.

[4] Pavana-suhṛd—"He whose friend is air"=Fire. When the wind blows, fire spreads.

plainly, sparks of light resembling sparks of fire appear before his mental vision above the triangle on which the Praṇava rests. It is by Yoni-Mudrā that the inner self (Antah-pūr) is restrained and detached from the outside world, the region of material sense. The Manas cannot be purified and steadied unless it is completely detached from the material sphere. It is therefore that the mind (Manas) should be completely detached by Yoni-Mudrā.

Yoni-Mudrā, which detaches the Manas from the outside world, is thus defined: "Place the left heel against the anus, and the right heel on the left foot, and sit erect with your body and neck and head in a straight line. Then, with your lips formed to resemble a crow's beak,[1] draw in air and fill therewith your belly. Next [2] close tightly your earholes with the thumbs, with your index-fingers the eyes, the nostrils by your middle fingers, and your mouth by the remaining fingers. Retain the air [3] within you, and with the senses controlled meditate on the Mantra whereby you realize the unity (Ekatvam) of Prāṇa and Manas.[4] This is Yoga, the favourite of Yogīs."

That steadiness of mind is produced by restraint of breath through the help of Mudrā, has been said by Śruti. "The mind under the influence of Haṁsa [5] moves to and fro, over different subjects; by restraining Haṁsa, the mind is restrained."

"*Closes the house*" (Puraṁ baddhvā).—This may also mean Khecarī Mudrā.[6] This latter also produces steadiness of mind.

As has been said, "As by this the Citta roams in the Brahman (Kha),[7] and as the sound of uttered word [8] also roams the Ether (Kha), therefore is Khecarī Mudrā honoured by all the Siddhas."

---

[1] That is, by Kākī-Mudrā. Śruti says that when Vāyu is drawn in by this Mudrā and stopped by Kuṁbhaka, steadiness of mind is produced.

[2] These and following verses occur in Śāradā-Tilaka, Ch. XXV, vv. 45, 46. The first portion of this passage describes Siddhāsana.

[3] That is, by Kuṁbhaka.

[4] That is, recite the Haṁsa or Ajapā-mantra, or breathing in Kuṁbhaka.

[5] The Jīvātmā manifesting as Prāṇa.

[6] One of the Mudrās of Haṭha-Yoga. See Introduction.

[7] Kha has three meanings—*viz.*,, Ether, Brahman, and space between eyebrows (Ājñā). Brahmānanda, the commentator of the Haṭha-yoga-pradīpikā, adopts the last meaning in interpreting this verse (Ch. III, v. 41), and in commenting on v. 55 of the Haṭha-yoga-pradīpikā gives it the meaning of Brahman.

[8] *Lit.*, tongue.

The Citta is Khecara [1] when, disunited from Manas and devoid of all attachment to all worldly things, it becomes Unmanī.[2]

As has been said,[3] "the Yogī is united with Unmanī; without Unmanī there is no Yogī." Nirālaṁba means that which has no support —namely, that from which the minds' connection with the world has been removed.

"*The knowledge whereof he has gained by the service of his Paramaguru*" (Parama-guru-sevā-suviditām).—Parama is excellent in the sense that he has attained excellence in Yoga practice (by instructions) handed down along a series of spiritual preceptors (Gurus), and not the result of book-learning.[4]

"*Serving the Guru*".—Such knowledge is obtained from the Guru by pleasing him by personal services (Sevā). *Cf.* "It can be attained by the instructions of the Guru, and not by ten million of Śāstras."

"*The abode of uninterrupted bliss*" (Su-sukha-sādhana)—*i.e.*, this is the place where one enjoys happiness that nothing can interrupt. This word qualifies *place* (Iha-sthāne—*i.e.*, Ājñā-Cakra.)

"*Sparks of fire distinctly shining*" (Pavana-suhṛdāṁ pravilasitarūpān kaṇān).—These sparks of Fire shine quite distinctly.

Elsewhere it is clearly stated that the Praṇava is surrounded by sparks of light: "Above it is the flame-like Ātmā, auspicious and in shape like the Praṇava, on all sides surrounded by sparks of light."

---

[1] What moves about in the sky or ether. It is Manas which deprives the Citta of freedom by causing attachment to the world. On being disunited from Manas it moves freely in the ether, going its own way.

[2] Unmanī is there where, to coin a word, the "Manasness" of Manas ceases. See note to v. 40. Ut=without, and manī is from Manas.

[3] This is from Jñānārṇava-Tantra, Ch. XXIV, v. 37.

[4] Which is well recognized to be insufficient in these matters.

Verse 37

Jvaladdīpākāraṁ tadanu ca navīnārkabahula-
prakāśaṁ jyotirvā gaganadharaṇīmadhyamilitaṁ
Iha sthāne sākṣād bhavati bhagavān pūrṇavibhavo-
'vyayaḥ sākṣī vahneḥ śaśimihirayormaṇḍala iva.

He then also sees the Light[1] which is in the form of a flaming lamp. It is lustrous like the clearly shining morning sun, and glows between the Sky and the Earth.[2] It is here that the Bhagavān manifests Himself in the fullness of His might.[3] He knows no decay, and witnesseth all, and is here as He is in the region of Fire, Moon, and Sun.[4]

Commentary

Yogīs such as these see other visions beside the sparks of light. After seeing the fiery sparks they see the light.[5]

"*Then*" (Tadanu)—*i.e.*, after seeing the sparks spoken of in the preceding Śloka.

He then describes this Light (Jyotiḥ).

"*Glows between the Sky and the Earth*" (Gagana-dharaṇī madhya-milita).—This compound adjective qualifies Jyotiḥ or Light.

---

[1] Jyotiḥ.

[2] See Commentary, *post.*

[3] Pūrṇa-vibhava, which, however, as Kālīcaraṇa points out *post,* may be interpreted in various ways. According to Viśvanātha, the second chapter of the Kaivalya-Kalikā-Tantra contains a verse which says that the presence of the all-pervading Brahman is realized by His action, as we realize the presence of Rāhu by his action on the sun and moon.

[4] That is, the triangle on Manipīṭha within the A-ka-tha triangle. See v. 4 of the Pādukāpañcaka.

[5] The practicle *vā* in the text is used in an inclusive sense.

Gagana (sky) is the sky or empty space above Śaṅkhinī-Nāḍī (see verse 40, *post*), and Dharaṇī (Earth) is the Dharā-maṇḍala in the Mūlādhāra. This light also extends from the Mūlādhāra to the Sahasrāra.

He next speaks of the presence of Parama-Śiva in the Ājñā-Cakra.

"*It is here*" (Iha sthāne)—*i.e.*, in the Ājñā-Cakra; Parama-Śiva is here, as in the Sahasrāra. Bhagavān is Parama-Śiva.

"*Manifests Himself*" (Sākṣād bhavati)—*i.e.*, He is here.[1]

"*In the fulness of his might*" (Pūrṇa-vibhava).—This compound word which qualifies *Bhagavān* is capable of various interpretations.

Pūrna-vibhava may also be interpreted in the following different ways:

(*a*) *Pūrna* may mean complete in Himself, and *vibhava* infinite powers, such as the power of creation, etc. In that case the word would mean: "One who has in Him such powers, who is the absolute Creator, Destroyer, and Supporter of the Universe."

(*b*) *Vibhava*, again, may mean "the diversified and limitless creation," and *pūrna* "all-spreading". In this sense *Pūrna-vibhava* means "He from whom this all-spreading and endless (vast) creation has emanated." *Cf.* "From whom all these originated, and in whom having originated they live, to whom they go and into whom they enter" (Śruti).[2]

(*c*) *Vibhava*, again, may mean: "omnipresence," and *Pūrna* "all-spreading". It would then mean: "He who in His omnipresence pervades all things."

(*d*) *Pūrna*[3] may also mean the quality of one whose wish is not moved by the result and is not attached to any object. *Pūrna-vibhava* would then mean one who is possessed of that quality.

All things except Ātmā pass away. The omnipresence of the ethereal region (Ākāśa), etc., is not ever-existent. The Nirvāṇa-Tantra (Ch. IX) speaks of the presence of Parama-Śiva in the Ājñā-Cakra in detail.

---

[1] He is seen here.

[2] Tait. Up., 3. I. I.

[3] Phalānupahita-viṣayitānāspadecchākatvaṁ: He whose wish is not moved by the result, and is not attached to any object; or, in other words, He whose ways are inscrutable to us, subject as we are to limitations (Māyā).

" Above this (*i.e.*, Viśuddha) Lotus is Jñāna Lotus, which is very difficult to achieve; it is the region [1] of the full moon, and has two petals." Again: " Inside it, in the form of *Haṁsah*, is the Bīja of Śaṁbhu "; and again: " Thus is *Haṁsah* in *Maṇi-dvīpa*,[2] and in its lap is Parama-Śiva, with Siddha-Kālī [3] on his left. She is the very self of eternal Bliss." By *lap* is meant the *space* within the *Bindus* which form the Visarga at the end of Haṁsah.[4]

So it has been said in describing the Sahasrāra: " There are the two Bindus which make the imperishable Visarga.[5] In the space within is Parama-Śiva." As It is in the Sahasrāra so It is represented here.[6]

We are to understand that these two, Śiva and Śakti, are here in union (Bandhana) in the form of Parabindu, as the letter Ma (Makārātmā), and that they are surrounded (Āccādana) by Māyā.[7] " She the Eternal One stays here (Ājñā-Cakra) in the form of a grain of gram,[8] and creates beings (Bhūtāni)." Here the Parama-Śiva as in the form of a gram dwells, and according to the Utkalādimata [9] also creates.

" *As He is in the region of Fire, Moon and Sun* " (Vahneh śaśimihirayor maṇḍalamiva)—As the presence of Bhagavān in these regions is well known, so is He here. Or it may be that the author means that as He in the shape of a grain of gram dwells in the regions of Fire, Moon, and Sun, in the Sahasrāra, so does He dwell here also. We shall describe the Arka,

---

[1] Pūrṇa-candrasya maṇḍalaṁ.

[2] The isle of gems in the Ocean of Ambrosia. The Rudra-Yāmala says that it is in the centre of the Ocean of nectar outside and beyond the countless myriads of world systems, and that there is the Supreme abode of Śrī-vidyā.

[3] A form of Śakti.

[4] *i.e.*, the two dots which form the aspirate breathing at the end of *Haṁsah.*

[5] Imperishable visarga—Visargarūpaṁ avyayaṁ.

[6] That is, the Para-bindu is represented in the Ājñā by the Bindu of the Oṁkāra, which is its Pratīka.

[7] Bindu is the nasal sound of Ma, which is a male letter. Bindu is here the unmanifest Ma.

[8] Caṇakākāra-rūpiṇī. See Introduction.

[9] Apparently a school of that name.

Indu, and Agni Maṇḍala in the Sahasrāra later. In Pīṭha-pūjā the Pūjā of Paramātmā and Jñānātmā should be performed on the Maṇḍalas of Sun (Arka), Moon (Indu), and Fire (Agni). By Paramātmā Parama-Śiva is meant, and by Jñānātmā Jñāna-Śakti. The Bindu should be meditated upon as like the grain of gram, consisting of the inseparable couple [1]—namely, Śiva and Śakti.

[1] The grain referred to is divided in two under its encircling sheath.

Verse 38

Iha sthāne viṣṇoratulaparamāmodamadhure
samāropya prāṇaṁ pramuditamanāḥ prāṇanidhane
Paraṁ nityaṁ devaṁ puruṣamajamādyaṁ trijagatāṁ
purāṇaṁ yogīndraḥ praviśati ca vedāntaviditaṁ.

This is the incomparable and delightful abode of Viṣṇu. The excellent Yogī at the time of death joyfully places his vital breath (Prāṇa)[1] here and enters (after death) that Supreme, Eternal, Birthless, Primeval Deva, the Puruṣa, who was before the three worlds, and who is known by the Vedānta.

Commentary

He now speaks of the good to be gained by giving up the Prāṇa by Yoga in the Ājña-Cakra.

This verse means: The excellent Yogī (Yogīndra) at the time of death (Prāṇa-nidhane) joyfully (Pramudita-manāh) places his Prāṇa (Prāṇam samāropya) in the abode of Viṣṇu in the Ājñā-Cakra (Iha sthāne Viṣṇoh—*i.e.*, in the abode of Bhagavān in the Bindu already described), and passes away, and then enters the Supreme Puruṣa.

"*At the time of death*" (Prāṇa-nidhane)—*i.e.*, feeling the approach of death.

"*Joyfully*" (Pramudita-manāh).—Glad in mind in the enjoyment of the blissful union with Ātmā. (Ātmānandena hṛṣta-cittaḥ.)

"*Viṣṇu*"=Bhagavān=Parama-Śiva (see previous Śloka).

"*Here*" (Iha sthāne—*i.e.*, in the Bindu in the Ājñā-Cakra spoken of above).

"*Places the Prāṇa here*" (Iha sthāne prāṇam samāropya)—*i.e.*, he places it on the Bindu already spoken of. He describes Puruṣa as Eternal.

---

[1] Compare, Bhagavad-Gītā, Ch. VIII, vv. 9 and 10, and the commentary of Śaṁkarācārya and Madhusūdana-Sarasvatī on those verses.

"*Eternal*" (Nityam).—Indestructible (Vināśarahitaṁ).

"*Birthless*" (Aja).

"*Primeval*" (Purāṇa).—He is the one known as the Purāṇa Puruṣa.[1]

"*Deva*" means he whose play is Creation, Existence, and Destruction.

"*Who was before the three worlds*" (Tri-jagatāṁ ādyaṁ).[2]—By this the implication is that He is the Cause of all as He preceded all.

"*Known by the Vedānta*" (Vedānta-vidita).[3]—Vedānta are sacred texts dealing with the inquiry concerning the Brahman. He is known by a Knowledge (Jñāna) of these.

The way the Prāṇa is placed (Prāṇāropaṇa-prakāra) in the place of Viṣṇu is described below: Knowing that the time for the Prāṇa to depart is approaching, and glad that he is about to be absorbed into the Brahman, the Yogī sits in Yogāsana and restrains his breath by Kuṁbhaka. He then leads the Jīvātmā in the heart to the Mūlādhāra, and by contracting the anus [4] and following other prescribed processes rouses the Kuṇḍalinī. He next meditates upon the lightning-like, blissful Nāda which is thread-like and whose substance is Kuṇḍalī (Kuṇḍalinī-maya). He then merges the Haṁsa which is the Paramātmā in the form of Prāṇa [5] in the Nāda, and leads it along with the Jīva through the different Cakras according to the rules of Cakra-bheda to Ājñā-Cakra. He there dissolves all the diverse elements from the gross to the subtle, beginning with Pṛthivī, in Kuṇḍalinī. Last of all, he unifies Her and the Jīvātmā with the Bindu whose substance is Śiva and Śakti (Śiva-Śakti-maya); which having done, he pierces the Brahma-randhra and leaves the body, and becomes merged in the Brahman.

---

[1] According to Śaṁkara, it is an adjective, and means "He who is the cause of Creation," and the like.

[2] That is, the three spheres Bhūh, Bhuvah, Svah, the Vyāhṛtis of the Gāyatrī.

[3] Śaṁkara reads Vedānta-vihita, and explains the expression to mean "'this is the teaching of the Vedānta".

[4] Gudaṁ ākuñcya—that is, by Aśvinī-Mudrā.

[5] Prāṇarupa-śvāsa-paramātmakaṁ. See Jñānārṇava-Tantra, Ch. XXI, vv. 13-18.

Plate VIII

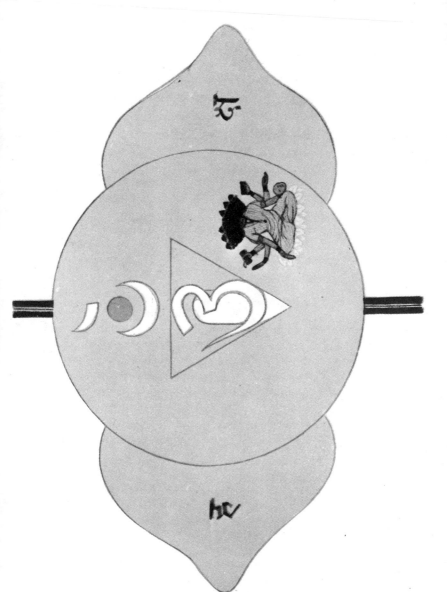

Summary of the Ājñā Cakra, Verses 32 to 38

The Ājñā Cakra has two petals and is white. The letters Ha and Kṣa, which are white,[1] are on the two petals. The presiding Śakti of the Cakra, Hākinī, is in the pericarp. She is white, has six red-coloured faces each with three eyes, and six arms, and is seated on a white lotus. With Her hands She displays Vara-mudrā and Abhaya-mudrā,[2] and holds a Rudrākṣa rosary, a human skull, a small drum, and a book. Above Her, within a Trikoṇa, is Itara-Liṅga, which is lightning-like, and above this again, within another Trikoṇa, is the inner Ātmā (Antar-ātmā), lustrous like a flame. On its four sides, floating in air, are sparks surrounding a light which by its own lustre makes visible all between Mūla and the Brahmarandhra. Above this, again, is Manas, and above Manas, in the region of the Moon, is Haṁsah, within whom is Parama-Śiva with His Śakti.

(Here ends the sixth section)

[Viśvanātha,[3] in the Commentary to the Ṣaṭcakra, gives under this verse a description, taken from the Svacchanda-saṁgraha, of the region beyond the Ājñā—that is, beyond the Samaṣṭi or collective or cosmic Ājñā: "Within the Bindu is a space a hundred million Yojanas[4] in expanse, and bright with the brightness of ten million suns. Here is the Lord of the State beyond Śānti (Śāntyatītcśvara), with five heads and ten arms and lustrous as a mass of lightning flashes. On His left is Śāntyatītā Manonmanī. Surrounding them are Nivṛtti, Pratiṣṭhā, Vidyā, and Śāntī.[5] Each of these is adorned with a moon and has five heads and ten arms. This is Bindu-Tattva. Above Bindu is Ardha-candra, with the Kalās of the latter—namely, Jyotsnā, Jyotsnāvatī, Kānti, Suprabhā, Vimalā. Above Ardha-candra is Nibodhikā, with the Kalās of the latter—Bandhatī,

---

[1] Karbura=white, and also means *variegated.*

[2] *V.* p. 337 *ante.*

[3] The portion in brackets is my note.—A. A.

[4] A Yojana is over eight miles.

[5] See, as to the Kalās, Introduction to Vol. III, Tāntrik Texts, ed. A. Avalon. See also Introduction to this volume; and *The Garland of Letters.*

Bodhinī, Bodhā, Jñāna-bodhā, Tamo'pahā. Above Nibodhikā is Nāda and its five Kalās—Indhikā, Recikā, Ūrdhvagā, Trāsā, and Paramā. On the lotus above this last is Īśvara, in extent a hundred million Yojanas, and lustrous as ten thousand moons. He is five-headed, and each head has three eyes. His hair is matted, and he holds the trident (Śūla). He is the one who goeth upwards (Ūrdhva-gāmini), and in His embrace (Utsaṅga) is the Kalā Ūrdhva-gāmini."]

Verse 39

Layasthānaṁ vāyostadupari ca mahānādarūpaṁ śivārdhaṁ
sirākāraṁ śāntaṁ varadamabhayaṁ śuddhabuddhiprakāśaṁ
Yadā yogī paśyed gurucaraṇayugāṁbhōjasevāsuśīlas-
tadā vācāṁ siddhiḥ karakamalatale tasya bhūyāt sadaiva.

When the actions of the Yogī are, through the service of the Lotus feet of his Guru, in all respects good, then he will see above it (*i.e.*, Ājña-cakra) the form of the Mahānāda, and will ever hold in the Lotus of his hand the Siddhi of Speech.[1] The Mahānāda, which is the place of dissolution of Vāyu[2] is the half of Śiva, and like the plough in shape,[3] is tranquil and grants boons and dispels fear, and makes manifest pure Intelligence (Buddhi).[4]

Commentary

He now wishes to describe the intermediate causal body (Kāraṇā-vāntara-śarīra)[5] situate above Ājñā-Cakra and below Sahasrāra and

[1] That is, all powers of speech.

[2] Vāyoh layasthānaṁ. Śaṁkara defines it by saying: Etat sthānaṁ vāyoh virāma-bhūtaṁ—this is the place where Vāyu ceases to be.

[3] That is, Śiva is Hakāra; and if the upper part of Ha is removed, the remaining portion of the letter has the form of an Indian plough.

[4] Śuddha-buddhi-prakāśa.

[5] Kāraṇāvāntara-śarīra, Kāraṇa=cause; Avāṇtara=secondary or intermediate or inclusive; Śarīra=body. Body is so called because it wastes and fades. It is derived from the root Śrī, to wane. Kāraṇāvāntara-śarīra would thus mean "the intermediate Śarīra of the Cause". The primary cause is the Great Cause. Its effects are also intermediate causes of that which they themselves produce; they are thus secondary or intermediate causal bodies. Taking the Sakala-Parameśvara to be the first cause, Mahānāda is one of its effects and a Kāraṇāvāntara-śarīra as regards that which it produces and which follows it.

says: When the actions of the Yogī are, through the service of the Lotus feet of his Guru, in all respects good—that is, when he excels by intense concentration of the mind in Yoga practice—he then sees the image of Mahā-nāda above it (above Ājñā-Cakra), and he becomes accomplished in speech (Vāk-siddha).

"*Actions in all respects good*" (suśīla).—The good inclination for Yoga practice rendered admirable by strong and undivided application thereto. This result is obtained by serving the Guru.

The author then qualifies Nāda, and says it is *the place of dissolution of Vāyu* (Vāyor laya-sthānaṁ). The Rule is "things dissolve into what they originate from." Hence, although in Bhūta-śuddhi and other practices it has been seen that Vāyu dissolves into Sparśa-tattva,[1] and the latter in Vyoma," [2] Vāyu dissolves in Nāda also. We have the authority of Revelation (Śruti) for this:

"Pṛthivī, the possessor of Rasa (Rasa-vatī), originated from Ī-kāra.[3] From Ka-kāra,[3] who is Rasa, the waters and Tīrthas [4] issued; from Repha (Ra-kāra) [3] originated Vahni-tattva [5]; from Nāda [3] came Vāyu [6] which pervades all life (Sarva-Prāṇamaya). From Bindu [3] originated the Void [7] which is empty of all things and is the Sound-container. And from all these [8] issued the twenty-five *Tattvas* which are Guṇa-maya. All this Universe (Viśva), which is the mundane egg of Brahmā, is pervaded by Kālikā."

---

[1] The "touch principle," also called Tvak-tattva. As to Bhūta-śuddhi, see the same described in Author's "Introduction to Tantra-Śastra".

[2] Ether.

[3] The Bīja Krīṁ is here being formed, Kakāra=Kālī; Ra-kāra=Brahmā as fire; Īkāra=Mahāmāyā. Anuśvāra or Candra-bindu (ṁ) is divided into two—*viz.*, Nāda, which is Viśvamātā, or Mother of the Universe; and Bindu, which is Duhkha-hara, or remover of pain (Bījakośa).

[4] Places of pilgrimage where the devotees bathe. It also means sacred waters.

[5] Fire.

[6] Air.

[7] Gagana or Ether.

[8] That is, from Krīṁ as composed of Ka+Ra+Ī+ṁ.

We should therefore realize in our mind that at the time the letters of the Kālī-mantra [1] are merged into that which is subtle, Vāyu is absorbed in Nāda.

"*Half of Śiva*" (Śivārdha).—By this is meant that here Śiva is in the form of Arddha-nārīśvara. Half is Śakti which is Nāda.

"*Like a plough*" (Sirākāra).—The word Sirā is spelt here with a short *i*, and in Amara-Kośa it is spelt with a long ī; but it is clearly the same word, as it begins with a dental *s*.

Cf. "Above it is Mahānāda, in form like a plough, and lustrous" (Īśvara-Kārtikeya-Saṁvāda).[2]

If the text is read as "Śivākāra instead of Sirākāra," then the meaning would be that the Nāda is Śiva-Śaktimaya.[3]

Cf. Prayoga-sāra: "That Śakti which tends towards seat of Liberation [4] is called male (Puṁrūpā—that is, Bindu) when, quickened by Nāda, She turns towards Śiva [5] (Śivon-mukhī)." It is therefore that Rāghava-Bhaṭṭa has said that "Nāda and Bindu are the conditions under which She creates".[6]

It has elsewhere been said: "She is eternal [7] existing as Cit (Cinmātrā) [8]: when being near the Light She is desirous of change, She becomes massive (Ghanī-bhūya) and Bindu."

---

[1] Krīn.

[2] *i.e.*, Sammohana-Tantra. Ed., R. M. Chattopādhyāya.

[3] That is, its substance is Śiva and Śakti.

[4] Nirāmaya-padōnmukhī=She who is turned to the place of Liberation: that is Śakti in the supreme state.

[5] Tending towards, intent on, or with face uplifted to, Śiva, that is here tending to creation. That is, the first state is Cit. Nāda is the Mithah-samavāya of Śakti or Bindu. The establishment of this relation quickens Her to turn to Śiva for the purpose of creation when She appears as male, or Bindu.

[6] Tasyā eva shakter nādabindū sriṣtyupayogyarūpau (Upayoga is capacity or fitness for creation).

[7] According to another reading this part would mean "She who is the Tattva".

[8] She is there, existing as Cit, with whom she is completely unified. She "measures Cit"—that is, co-exists with and as Cit, and is also formative activity. The above translation is that of the text, but the verse has been quoted elsewhere as if it were Cinmātrajyotiṣah, and not Cinmātrā jyotiṣah, in which case the translation would be: "She who when near Jyotih, which is mere consciousness, becomes desirous of change, becomes massive and assumes the form of Bindu."

So in the word of the honoured (Śrīmat) Ācārya:[1] "Nāda becomes massive and the Bindu." Now, taking all these into consideration, the conclusion is that Śakti manifests Herself as Nāda-bindu, like gold in ear-rings made of gold.[2]

Nāda and Bindu again are one—that is the deduction.

---

[1] Śaṁkarācārya.

[2] That is, they are both gold in the form of an ear-ring.

Cf. Chāndogya Up., 6. 1. 4.

"Gentle One, by one lump of clay all things made up of clay are known. The variation is in the names given to it when spoken about. The clay alone is real."

Verse 40

Tadūrdhve śaṅkhinyā nivasati śikhare śūnyadeśe prakāśaṁ
visargādhaḥ padmaṁ daśaśatadalaṁ pūrṇacandrātiśubhraṁ
Adhōvaktraṁ kāntaṁ taruṇaravikalākāntikiñjalkapuñjaṁ
ḷakārādyairvarṇaiḥ pravilasitavapuḥ kevalānandarūpaṁ.

Above all these, in the vacant space[1] wherein is Śaṅkhinī Nāḍī, and below Visarga is the Lotus of a thousand petals.[2] This Lotus, lustrous and whiter than the full Moon, has its head turned downward. It charms. Its clustered filaments are tinged with the colour of the young Sun. Its body is luminous with the letters beginning with A, and it is the absolute bliss.[3]

Commentary

The Ācārya enjoins that Sādhakas who wish to practise Samādhi Yoga " should before such time with every consideration and effort dissolve all things in their order from the gross to the subtle in Cidātmā ".[4] All things, both gross and subtle, which make up creation should first be meditated upon. As the knowledge thereof is necessary, they are here described in detail.

The five gross elements—Pṛthivī[5] and so forth—have been spoken of as being in the five Cakras from Mūlādhāra to Viśuddha. In the

---

[1] This place is called the Supreme Ether (Parama-vyoma) in the Svacchanda-saṁgraha, cited by Viśvanātha. Parama-vyoma is the name given in the Pañcarātra to the Highest Heaven or Vaikuṇṭha. See Ahirbhudhnya, 49.

[2] The Sahasrāra is called Akula, according to the Svacchanda-saṁgraha, cited by Viśvanātha.

[3] Kevalānanda-rūpam, *i.e.*, Brahman Bliss.

[4] The Ātmā considered as Cit.

[5] Earth, Water, Fire, Air, Ether.

Bhūmaṇḍala [1] in the Mūlādhāra there are the following—*viz.*, feet, sense of smell, and Gandha-tattva, [2] for this is their place. In the Jala-maṇḍala,[3] similarly, are the hands, sense of taste, and Rasa-tattva.[4] In the Vahni-maṇḍala [5] are the anus, the sense of sight, and Rūpa-tattva.[6] In the Vāyumaṇḍala,[7] are the penis, sense of touch, and Sparśa-tattva.[8] In the Nabho-maṇdala [9] are speech, the sense of hearing, and Śabda-tattva.[10] These make fifteen tattvas. Adding these fifteen to Pṛthivī and so forth we get twenty gross tattvas.

We next proceed to the subtle forms. In the Ājñā-Cakra the subtle manas has been spoken of. Others have been spoken of in the Kaṅkāla-mālinī-Tantra (Ch. II) when dealing with the Ājñā-Cakra: "Here constantly shines the excellent Manas, made beautiful by the presence of the Śakti Hākinī. It is lustrous, and has Buddhi,[11] Prakṛti,[12] and Ahaṁkāra [13] for its adornment."

From the above the presence of the three subtle forms—*viz.*, Buddhi, Prakṛti, and Ahaṁkāra—in this place becomes clear. We must, however, know that Ahaṁkāra is not placed in the order shown in the above quotation. We have seen that from the Mūlādhāra upwards the generated is below the generator; that which is dissolved is below what it is dissolved into, and we also know that the Śābda-krama is stronger than Pāṭa-krama.[14] We must remember that Vyoma is dissolved in Ahaṁkāra, and hence the latter is next above Vyoma. *Cf.* "In Ahaṁkāra, Vyoma with

---

[1] Region of the Earth Element, or Mūlādhāra-Cakra.

[2] Smell principle or Tanmātra.

[3] Svādhiṣṭāna, which is the region of Water (Jala).

[4] Principle of taste.

[5] Maṇi-pūra, which is the region of Fire (Vāhni).

[6] Principle of sight.

[7] Anāhata, which is the region of Air (Vāyu).

[8] Principle of touch.

[9] Viśuddha, which is the region of Ether (Nabhas).

[10] Principle of sound.

[11] See next note.

[12] See Introduction, and *post*, Commentary.

[13] Egoism—self-consciousness.

[14] That is, the actual arrangement of things as compared with the order in which they are stated.

sound should be dissolved, and Ahaṁkāra again in Mahat." Ahaṁkāra, being the place of dissolution, comes first above Vyoma, and above it are Buddhi and Prakṛti.

The Śāradā-tilaka (I. 17, 18) speaks of their connection as Janya (effect, generated) and Janaka (cause, generator).

" From the unmanifest (Avyakta) Mūla-bhūta, Para-vastu [1] when Vikṛta originated Mahat-tattva,[1] which consists of the Guṇas and Antahkaraṇa. From this (Mahat-tattva) originated Ahaṁkāra, which is of three kinds according to its source of generation." [2] By Vikṛti which means change is here meant reflection or image (Prati-bimba) [3] of the Para-vastu, and as such reflection it is Vikṛti; but as it is the Prakṛti of Mahat-tattva, etc., it is also called Prakṛti.[4] *Cf.* " Prakṛti is the Paramā

---

[1] Mahat-tattva is a Vikṛti of Prakṛti. The Mūlabhūta avyakta (unmanifested root-being) corresponds with the Sāṁkhyan Mūla-prakṛti. Here, as Rāghava-Bhaṭṭa says, Tattvasṛṣṭi is indicated (Comm. to Ch. I, vv. 17, 18 of Śāradā), and interprets (Ch. I. vv. 17, 18) thus: Unmanifest Mūlabhūta Para-vastu may mean either the Bindu or Śabda Brahman. By Vikṛta is meant readiness or proneness to create (Sṛṣṭyunmukha). From this Bindu or Śabda-Brahman emanates Mahat-tattva by which is meant the Padārtha Mahat: which is known as Buddhi-tattva in Śaiva-mata. This Mahat or Buddhi-tattva consists of the three Guṇas—Sattva, Rajas and Tamas. That is, it includes Manas, Buddhi, Ahaṁkāra and Citta. These four are the product (Kārya) of the Guṇas as cause (Kāraṇa), and the cause (Kāraṇa) inheres (Upacāra) in the effect (Kārya). After quoting the words of Īśāna-Śiva, Rāghava remarks that Vāmakeśvara-Tantra also says that from the Unmanifest Śabda-Brahman originates Buddhi-tattva wherein Sattva Guṇa is manifest. He then distinguishes the Sāṁkhya view according to which the state of equilibrium of Sattva, Rajas and Tamas is Prakṛti, which is also called Pradhāna and Avyakta. This is the Supreme (Para-vastu). From a disturbance in the equilibrium of the Guṇas arises Mahat. This Mahat consists of Guṇas and is the cause of the Antahkaraṇas. By Guṇas according to this are meant the five Tanmātras, Śabda, Sparśa, etc. According to this view also from Prakṛti comes Mahat and from the latter Ahaṁkāra.

Rāghava thus shows the different ways in which the text of Śāradā can be interpreted from the Śākta, Śaiva and Sāṁkhya points of view.

[2] Sṛṣṭi-bheda—that is, one Ahaṁkāra is the result of the predominance of Sattva, another of Rajas, and a third of Tamas.

[3] That is in the sense of product. In Śaiva-śākta-darśana, Mūla-prakṛti is itself a product of the Śiva-śakti-tattva, for the Self becomes object to itself.

[4] That is, as regarded from the point of view of the Para-vastu it is an effect, but regarded in relation to that which it produces it is a cause.

(Supreme) Śakti, and Vikṛti is the product thereof." [1] It has also been shown before that the Prakṛti of the Para Brahman is but another aspect of Him (Pratibimba-svarūpiṇī).

According to Śāradā-tilaka, Mahat-tattva, is the same as Buddhi.[2] Īśāna-Śiva says: "The objective Prakṛti,[3] which is evolved by Śakti, is, when associated with Sattva-Guṇa, Buddhi-tattva. It is this Buddhi that is spoken of as Mahat in Sāṁkhya."

Mahat-tattva consists of the Guṇas and the Antah-karaṇa. The Guṇas are Sattva, Rajas and Tamas. The Śāradā-tilaka says: "Antah-karaṇa is the Manas, Buddhi, Ahaṁkāra and Citta, of the Ātmā.[4] All these are comprised in the term Mahat-tattva.

Now, a question may be raised—namely, if Manas be within Mahat-tattva, what of that which has been said in v. 33, where Manas has been spoken of as having an independent existence? But the answer to that is, that that Manas is the product of Ahaṁkāra, and Rāghava-Bhaṭṭa quotes a text which says: "In so much as the other Manas is the one which selects and rejects (Sa-saṁkalpa-vikalpaka),[5] it is known to be the product of Tejas." [6] Thus it is that, as Manas and other Tattvas in the Ājñā-Cakra are placed in their order, Ahaṁkāra and others should be known as being placed above them. In the Ājñā-Cakra are Hākinī, Itara-Liṅga, Praṇava, Manas, Ahaṁkāra, Buddhi, and Prakṛti placed consecutively one above the other. No place being assigned to Candra-maṇḍala, which has been spoken of before, it should be taken to be placed above all these. If it be asked, why is it not below all these? then the reply is that it has been said in the Sammohana-Tantra: "Moon (Indu) is in the forehead, and above it is Bodhinī Herself." From this it would appear that Indu and Bodhinī are above Ājñā-Cakra, placed one above the other without anything intervening between them. Bodhinī is above all the rest.

The Sammohana-Tantra speaks of the Cause (Kāraṇarūpa) as above Ājñā-Cakra: "Indu (the Moon, here—Bindu) is in the region of

---

[1] Vikṛtih pratibimbatā—in a mirror one is seen but the image is not oneself.

[2] Rāghava-Bhaṭṭa says that this is so according to Śaiva doctrine.

[3] Boddhavya-lakṣaṇā—that is, that which can be known (Jñeya); the objective or manifested Prakṛti.

[4] See Introduction.

[5] As to Sa-saṁkalpa-vikalpa, see Introduction.

[6] That is, Taijasa ahaṁkāra, which is the source of the Indriyas.

the forehead, and above it is Bodhinī Herself. Above Bodhinī shines the excellent Nāda, in form like the half (crescent) moon; above this is the lustrous Mahā-nāda, in shape like a plough; above this is the Kalā called Āñjī, the beloved of Yogīs. Above this last is Unmaṇi,[1] which having reached, one does not return."

In the above passage, in the words "above it is Bodhinī," the word "it" stands for the forehead or Ājñā-Cakra.

The Bhūta-śuddhi-Tantra speaks of the existence of the Bindu below Bodhinī: "Devī, above Bindu and Mātrārdhā is Nāda, and above this, again, is Mahā-nāda, which is the place of the dissolution of Vāyu." Mātrārdhā is Mātrārdhā-Śakti.[2]

The following passage from Bṛhat-tri-vikrama-saṁhitā proves that the Ardha-mātrā means Śakti: "Lustrous like the young Sun is Akṣara, which is Bindumat (Bindu itself); above it is Ardha-mātrā, associated with the Gāndhārarāga."[3]

As both the above passages point to the same thing, we must take it that Ardha-mātrā and Bodhinī are identical. Bindu, Bodhinī, and Nāda, are but different aspects of the Bindu-maya-para-śakti.

---

[1] In this passage Āñjī is Samanī. The Bhūta-śuddhi (see *post*), makes a distinction too between Ājñī and Samanī. These are the Avāntara-śarīras of the First Cause enumerated in Laya-krama. The text quoted from the Śāradā gives the Sṛṣṭi-krama.

[2] Mātrārdhā. In the Devī Bhāgavata there occurs the expression Ardhamātrā (which is a name for Nāda) in I, 1, v. 55, and III, 5, v. 29, and Nīlakaṇṭha defines it to mean Paraṁ padaṁ=the supreme state, or the Brahman. The expression Ardha-mātrā also occurs in Caṇḍī, I, 55, in practically the same sense. Gopāla Chakravartī quotes a passage which says: "Ardha-mātrā is attributeless (Nirguṇa), and realizable by the Yogi." He quotes another passage which says: "Oṁ—this is the three Vedas, three Lokas, and after the three Lokas, Mātrārdhā is the fourth—the Supreme Tattva." See Caṇḍī "Tvamudgīthe ardhamātrāsi" and Devībhāgavata, I, 5, v. 55. Śruti says: "Thou art the Ardhamātrā of Praṇava, Gāyatrī, and Vyāhṛti." Here the unity of Devī and Brahman is shown. She is Brahman united with Māyā (Māyā-viśiṣṭa-brahmarūpiṇī). The Nāda-bindu Upaniṣad (v. 1) says: "A-kāra is the right wing (of Oṁ figured as a bird), U-kāra is the other (left) wing, Ma-kāra the tail, and Ardhamātrā the head. Sattva is its body, and Rajas and Tamas are its two feet. Dharma is its right eye and Adharma is its left eye. The Bhūrloka is its feet; the Bhuvarloka its knees; the Svarloka is its middle; the Maharloka its navel; Janaloka is the heart; Tapoloka its throat, and Satyaloka the place between the eyebrows." See also Brahmavidyā Up., v. 10.

[3] The third of the seven primary subtle tones.

The Śāradā-tilaka says: "From the Sakala Parameśvara,[1] who is Sat, Cit, and Ānanda, Śakti emanated; from Śakti, again, emanated Nāda; and Bindu has its origin from Nāda. He who is Para-Śakti-maya manifests Himself in three different ways. Bindu and Nāda and Bīja are but His different aspects. Bindu is Nādātmaka,[2] Bīja is Śakti, and Nāda, again, is the union or relation of the one to the other.[3] This is spoken of by all who are versed in the Āgamas." [4]

"Para-Śakti-maya": Para=Śiva; hence Śiva-Śakti-maya=Bindu. The Bindu who is above the forehead is Nādātmaka—that is, Śivātmaka.[5] Bīja is Śakti as Bodhinī (Bodhinī-rūpaṁ). Nāda is the connection between the two whereby the one acts upon the other; hence it is Kriyā-Śakti. Above these three is Mahā-nāda. This has already been shown.

"Above this is Kalā," etc.: Kalā=Śakti. Āñjī=a crooked, awry, bent, line. This is in shape like a bent or crooked line over a letter. This Śakti appeared in the beginning of creation, *Cf.* Pāñcarātra: "Having thus seen, the Supreme Male in the beginning of creation makes manifest the eternal Prakṛti who is the embodiment of Sat, Cit and Ānanda, in whom [6] are all the Tattvas, and who is the presiding (Adhiṣṭātrī) Devī of creation.

Also elsewhere: "From the unmanifested (Avyakta) Parameśvara, the united Śiva and Śakti, emanated the Ādyā (first) Devī Bhagavatī, who is Tripura-sundarī, the Śakti from whom came Nāda, and thence came Bindu."

---

[1] Śāradā, Ch. I, vv. 7-9, Sakala, as opposed to Niṣkala, or Nirguṇa, means united with Kalā, which according to Sāṁkhya is Sāmyāvasthā of the Guṇas which is Prakṛti. According to the Vedāntists of the (Māya-Vāda), Kalā is Avidyā, in the Śaiva-Tantra Kalā is Śakti (Rāghava-Bhaṭṭa).

[2] Another text has Śivātmaka—that is, Bindu is the Śiva aspect.

[3] Samavāya=kṣobhya kṣobhaka-sambandha—lit., connection which is the connection of reciprocity.

[4] See Introduction.

[5] In the Benares edition as also in Rasika Mohana Chattopādhyāya's edition of the Śāradā-tilaka the text reads Śivātmaka, as if qualifying Bīja, which seems erroneous.

[6] Rāghava reads: "Samasta-tattva-saṁghātma-spūrtyadhiṣṭhatrīrūpiṇīṁ"—which means "who is the Devī presiding over or directing the evolution or manifestation of all the mass of Tattvas".

"Above it is Unmanī," etc.: *Cf.* 'By going where 'Manasness' (Manastva) of Manas ceases to be called Unmanī, the attainment of which is the secret teaching of all Tantras." [1]

The state of Unmanī is the Tattva which means the dispelling of the attachment prompted by Manas towards worldly objects.

Unmanī, again, is of two kinds: (1) Nirvāṇa-kalā-rūpā which also has its place in the Sahasrāra [2]; (2) Varṇāvali-rūpā, which also has its place in this region. *Cf.* Kankāla-mālinī: "In the pericarp of the Sahasrāra, placed within the circle of the moon, is the seventeenth Kalā, devoid of attachment.[3] The name of this is Unmanī, which cuts the bond of attachment to the world."

Cf. also: "By mental recitation of the Mālā-varṇa (rosary of letters) is Unmanī the granter of Liberation (attained)." Mālā-varṇa=Varṇāvalī-rūpa.

The Bhūta-śuddhi speaks of the Samanī below Unmanī. "Next is the Vyāpikā-Śakti (Diffusive Energy) which people know as Āñjī. Samanī [4] is over this, and Unmanī is above all." This (Samanī) also is an intermediate aspect (Avāntara-rūpa) of Paraśakti.

We now get the following:

Above Ājñā-Cakra is the second Bindu—which is Śiva (Śiva-svarūpa). Above Bindu is the Śakti Bodhinī in shape like an Ardhamātrā; next is Nāda which is the union of Śiva and Śakti, in shape like a half (crescent) moon; next (above this) is Mahānāda, shaped like a plough; above Mahānāda is the Vyāpikā Śakti, crooked (Āñjī) in shape; above this last is Samanī and highest of these all is Unmanī. This is the order in which the seven causal forms (Kāraṇa-rūpa) are placed.

---

[1] Viśvanātha, quoting Svacchanda-saṁgraha, which speaks of Unmanī as above Samanā, says that in the Unmanī stage there is no cognition of and no distinction is made between Kāla and Kalā; there is no body, and no Devatās, and no cessation of continuity. It is the pure and sweet mouth of Rudra. *Cf.* Vṛttīnaṁ manah in the Śiva-Saṁhitā, V, 219.

[2] Sahasrārādharā. See introduction.

[3] Sarva-saṁkalpa-rahitā—*i.e.*, who is free from all attachment, not prompted by anything in any action. The passages quoted are from ch. v, Kaṇkāla-mālinī.

[4] Viśvanātha speaks of it as Samanā, and says that She is Cidānanda-svarūpā (that is, Cit and Ānanda), and the cause of all causes (Sarva-kāraṇa-kāraṇaṁ).

There is no need to go into further detail. Let us then follow the text.

Wishing to describe the Sahasrāra he speaks of it in ten more verses.

"*Above all these*" (Tadūrdhve).—Above every other that has been described or spoken before.

"*Over the head of the Śaṅkhinī-Nāḍī*"—a sight of which has been given to the disciple.

"*Vacant space*" (Śūnya-deśa)—that is, the place where there are no Nāḍīs; the implication is that it is above where Suṣumṇā ends.

"*Below Visarga is the lotus of a thousand petals.*"—This is the purport of the Śloka. Visarga is in the upper part of the Brahma-randhra. *Cf.* "(Meditate) in that aperture on Visarga the ever blissful and stainless." There are other similar passages.

"*Its body is luminous with,*" *etc.* (Lalāṭādyaih varṇaih pravilasita-vapuh).—The word Lalāṭa stands for the first vowel, A. By this we are to understand that the second Lakāra (L) is to be left out in counting the letters of the Alphabet. In counting the fifty letters, the second Lakāra [1] is always left out.

If the text is read as "Lakārādyaih varṇaih," as is done by some, we must leave Kṣa-kāra out in counting the letters. The fifty-one letters cannot be taken to be in the petals of the Sahasrāra.[2] With fifty-one letters repeated twenty times, the number is 1,020, and repeated nineteen times is 969. By leaving out Kṣakāra we are freed of this difficulty. By "Lakārādyaih" is it not meant that the letters are to be read Viloma.[3] The Kaṅkālamālinī in the following passage distinctly says that it is to be read Anuloma [4]: "The Great Lotus Sahasrāra is white and has its head downward, and the lustrous letters from A-kāra (A), ending with the last letter before Kṣakāra (Kṣa), decorate it." Here it is distinctly stated that the letter Kṣa is left out.

Akārādi-kṣa-kārāntaih: This compound, Kṣa-kārānta, if formed by Bahu-vrīhi-samāsa,[5] would mean that Kṣakāra is left out of calculation.

---

[1] Vaidika Lakāra (La).

[2] *i.e.*, fifty-one letters cannot be arranged in the Sahasrāra.

[3] *i.e.*, from end to beginning.

[4] From beginning to end.

[5] A form of Sanskrit verbal compound.

There is nothing said of the colour of the letters, and, as the Mātṛkā (letters) are white, they are to be taken as being white on the Sahasrāra petals. These letters go round the Sahasrāra from right to left.[1]

Some read Pravilasita-tanuh in place of pravilasita-vapuh, and say that, as the word *padma* alternatively becomes masculine in gender (vā pumsi padmaṁ), therefore the word Tanu, which qualifies a word in the masculine gender, is itself masculine. That cannot be. The verb Nivasati (=is, dwells) has for its nominative Padmaṁ, and, as it ends with the *Bindu* (m), it is in the neuter gender and not masculine. For in that case it would have ended with *visarga* (*i.e.*, *h*), and its adjective *tanu*, would also end with a *visarga*. The word *tanu* (if their reading is accepted) would be in the neuter; therefore it cannot end with a *Bindu*. And if there is no Bindu the metre becomes defective. Therefore the correct reading is Pravilasita-vapuh.

The rest is clear.

[1] Dakṣināvarta—the opposite way to that in which the hands of a clock work.

Verse 41

Samāste tasyāntaḥ śaśaparirahitaḥ śuddhasaṁpūrṇacandraḥ
sphurajjyotsnājalaḥ paramarasacayasnigdhasaṁtānahāsī.
Trikoṇaṁ tasyāntaḥ sphurati ca satataṁ vidyudākārarūpaṁ
tadantaḥśūnyaṁ tatsakala-suragaṇaiḥ sevitaṁ cātiguptaṁ.

Within it (Sahasrāra) is the full Moon, without the mark of the hare,[1] resplendent as in a clear sky. It sheds its rays in profusion, and is moist and cool like nectar. Inside it (Candra-maṇḍala), constantly shining like lightning, is the Triangle[2] and inside this, again, shines the Great Void[3] which is served in secret by all the Suras.[4]

Commentary

He here speaks of the existence of the Candra-maṇḍala in the pericarp of the Sahasrāra.

"*Resplendent as in a clear sky*" (Śuddha)—seen in a cloudless sky (*nirmalo-daya-viśiṣta*).

"*Is moist and cool,*" *etc.* (Parama-rasa-cāya-snigdha-santāna-hāsī). —Snigdha which means moist here implies the moisture of the nectar.

---

[1] The man in the moon.

[2] The A-ka-thādi triangle according to Viśvanātha.

[3] Śūnya=Bindu—that is, the Para-bindu, or Īśvara, having as its centre the abode of Brahman (Brahmapada). In the northern Śaiva and Śākta schools Sadāśiva and Īśvara are the Nimeṣa and Unmeṣa aspects of the experience intermediate between Śiva-Tattva and Śuddha-vidyā, the former being called Śūnyātiśunya. The positions of the Sun and Moon circles in the Śahasrāra and of the twelve-petalled lotus with the Kāmakalā are given in the Text.

[4] *i.e.*, Devas.

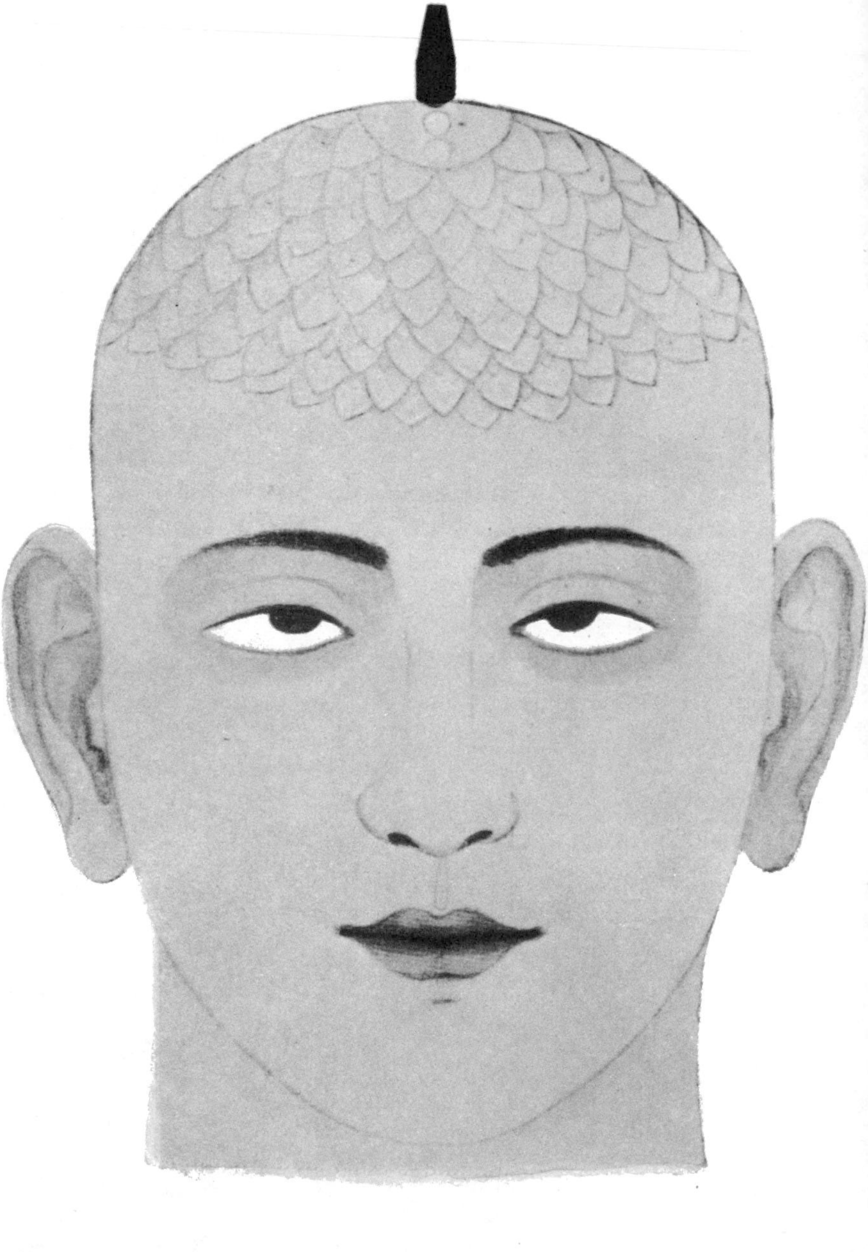

Plate VIII] Sahasrāra [To face Page 429

Parama-rasa (Amṛta) is free from heat. Hence the meaning of this compound word: Its rays are cool and moist, and produce a feeling of smiling gladness.

The Kaṅkāla-mālinī speaks of the presence of Antarātmā, etc., in the upper portion of the space below Candra-maṇḍala. In dealing with the Sahasrāra, it says: " In its pericarp, O Deveśī, is the Antarātmā. Above it is the Guru. The Maṇḍalas of Sūrya and Candra are also there. Above this is Mahā-vāyu, and then the Brahmarandhra. In this aperture (Randhra) is Visarga, the ever blissful Brahman. Above this (Tadūrdhve) last is the Devi Śaṅkhinī, who creates, maintains, and destroys."

" *Within Candra-maṇḍala constantly shines, like lightning, the triangle* " (Trikoṇaṁ tasyāntaḥ vidyudākāra-rūpam).—That is, the shining triangle is there.

" *Inside this shines the Great Void* " (Tadantah śūnyam sphurati).—That which as a void within is, the body of the Para-bindu (Para-bindu-śarīraṁ). Within the triangle the excellent Bindu (Śūnya) shines, or within the triangle the Śūnya which is the excellent Bindu shines.

Cf. Toḍala-Tantra, 6th Ullāsa: " The Supreme Light is formless (Nirākāra), and Bindu is imperishable. Bindu means the void (Śūnya) and implies Guṇa also." [1]

" *Served in secret* " (Sevitaṁ cātiguptaṁ).—The rule is, " Eating (Āhāra), evacuation (Nirhāra), sexual intercourse (Vihāra), and Yoga, should be done in secret by him who knows the Dharma." Hence Suras (Devas) serve or worship It in secret.

---

[1] When it assumes the form of Bindu, It is with the operating Guṇas, or then It is Sakala.

VERSE 42

Suguptaṁ tadyatnādatiśayaparamāmoda-saṁtānarāśeḥ
paraṁ kandaṁ sūkṣmaṁ sakalāśaśikalasuddharūpaprakāśaṁ
Iha sthāne devaḥ paramaśivasamākhyānasiddhaḥ prasiddhaḥ
svarūpī sarvātmā rasavirasanutoऽiñānamohāndhahaṁsaḥ

WELL concealed, and attainable only by great effort, is that subtle Bindu (Śūnya) which is the chief root of Liberation and which manifests the pure Nirvāṇa-Kalā with Amā-Kalā.[1] Here is the Deva who is known to all as Parama-Śiva. He is the Brahman and the Ātmā of all beings. In Him are united both Rasa and Virasa,[2] and He is the Sun which destroys the darkness of nescience[3] and delusion.[4]

COMMENTARY

The sense is that the void (Śūnya) is very secret and subtle, being, as described later, like the ten millionth part of the end of a hair. It is attainable only by great effort consisting of long and incessant performance of Dhyāna and like practices. It makes manifest the purity of the sixteenth Kalā of the moon along with Nirvāṇa-Kalā—*i.e.*, the void (Antah-śūnya) along with the Amā Kalā and Nirvāṇa-Kalā within the triangle is realized (Prakāśam bhavati) by meditation (Dhyāna). It is the source of all the mass of great Bliss, which is Liberation. Some, however, read Sakala-śaśi-kalā-śuddha-rūpa-prakāśaṁ as qualifying the great Void within the

[1] There are seventeen Kalās (digits) of the Moon, but the nectar-dropping Amā and the Nirvāṇa-kalā are only at this stage revealed. The other Kalās are mentioned in Skānda-Purāṇa Prabhāsa-Khaṇḍa.

[2] The Bliss of liberation and that arising from the union of Śiva and Śakti: *vide post.*

[3] Ajñāna.

[4] Moha. This verse occurs in Tripurā-sāra-samuccaya, ch. V. 40.

triangle, and read '*sakala*' to mean with all the sixteen kalās and say that the Para Bindu manifests the moon with such kalās. This requires consideration. When it was said that the Trikoṇa (triangle) is within the full moon, the repetition of it is useless. Furthermore, in the previous verse we have got "served by the Suras". The term "service" as applied to a void is inappropriate. The object of service is the Bindu within the triangle. If it be said that the void should be worshipped by reason of the presence of the Para-Bindu, then the Para-Bindu being there present there is no void.

"*Well concealed*" (Suguptaṁ).—By reason of its being like the ten millionth part of a hair.

"*By great effort*" (Yatnāt)—*i.e.*, by long-continued practice of meditation (Dhyāna) and so forth.

"*Chief root*" (Paraṁ kandaṁ).[1]—Para usually means supreme, excellent; here chief, principal. Kanda=Mūla.

"*Liberation*," *etc.*, (Atiśaya-paramāmoda-saṁtāna-rāśi).—The compound word means, literally, continuity of all the mass of great and supreme bliss, and this is Liberation (Mokṣa).

"*Manifests, etc., Amā-kalā*" (Sakala-śaśi-kalā-śuddha-rūpa-prakāśaṁ).—This compound word is to be broken up as follows:

Sakala=with the Kalā: Kalā here meaning Nirvāṇa-Kalā. In the word Śaśi-kalā the Kalā means Amā-kalā, the sixteenth Kalā, or digit, of the moon. *Śuddha*=pure; the lustre is not obscured by anything.

The sense is that the Para-bindu, though subtle and otherwise imperceptible, is seen by meditation (Dhyāna) with the Amā-Kalā and Nirvāṇa-Kalā in the Trikoṇa. If Sugopyaṁ be read in place of Suguptaṁ, then it would be qualified by Yatnāt.

Some read Sakala-śaśi-kalā-śuddha-rūpa-prakāśaṁ to qualify Śūnya in the previous verse, and say Śūnya means "vacant space" but that is absurd."[2]

Next he speaks of the presence of Parama-Śiva in the pericarp of the Sahasrāra.

---

[1] Kanda means bulb or root. The Yoginī-hṛdaya says that this Kanda is the subtle Parānanda-kanda-bindu-rūpa, or the root of supreme Bliss in Bindu form (Viśvanātha).

[2] According to the Commentator, it qualifies Kanda. Bindu is the circle O, the void is the Brahmapada or space within.

"*Paramaśiva*"[1] (Paramaśhiva-samākhyāna-siddha).—He who is known by the name Parama Śiva.

"*The Brahman*" (Kharūpī).[2]—Kha=Ātmā, the spirit.

"*The Ātmā of all beings*" (Sarvātmā).—Sarva=all (beings). He is the Jīvātmā, but in fact there is no distinction between Jīvātmā and Paramātmā. The Ātmā is the Jīva. The Adhyātma Rāmāyaṇa says: "The Jīvātma is merely another name (Paryāya) for the Paramātmā. When by the instruction of the Ācārya and the Śāstras their oneness is known, then the disciple possesses Mūlavidyā concerning Jīvātmā and Parammātā."

The Śruti also, when it says "That thou art"—*Tat tvam asi*,[3]—identifies the *Tvam* (Thou) with the *Tat* (That).

"*Rasa and Virasa*" (Rasa-virasamita).—Rasa is Paramānandarasa —*i.e.*, the experience of Supreme Bliss.[4] Virasa is the bliss which is the product of the union of Śiva and Śakti. He is both. Or Rasa may mean the natural attachment to worldly enjoyment, and Virasa detachment from it. The meaning would then be: in Him is the Supreme Bliss arising from his detachment from worldly enjoyment.[5]

"*The Sun*"=Haṁsa. As the sun dispels darkness, so does He dispel nescience (Ajñāna) and delusion (Moha).

---

[1] Viśvanātha says that this Śiva is the Saguṇa-Śiva.

[2] *Cf.* Śruti "Khaṁ Brahma" Chā. 4—10—5; Bṛ. 5—1—1.

[3] "That thou art." See Introduction.

[4] *i.e.*, Mokṣa.

[5] That is, the Rasa in Him has become Virasa.

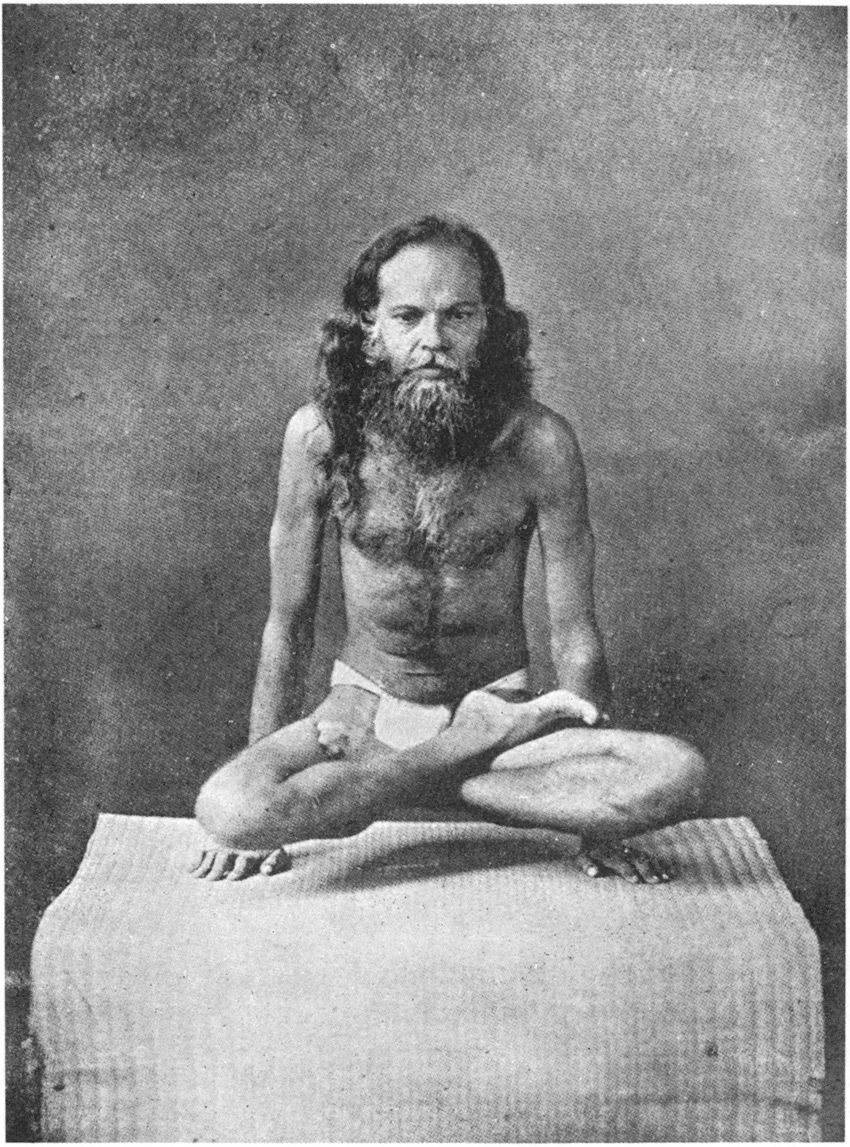

Plate IX] Mahābedha [To face Page 433
According to Haṭhayogapradīpika and Yāmala

Verse 43

Sudhādhārāsāraṁ niravadhi vimuñcannatitarāṁ
yateḥ svātmajñānaṁ diśati bhagavān nirmalamateḥ.
Samaste sarveśaḥ sakalasukhasaṁtānalaharī
parivāko haṁsaḥ parama iti nāmnā paricitaḥ.

By shedding a constant and profuse stream of nectar-like essence,[1] the Bhagavān[2] instructs the Yati[3] of pure mind in the knowledge by which he realizes the oneness of the Jīvātmā and the Paramātmā. He pervades all things as their Lord, who is the ever-flowing and spreading current of all manner of bliss known by the name of Haṁsah Parama (Paramahaṁsah).

Commentary

"*Constant and profuse*" (Niravadhi atitarāṁ).

"*By shedding a stream of nectar-like essence*" (Sudhā-dhārāsāraṁ vimuñcan).—The compound word can be made up and interpreted in four different ways:

1. Shedding a stream of nectar-like essence.

2. The Ādhāra (receptable) of Sudhā (nectar) is Sudhādhāra, by which is meant the Moon; Āsāra is what flows therefrom, a stream. Now, what flows from the Moon is Nectar, which is silvery; hence the whole

---

[1] As appears from the Commentary *post*, this may be variously translated as follows: "By shedding a constant and profuse stream of nectar resembling the silvery beam of the Moon," *or* "By unremitting and nectar-like words strong for the destruction of the darkness of delusion," *or* "By constant repetition of the word which is nectar-like in its mercy and contains the essence of the Brahma-mantra."

[2] That is, the Lord as the possessor of the six forms of Aiśvarya.

[3] Self-controlled, whose mind is unified with the object of worship.

word means " the silvery beams of the moon ". This adjective proves that the qualified noun is white or transparent like the moon. Shedding =Vimuñcan.

3. Āsāra may, again, mean " what is uttered," " word ". Sudhādhāra=receptacle of sweetness, which is a quality of nectar; hence Sudhādhārāsāraṁ=nectar-like or ambrosial word. The meaning of Niravadhi would then be " at all times," and Atitarām would mean " powerful in destroying the darkness, ignorance or delusion." Vimuñcan should then mean " uttering ".

4. Sudhā, again, may mean " nectar of mercy," and Sāre is " essence "—*i.e.*, the essence of Brahma-mantra; and Dhārā is a stream (continuous repetition) of the merciful word containing the essence of the Brahma-mantra.

" *Instructs the Yati*," *etc.*, (Bhagavān nirmala-mater yateh svātma-jñānaṁ diśati).

" *Yati*."—He whose mind intently rests upon the Devatā of his worship.

Knowledge by which, etc., Paramātmā (Svātma-Jñāna): Svam=Jīvātmā and Ātmā=Paramātmā; and Jñāna [1] that by which one knows—namely, the Tāraka-brahma-mantra, which leads to a knowledge of the Paramātmā, and thereby helps the worshipper to realise the oneness of the Jīvātmā and Paramātmā. Diśati=Upadiśati (instructs). The above qualifying expressions imply that the qualified noun is the Guru, as instructions regarding Tāraka-brahma-mantra proceed from Him. So it qualifies " Parama-Śiva " in the preceding verse, as He is the Guru. *Cf.* Gurus-tattva-nirūpaṇa in Lalitā-rahasya.

After describing Guru as " the well-known and excellent Puruṣa who is ever fond [2] of enjoyment with the Self (Ātma-rati-priya)," it goes on to say: " His beloved is the lustrous One who may be gained with difficulty by the Brahma-vartma (Brahman road). The Para-Brahman is but the effulgence of Her lotus feet."

By the above passage is meant that the great beauty of Her lotus feet overspreads the heart-lotus of Parama-Śiva who is Para-Brahman. The place for the feet of the lustrous (Tejo-rūpa) Beloved (Śakti) of the

[1] Jñāna is spiritual knowledge or wisdom, and Vijñāna is the knowledge of the material world (science).

[2] *i.e.*, who is engrossed in.

Guru is on the breast of the Guru,[1] and not on that of any other Puruṣa. Hence Parama-Śiva and the Guru are one and the same.

The Nirvāṇa-Tantra also says[2]: "In the Lotus in the head is Mahādeva—the Parama-Guru: there is in the three worlds no one, O Deveśī, who is so deserving of worship as He. O Devī, meditate on His form,[3] which includes all the four Gurus."[4]

This Parama Śiva is outside the triangle in the pericarp, and above the Haṁsah of which we speak below.

The Kaṅkāla-mālinī Tantra[5] says: "In the pericarp of this Lotus, O Deveśī, is the Antarātmā, and above it the Guru. The Maṇḍalas of Sun and Moon are also there." And after having spoken of the presence of different things in their order up to Mahā-śaṅkhinī, it then proceeds: "Below it, O Deveśī, is the Trikoṇa (triangle), placed in the Maṇḍala of Moon; and having meditated there on the undecaying Kalā, (one should

---

[1] This is in praise of Śakti, without whom Śiva is Śava (a corpse, and unable to move.)

[2] This passage occurs in the 3rd Paṭala of the Nirvāṇa-Tantra (Rasika Mohana Chaṭṭopādhyāya's Edition, p. 9), and is in answer to the following question of the Devī: "The Deva who is in the Turīyadhāma (the fourth state) is unquestionably the Paramātmā; if he be placed in the Lotus in the head, how can obeisance be made to him outwardly?" That is, How can the Sādhaka bow to him who is in the head which is itself bowed?

[3] The passage as quoted by the Commentator reads "Tadaṁśaṁ" (his part); in R. M. Chaṭṭopādhyāya's Edition it reads "Tadrūpaṁ" (his form), which reading is here adopted.

[4] *i.e.*, Guru, Parama-Guru, Parāpara-Guru, and Parameṣṭi-Guru.

[5] This passage occurs in Paṭala II (p. 3 of R. M. Chaṭṭopādhyāya's Edition), which in its entirety runs thus: "In it (Sahasrāra), O Deveśī, is the Antarātmā, and above it Vāyu, and above Mahānāda is Brahmarandhra. In the Brahmarandhra is Visarga, which is Eternal Peace and Bliss. (Peace—Nirañjana, which also means stainless, free from delusion). Above it is the Devī Śaṅkhinī, the Creatrix, Maintainer, and Destructress. Having meditated on the Triangle placed below, He thinks that Kailāsa (the paradise of Śiva) is there. O Mahādevī, by placing the undisturbed Cetas (heart or mind) here one lives in bliss to the full term of one's life (Jīva-jīvī) free from all ills, and for such a one there is no rebirth. Here constantly shines Amā Kalā which knows neither increase nor decay, and within it, again, is the seventeenth digit, known as Nirvāṇa-Kalā. Within Nirvāṇa-Kalā is the fiery Nibodhikā. Above it is unmanifested Nāda, effulgent as ten million suns. It is the excellent Nirvāṇa Śakti, the cause of all. In this Śakti it should be known that Śiva who is changeless and free from illusion abides."

meditate) within upon the seventeenth Kalā, by name Nirvāṇa which is like a crescent " (Kuṭilā).[1]

The above passage speaks of the presence of Amā-Kalā, and so forth, within the triangle in the Candra-Maṇḍala. The Guru therefore is below them and above Antarātmā. Now, if it be asked how it is that, the Kaṅkāla-mālinī having placed the Guru over the Antarātmā, the Guru is spoken of as placed above Haṁsah, the answer is that the Antarātmā and the Haṁsah are one and the same.

Cf. Guru-dhyāna in Kaṅkāla-mālinī[2]: " Meditate on your Guru seated on a shining throne (Simhāsana) placed on the excellent Antarātmā between Nāda and Bindu," etc. Also elsewhere: " Meditate on your Guru, who is the image of Śiva Himself, as seated on the Haṁsa-pīṭa which is Mantramaya." Also *cf.* the Annadā-kalpa-Tantra[3]: " Meditate on your Guru in the white Lotus of a thousand petals in the head; He is Parama-Śiva seated on the Haṁsa among the filaments."

On a careful consideration of the above authorities, the identity of Haṁsa with Antarātmā becomes clear. By the expression " one's own Guru, who is Parama-Śiva," it is to be understood that Parama-Śiva Himself is the Guru.

The following passage, which relates to the Sahasrāra, shows that Parama-Śiva is in the triangle: " Within (or near) it (Sahasrāra) is the lightning-like Triangle, and within the Triangle are the two Bindus which make the imperishable Visarga. There in the empty void is Parama-Śiva."

These conflicting views lead to the conclusion that the Guru is within the triangle in the pericarp of the upturned Lotus of twelve petals, below the pericarp of the Sahasrāra and inseparable from it. This has been made clear in the Pādukā-pañcaka-Stotra.[4] From these passages it is not to be inferred that the Guru is within the triangle in the pericarp of the Sahasrāra. The triangular Haṁsa is below the middle triangle; otherwise it would conflict with the authority of the Kaṅkāla-mālinī-Tantra.

" *He pervades all things as their Lord* "—(Samāste sarveśah)—*i.e.*, in this pericarp dwells He who is the Lord of All. Now, by saying

---

[1] See Jñānārṇava-Tantra, XXIV, 36.

[2] Paṭala III.

[3] This quotation is not traceable in Prasannakumāra Śāstrī's Edition of this Tantra.

[4] See notes to v. 7 of the Pādukā-Pañcaka.

that Parama-Śiva is there, it has been said that Īśvara (Lord) is there; then why this repetition? But there is an object in so doing, as the following qualifying expressions will show. The Sarveśa (Lord of All) is the Haṁsa—*i.e.*, He is the Mantra " Haṁ-Sah ".

Cf. Prapañca-sāra: " She whose name is Tattva is Cinmātrā [1]: when by proximity to the Light she wishes to create,[2] She becomes massive (Ghaṇībhūya) and assumes the form of Bindu. Then in time She divides Herself in two: the one on the right is Bindu, and that on the left side is Visarga. The right and left are respectively distinguished as *male* and *female*. Ham is the Bindu, and Sah is the Visarga; Bindu is Puruṣa, and Visarga is Prakṛti; Haṁsah is the union of Prakṛti and Puruṣa, who pervade the Universe."

The Mahākālī-Tantra speaks clearly on the subject (Paṭala I): " In the empty space [3] in the Candra-Maṇḍala [4] which is within the Sahasrāra, adorned with a celestial gateway, are the letters Haṁ and Sah, over which (meditate on) Him who is pure like rock crystal and dressed in pure white silken raiment, and so forth." Here the letters Haṁ and Sah are explicitly spoken of.

Or if Haṁsa and Parama be read separately as Haṁsa and Parama it would mean " He who is known as Haṁsa and Parama ". The Author himself speaks of Him as Haṁsa in the forty-ninth verse. Or if the two words be read together, then the meaning would be " He who is known by the name of Parama-haṁsa," by one of the exceptional rules of Karmadhāraya-Samāsa this word having been formed, the word ' antah ' being omitted. *Cf.* Āgama-kalpa-druma: He is called Parama-haṁsah, pervading all that is moving and motionless."

" *Who is the ever flowing*," *etc.*, (Sakala-sukha-santāna-laharī-parīvāha)—*i.e.*, in Him becomes manifest in every possible way all kinds of imperishable and increasing happiness; that is, He is, as it were, an interminable chain of happiness.

It has previously been said that this Haṁsa is below Parama-Śiva.

---

1 *Vide ante*, v. 39. The text quoted here differs from that of the edition published by me (See ch. I, vv. 41-44, Tāntrik Texts, Vol. III).

2 Vicikīrṣu—" wishes to distort herself." Here " distortion," or stress, is creation. See Introduction.

3 Śūnya. The Śūnya is the empty space within the Bindu.

4 The locative is to be read Sāmīpye-saptamī—that is, the space is not in, but near, the Candra-Maṇḍala; otherwise there appears to be a contradiction.

Verse 44

Śivasthānaṁ śaivāḥ paramapuruṣaṁ vaiṣṇavagaṇā
lapantīti prāyo hariharapadaṁ kecidapare.
Pabaṁ devyā devicaraṇayugalāṁbhojarasikā
munīndrā apyanye prakṛtipuruṣasthānamamalaṁ.

The Śaivas call it the abode of Śiva [1]; the Vaiṣṇavas call it Parama Puruṣa [2]; others again, call it the place of Hari-Hara. [3] Those who are filled with a passion for the Lotus feet of the Devī [4] call it the excellent abode of the Devī; and other great sages (Munis) call it the pure place of Prakṛti-Puruṣa. [5]

Commentary

As Haṁsah, who has in Him all the Devatās (Sarvadevatāmaya), and others, are in this pericarp, it is the place of the Devatās of worship of all classes of worshippers, such as Śaivas, Śāktas, etc.

"*The Śaivas*"—*i.e.*, the worshippers of Śiva—call it the place of Śiva.

"*The Vaiṣṇavas* [6] *call it Parama-Puruṣa*"—*i.e.*, the place of the Parama-Puruṣa, or Viṣṇu.

"*Others, again*" (Kecid apare)—*i.e.*, others who are worshippers of Hari-Hara, or, in other words, United Viṣṇu and Śiva and not of Śiva alone or Viṣṇu alone—call it the place of Hari-Hara.[7] They do not call

[1] Śiva-sthānaṁ.
[2] *i.e.*, the place of Parama-Puruṣa—Viṣṇu.
[3] Viṣṇu and Śiva.
[4] Śakti, or the Goddess.
[5] Śakti-Śiva.
[6] Worshippers of Viṣṇu.
[7] Hari-Hara-padaṁ.

it either the place of Hari (Viṣṇu) or of Śiva (Hara) but the place of their united selves.

" *Other great sages* [1] " (Munīndrā apyanye).—By this the author here means the worshippers of the " Haṁsah " Mantra who call it the pure place of Prakṛti-Puruṣa. Haṁsah is the union of Prakṛti and Puruṣa,[2] hence it is the place of Prakṛti and Puruṣa.

The above shows that, as this Lotus is the dwelling-place of the Para Bindu, in which are all the Devatās, each worshipper calls it the place of the Devatā of his own separate worship.

---

[1] Muni means " knower " and whose Mind is therefore always in a state of Meditation.

[2] Haṁsasya prakṛti-puruṣobhayarūpatvāt. Haṁ is the Puruṣa, and Sah is Prakṛti.

VERSE 45

Idaṁ sthānaṁ jñātva niyatanijacitto naravaro
na bhūyāt saṁsāre punarapi na baddhastribhuvane.
Samagrā śaktiḥ syānniya mamanasastasya kṛtinaḥ
sadā kartuṁ hartuṁ khagatirapi vāṇi suvimalā.

THAT most excellent of men who has controlled his mind [1] and known this place is never again born in the Wandering, [2] as there is nothing in the three worlds which binds him. His mind being controlled and his aim achieved, he possesses complete power to do all which he wishes, and to prevent that which is contrary to his will. He ever moves towards the Brahman. [3] His speech, whether in prose or verse, is ever pure and sweet.

COMMENTARY

In this verse he speaks of the fruit of a complete knowledge of the Sahasrāra. The idea sought to be conveyed is that a knowledge of this place should be gained as a whole and in detail.

" *Who has controlled his mind* " (Niyata-nija-citta)—*i.e.*, he who has controlled and concentrated the inner faculties on this place. Such an one becomes free from Saṁsāra, or, in other words, he is released from bondage, as there is nothing to bind or attract him in these worlds. By bondage is meant the Māyik bonds of virtue (Puṇya) and sin (Pāpa).

---

[1] Citta.

[2] Saṁsāra, the world of birth and rebirth to which men are impelled by their Karma.

[3] The interpretation of Viśvanātha is here adopted, according to which Kha=Brahman. As the term also means the " air " or " ether," the text is capable of translation as " He is able to roam the sky ".

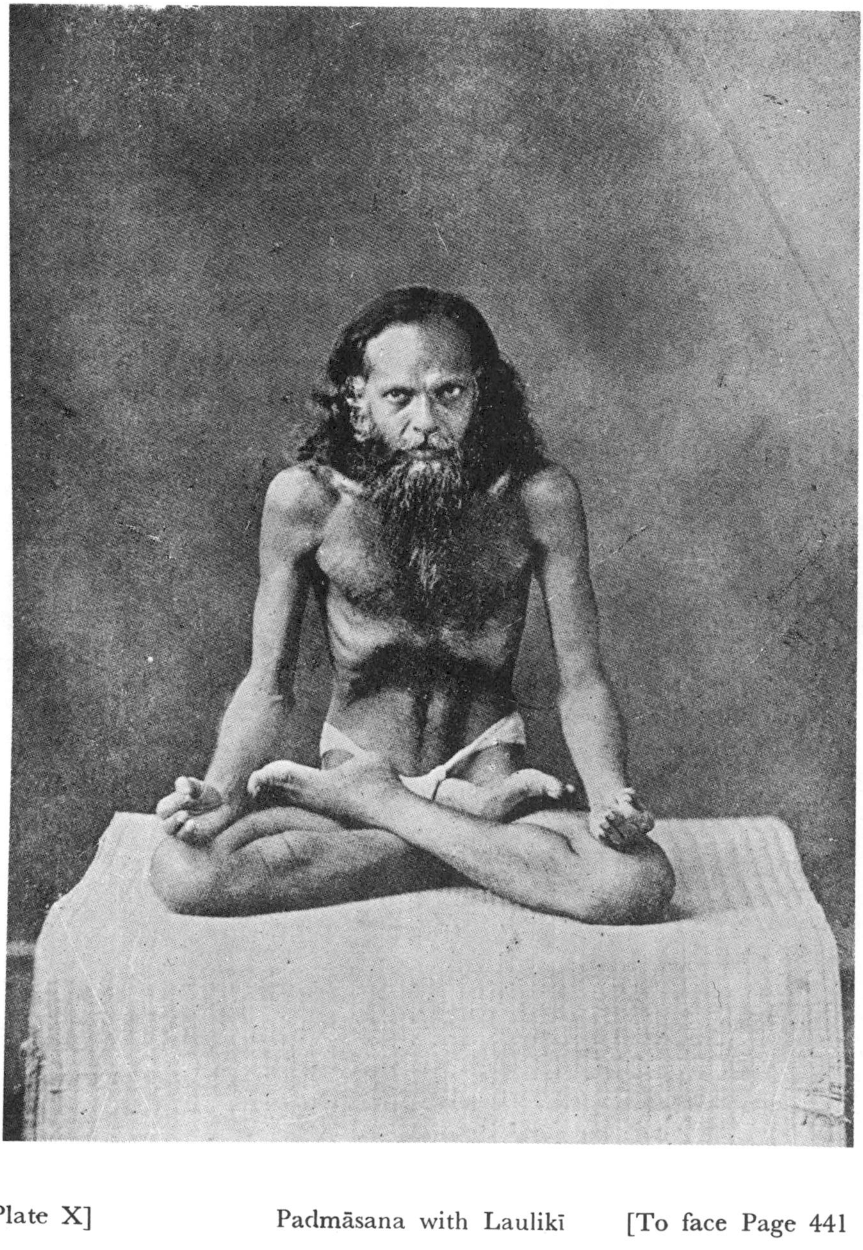

Plate X] Padmāsana with Laulikī [To face Page 441

The Bhāgavata says: " If the action which is the product of the operation of the Guṇas is attributed to the self, then such (false) attribution is bondage and Saṁsāra and servitude." Also *cf.* Bhagavad-Gītā: " O Son of Kuntī, Man is bound by action which is the product of his own nature (Sva-bhāva)." [1]

To inhabit this body for the purpose of undergoing Pāpa (sin) and Puṇya (virtue) is bondage. In heaven one enjoys (the fruit of) Puṇya, and in the nether world (Pātāla) one suffers sorrow, and on earth man is subject to both Pāpa and Puṇya. For the Tattva-jñānī (him who knows the truth) there is neither Puṇya nor Pāpa, which are the causes of bondage; his accumulated (Saṁcita) Karma of merit (Puṇya) and demerit (Pāpa) is also destroyed. He is in consequence under no bondage whether in heaven (Svarga), earth (Martya), or nether world (Pātāla), and he is not truly embodied.[2] Such a one stays on earth so long only as he has not worked out what he has begun. He is liberated though living (Jīvanmukta), and attains complete Liberation on the dissolution of the body.

The Kulārṇava Tantra says: " Those who have the Brahman in the heart can acquire neither merit by performing a hundred horse sacrifices, nor demerit by killing a hundred Brāhmaṇas." The Gītā (III, 18) also says: " For him there is nothing in this world that should or should not be done. For such an one there is no dependence on any being." [3]

The Subodhinī [4] interprets this verse to mean that the " knower " (Tattvajñānī) acquires no merit by the performance of actions nor demerit by the omission thereof.

Śruti [5] speaks of the destruction of accumulated (Saṁcita) Puṇya and Pāpa: " When Manas, which is now selecting and now rejecting, is dissolved in That; when Pāpa and Puṇya are destroyed (lit., burnt),

---

[1] Ch. XVIII, v. 60.

[2] Na śarīrī bhavati—though he has a body, he is not of it.

[3] Telang's Translation: " He has no interest at all in what is done, and none whatever in what is not done, in this world; nor is any interest of his dependent on any being " (p. 54, Sacred Books of the East, Vol. VIII).

[4] That is, Śrīdhara-svāmī's Commentary on the Gītā.

[5] The text quoted is from Haṁsa Upaniṣad but differs slightly from the published texts of that Upaniṣad.

Sadāśiva, who is Śakti and Ātmā (*cf.* Haṁsah, *ante*), is Śānta."[1] *Cf.* Bhagavad-Gītā: " And so the fire of knowledge destroys all actions."[2]

"*Complete power*" (Samagrā-śaktī)—*i.e.*, power which enables him to do everything. By power, or Śakti, is meant ability to do all he desires to do[3] and counteract all harm, to fly across the air,[4] and to become possessed of great powers of speech and of poetic composition.

---

[1] That is, peace and quietude like the still surface of an ocean characteristic of the Supreme State.

[2] IV, 37.

[3] Such an one may have such a power but will not wrongly exercise it.

[4] Khagati; this is Kālīcaraṇa's interpretation.

Verse 46

Atrāste śiśusūryasodarakalā candrasya sā ṣodaśī
śuddhā nīrajasūkṣmatantuśatadhābhāgaikarūpā parā.
Vidyutkoṭisamānakomalatanūrvidyotitādhomukhī
[1] *nityānandaparamparātivigalat-pīyūṣadhārādharā.*

HERE is the excellent (supreme) sixteenth Kalā of the Moon. She is pure, and resembles (in colour) the young Sun. She is as thin as the hundredth part of a fibre in the stalk of a lotus. She is lustrous [2] and soft like ten million lightning flashes, and is down-turned. From Her, whose source is the Brahman, flows copiously the continuous stream of nectar [3] (or, She is the receptacle of the stream of excellent nectar which comes from the blissful union of Para and Parā). [4]

Commentary

Verses 41 and 42 speak of the presence of Amā-kalā, Nirvāṇa-kalā, and Para-Bindu, within the triangle in the pericarp of the Sahasrāra. He now desires to describe them by their distinctive attributes, and speaks in this verse of the distinctive features of Amā-kalā.

---

[1] पूर्णा इति वा.

[2] Kālīcaraṇa reads "Vidyotitā," but Śaṁkara reads "Nityoditā," "constantly shining".

[3] Alternative reading of Commentator: "Nityānanda-paramparātivigalat-pīyūṣa-dhārā-dharā." Paramparā may mean "in a continuous course," or Paraṁ may mean Śiva and Parā-Śakti. This difference in meaning is due to the different ways in which these words may be read.

[4] Parā, according to Śaṁkara, may mean Parā, Paśyantī, Madhyamā, and Vaikharī collectively. Para and Parā are the Bindu-rūpa Śiva and Śakti.

"*Excellent or supreme*" (Parā)—*i.e.*, She is Cit-Śakti. In the Prabhāsa-khaṇḍa occurs the following passage: "The excellent Māyā who maintains the bodies of all that have bodies." This is attributive of Amā.

"*The sixteenth Kalā of the Moon*" (Candrasya ṣodaśī).—By this we are to understand that he is speaking of Amā-kalā.[1]

"*Pure*" (Śuddhā)—*i.e.*, stainless.

"*She resembles,*" *etc.*, (Śiśu-sūrya-sodara-kalā).—By this the redness of this Kalā is indicated.

"*Thin as the hundredth part of a fibre in the stalk of the lotus*" (Nīraja-sūkṣma-tantu-śatadhā-bhāgaika-rūpā).—Thin like a hundredth part of the fibre in the lotus-stalk split length-wise.

"*Whose source is the Brahman*" (Nityānanda-paramॅpara).—Nityānanda=Pūrṇānanda=Brahman.

"*Flows,*" *etc.*, (Ati-vigalat-pīyūṣa-dhārā-dharā).—If the last two compound words be read as one long compound word, as follows, Pūrṇānanda-paraṁparāti-vigalat-pīyūṣa-dhārā-dharā, the meaning, of it will be as given within brackets at the end of the verse. Ānanda will then mean the joy of union, and Paraṁ-Parā will then mean Śiva and Śakti.

Para=Bindu-rūpa, Śiva; Parā=Prakṛti, Śakti. Ānanda is the joy which arises from the union of the two, and from such union flows the nectar of which Amā-kalā is the receptacle.

---

[1] Viśvanātha says that this Amā-kalā is Urdhva-śakti-rūpā, or the upward (towards the Brahman) moving Śakti.

Verse 47

Nirvāṇākhyakalā parā paratarā sāste tadantargatā
keśāgrasya sahasradhā vibhajitasyaikāṁśarūpā satī.
Bhutānāmadhidaivataṁ bhagavati nityaprabodhodayā
candrārdhāṅgasamānabhaṅguravatī sarvārkatulyaprabhā.

Inside it (Amā-kalā) is Nirvāṇa-kalā, more excellent than the excellent. She is as subtle as the thousandth part of the end of a hair, and of the shape of the crescent moon. She is the ever-existent Bhagavatī, who is the Devatā who pervades all beings. She grants divine knowledge, and is as lustrous as the light of all the suns shining at one and the same time.

Commentary

In this verse the Nirvāṇa-kalā is described.

"*Inside it*" (Tadantargatā)—*i.e.*, placed in the lap [1] of Amā-kalā. The Kalā has already been described [2] as the "crescent seventeenth Kalā placed within Amā, and known by the name of Nirvāṇa-kalā."

"*More excellent than the excellent*" (Parā-paratarā).—The Amā-kalā is excellent; this is more excellent than Amā. If "Parātparatarā" be accepted for 'Parā-paratarā,' then the meaning will be that She is the most excellent.

"*She is as subtle . . . hair*" (Keśāgrasya sahasradhā vibhajitasyaikāṁśa-rūpā).—She is equal in dimension to the thousandth part of the end of a hair, so very subtle is She.

"*Of the shape of the crescent Moon*" (Candrārdhānga-samāna-bhanguravatī)—like Amā-kalā she is in shape like the crescent.

---

[1] That is, within the curve of Amā-kalā. Viśvanātha says, not within Amā-kalā, but within the Candra-Maṇḍala, of which the Amā-kalā is one of the digits, Nirvāṇa-kalā is, he says, Vyāpinī-tattva.

[2] See p. 436, *ante*.

"*That Devatā who pervades all beings*" (Bhūtānām adhidaivataṁ).—Adhi-daivataṁ=Hārdda-caitanyaṁ,[1] and this Kalā is Hārdda-caitanya-svarūpā of all beings.

"*She grants divine knowledge*" (Nitya-prabodhodayā).—*i.e.*, She grants Tattva-jñāna, or knowledge of the Brahman.

"*And is lustrous,*" *etc.* (Sarvārka-tulya-prabhā).—There are twelve suns (Dvādaśāditya). "When all the twelve suns are shining"—such is Her lustre. This adjective also implies that She is red.

---

[1] Hārdda-caitanyaṁ. Amara defines Hārdda to mean Prema, Sneha—*i.e.*, affection, love. That is, the Iṣṭadevatā worshipped in the heart; the Śakti who is Herself the heart of the Lord. The word is derived from hṛd=heart. The Devatā also exists as what is called the Hārdda-kalā. See Introduction.

Verse 48

Etasyā madhyadeśe vilasati paramāpūrvanirvāṇaśaktiḥ
koṭyādityaprakāśā tribhuvanajananī koṭibhāgaikarūpā.
Keśāgrasyātisūkṣmā niravadhi vigalatpremadhārādharā sā
sarveṣaṁ jīvabhūtā munimanasi mudā tattvabodhaṁ vahanti.

Within its middle space (*i.e.*, middle of the Nirvāṇa-kalā) shines the Supreme and Primordial Nirvāṇa-Śakti [1]; She is lustrous like ten million suns, and is the Mother of the three worlds. She is extremely subtle, and like unto the ten-millionth part of the end of a hair. She contains within Her the constantly flowing stream of gladness, [2] and is the life of all beings. She graciously carries the knowledge of the Truth (Tattva) [3] to the mind of the sages.

Commentary

He now speaks of the Para-Bindu.

"*Its*" (Etasyāh)—*i.e.*, of the Nirvāṇa-kalā.

"*Middle*" (Madhya-deśe).—Within the lap.[4]

"*The Supreme and Primordial Nirvāṇa-Śakti*" (Paramā-pūrva-nirvāṇa-śakti=paramā apūrva-nirvāṇa-śakti).—Parama [5]—*i.e.*, the Supreme

---

[1] This is, according to Viśvanātha, the Samanāpada or Samanī Śakti. This state is not free from the multitude of bonds (Pāśajāla).

[2] Prema. See notes, *post.*

[3] This word "Tattva" has by Viśvanātha been said to be Śivābheda-jñānaṁ—*i.e.*, the non-distinction between Śiva and Śivé.

[4] That is, within the crescent. According to Viśvanātha the locative indicates proximity and means near the middle but slightly above it.

[5] This word has been defined by Śaṁkara to mean "She who is as great as the Para or Supreme". Viśvanātha says it means "She who measures futurity (Para=Uttara-kāla)"—that is, all future time is in Her control.

Brahman as śakti. Apūrva—*i.e.*, She before whom there was nothing, She having appeared at the beginning of creation.

"*Shines*" (Vilasati paramā) [1]—*i.e.*, dwells resplendent.

"*Mother of the three worlds*" (Tri-bhuvana-jananī)—*i.e.*, She is the origin of the Universe which comprises Svarga, Martya, and Pātāla and the like.[2]

"*She is extremely subtle, like unto the ten-millionth part of the end of a hair*" (Keśāgrasya-koṭi-bhāgaika-rūpā-tiśukṣmā).—As She is like the ten-millionth part of the end of a hair, She is extremely subtle.

"*She contains within her the constantly flowing stream of gladness*" (Niravadhi-vigalat-prema-dhārā-dharā).—Prema is the tenderness of mind produced by feeling of gladness; that is, She holds within Her the stream of excellent nectar which has its origin in the blissful union of Śiva and Śakti, and which flows incessantly.

"*Is the life of all beings*" (Sarveṣāṁ jīva-bhūtā)—*i.e.*, animated being is but a part of Her.

Cf. "O Devī, as sparks fly forth from a flame, so does the Parabindu (as Jīva) issue from Her (Nirvāṇa-Śakti), and becomes knowing [3] when it touches the Earth." [4]

By "Her" is meant the Śakti who is in the Para-bindu, who is both Śiva and Śakti; and from Her emanates the Jīva.

Nirvāṇa-Śakti is situated below Nirvāṇa-kalā, and over Nibodhika,[5] which is Nāda-rupā.[6] *Cf.* "Placed within Nirvāṇa (Kalā) is the fiery (Vahni-rūpā) Nibodhikā, who is unmanifested Nāda [7]; above it is the supreme Nirvāṇa-Śakti, who is the cause of all and is possessed of the

---

[1] Paramā—She who is co-existent or of equal degree with the Supreme (Para) or she who knows the Supreme. This is as applied to Māyā.

[2] Heaven, Earth, and Netherworld.

[3] Saṁjñāyuktah, *i.e.*, Jīva-consciousness. It may also mean 'becomes endowed with a name'. Name and form characterise the world as Sat, Cit and Ānanda do Brahman.

Cf. Asti bhāti priyaṁ rūpaṁ nāma cetyaṁśa-pañcakaṁ.

Ādyaṁ trayaṁ Brahma-rūpaṁ jagadrūpaṁ tato dvayaṁ.

[4] Yadā bhūmau patati tadā saṁ ñāyukto bhavati. The creation of Jīva is here spoken of. The Text quoted is from Nirvāṇa-tantra I.

[5] See Introduction, and note to v. 40, particularly the portion dealing with Nāda, Bodhinī and Bindu.

[6] That is Śakti, as Nāda.

[7] Avyakta-nāda—unmanifested sound.

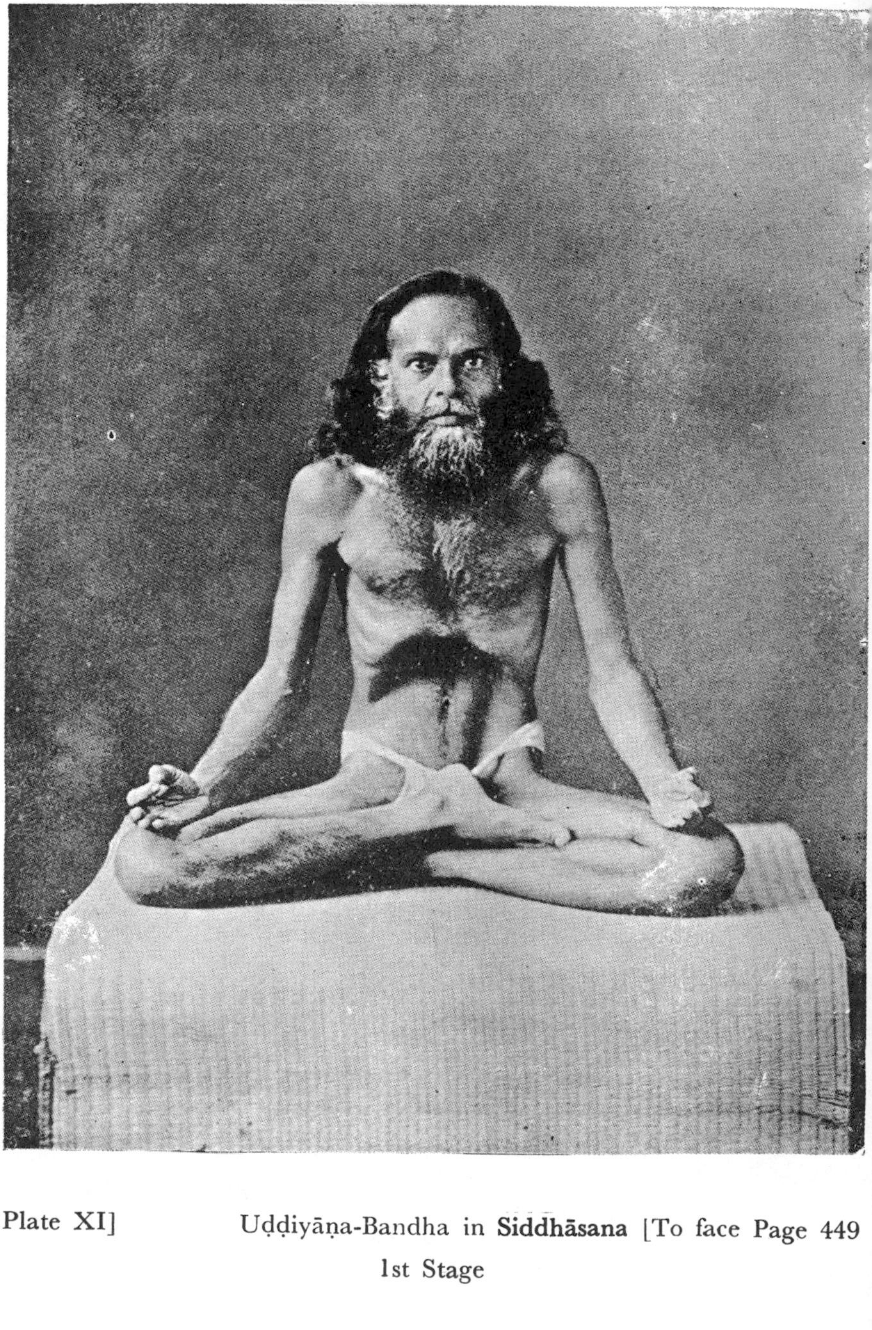

Plate XI] Uḍḍiyāṇa-Bandha in **Siddhāsana** [To face Page 449
1st Stage

lustre of ten million suns. It is in Her that there is the Brahman [1] who is the changeless Śiva [2]; it is here that Kuṇḍalī-Śakti enjoys with Paramātmā."

Nibodhikā is a phase of Avyakta-nāda (Avyakta-nādātmikā), and is fire-like. Rāghava-bhaṭṭa says: "Nāda exists in three states. When Tamo-guṇa is dominant, it is merely sound unmanifest (Avyakta-nāda) [3] in the nature of Dhvani; when Rajo-guṇa is more dominant, there is sound in which there is somewhat of a placing of the letters [4]; when the Sattva-guṇa preponderates, Nāda assumes the form of Bindu." [5] Hence Nāda, Bindu, and Nibodhikā, are respectively the Sun, the Moon, and Fire,[6] and their activities are Jñāna, Icchā, and Kriyā. Jñāna, again, is Fire, Icchā the Moon, and Kriyā the Sun. This has been said in the Śāradā. Therefore, insomuch as it has been said that Nirvāṇa Śakti is above the fiery (Vahni-rūpā) Nibodhikā, the wise should conclude that Nirvāṇa-Śakti is placed above the Maṇḍalas of the Sun, the Moon, and Fire.

This has been clearly stated in the Kulārṇava-Tantra, in the Para-Brahma-dhyāna, which begins, "The Bindu-rūpa Para-Brahma in the Sahasrāra," and ends, "Beautified by the three Maṇḍalas within the triangle in the pericarp." By three Maṇḍalas are meant the Maṇḍalas of Sun, Moon, and Fire. We shall show that the Nirvāṇa-Śakti is in the form of Para-bindu (Para-bindu-rūpā).

---

1 Nirañjana. This word may either be equal to Nir+añjana (*i.e.*, stainless) or Nih+añjana (unaffected by pleasure or pain, unmoved). It is one of the aspects of the Brahman.

2 Nirvikāra. Some read Nirvikalpa, or of unconditioned, consciousness. Nirvikalpa is also the last stage of Samādhi, in which there are no (Nir) specific distinctions (Vikalpa); and no "this" and "that".

3 Tamo-guṇādhikyena kevala-dhvanyātmako'vyakta-nādah.

4 Raja ādhikyena kiṁcidvarṇa-baddha-nyāsātmakah. The sense appears to be that the letters exist anyhow together in massive undifferentiated form.

5 Sattvādhikyena bindu-rūpah.

6 Tatash cha nāda-bindu-nibodhikā arkendu-vahni-rūpah. Jñāna is Fire, because it burns up all actions. When the result of action is realized, action ceases (see note to v. 45). Icchā is the Moon, because Icchā is the precursor of creation and is eternal. The Moon contains the Amā-kalā, which knows neither increase nor decay. Kriyā is the Sun, because like the Sun it makes everything visible. Unless there is striving there cannot be realization and manifestation. *Cf.* "As one Sun makes manifest all the Lokas" (Gītā).

The Text will be made clearer if an arrangement be made in the following groups: (1) Nāda, Sun, Kriyā; (2) Bindu, Moon, Icchā; (3) Nibodhikā, Fire, Jñāna. But see Introduction.

Verse 49

Tasyā madhyāntarāle śivapadamamalaṁ śāśvataṁ yogigamyaṁ
nityānandābhidhānaṁ sakalasukhamayaṁ śuddhabodhasvarūpaṁ.
Kecidbrahmābhidhānaṁ padamiti sudhiyo vaiṣṇavaṁ tallapanti
keciddhaṁsākhyametatkimapi sukṛtino mokṣamātma-prabodhaṁ

Within Her is the everlasting place called the abode of Śiva,[1] which is free from Māyā, attainable only by Yogīs, and known by the name of Nityānanda. It is replete with every form of bliss,[2] and is pure knowledge itself.[3] Some call it the Brahman; others call it the Haṁsa. Wise men describe it as the abode of Viṣṇu, and righteous men[4] speak of it as the ineffable place of knowledge of the Ātmā, or the place of Liberation.

Commentary

He speaks of the Para-Brahma-sthāna (place of Para-Brahma) in the Void within Nirvāṇa-Śakti.

---

[1] Śiva-padam or state of Śiva. This, Viśvanātha says, is the Unmanī state of Śakti where there is neither Kāla nor Kalā, time nor space. It is the body of Śiva (Śiva-tanu). It is then said Unmanyante Para-śivah. The following verse which occurs in Padma-Purāṇa (Uttara-Khaṇḍa, ch. 78, v. 43) puts the idea in a more popular form. It says:

Śaivāh Saurāsh ca Gāṇeśāh Vaiṣṇavāh Śakti-pūjakāh.
Māmeva prāpnuvantī hi varṣāṁbhah sāgaraṁ yathā.

" Śaivas, Sauras, Gāṇeśas, Vaiṣṇavas and Śāktas, all verily come to me like rain water to the ocean."

[2] Sakala-sukhamayam. Viśvanātha reads here Parama-kulapadaṁ, which he interprets as Param Akula-padaṁ, or the abode of the Supreme Śiva, who is known as Akula, as Kula is Śakti. It is so called because it is here that the universe finds its rest.

[3] Śuddha-bodha-svarūpaṁ.

[4] Sukṛtinah.

"*Within Her*" (Tasyāh madhyāntarāle)—*i.e.*, within Nirvāṇa[1] Śakti in Her form of Paraṁ Bindu, *i.e.*, the empty space within the Bindu.

"*Abode of Śiva*" (Śiva-padaṁ).—This is the place of the Brahman.

"*Free from Māyā*" (Amalaṁ)—*i.e.*, free the impurity of Māyā.

"*Called*"—*i.e.*, called by those who know the Tattva.

"*Attainable only by Yogīs*" (Yogi-gaṁyam).—On account of its extreme subtlety, it is beyond the scope of word and mind, is attainable by Yogīs by pure Jñāna[2] only.

"*Some call it*"—*i.e.*, the Vedāntists (Vaidāntikas) call it.

"*Ineffable*" (Kimapi)—*i.e.*, wonder-inspiring.

"*Place of the knowledge of the Ātmā*" (Ātmā-prabodham).—The place where the Ātmā is seen or realized.

"*Liberation.*" (Mokṣa)—*i.e.*, where one is liberated from Māyā by which one is surrounded.

Now be good enough to mark the following: the Para-bindu which is Prakṛti and Puruṣa is surrounded[3] by Māyā, and is within the triangle in the pericarp of the Lotus of a thousand petals. So it has been said:

"In the Satya-loka is the formless and lustrous One; She has surrounded Herself by Māyā, and is like a grain of gram; devoid of hands, feet, and the like. She is Moon, Sun, and Fire. When casting off (Utsṛjya) the covering (Bandhana) of Māyā, She becomes of two-fold aspect (Dvidhā bhitvā) and Unmukhī,[4] then on the division or separation of Śiva and Śakti[5] arises creative ideation."[6]

The word "Satya-loka" in the above passage means Sahasrāra.

Also *cf.* "The attributeless Bindu is without doubt the Cause (of the attainment) of Siddhis. Some say that the Deva who is one, stainless

---

[1] Viśvanāthā says Samanā.

[2] Spiritual knowledge, as it is said: Mokṣe dhīr jñānam anyatra vijñānaṁ shilpa-śāstrayoh. The knowledge which gains Mokṣa (Liberation) is called Jñāna, other forms of knowledge, such as fine arts, and the Śāstras being Vijñāna.

[3] Māyā-bandhanā-cchādita-prakṛti-puruṣātmaka-para-bindu.

[4] By Unmukhī is meant that She becomes intent on creation.

[5] Śiva-Śakti-vighāgena. By division or separation is not meant that Śiva is really divided or separated from Śakti—for the two are ever one and the same—but that Śakti, who exists latently as one with the Brahman in dissolution, appears to issue from It on creation as the manifested universe.

[6] Sṛṣṭi-kalpanā. That is, the subject knows itself as object.

(Nirañjana), all-embracing (Mahā-pūrṇa) and united with the primordial Śakti as in the form of a grain of gram [1] is Brahmā, and by some, again, He is called Viṣṇu: by others, again, He is called the Deva Rudra."

The luminous empty space within the Nirvāṇa-Śakti (*i.e.*, the outer circle of the Para-bindu), which is more minute than the ten-millionth part of the end of a hair, is according to the author, the abode of Brahman (Brahma-pada). *Cf.* "Within it [2] is Para-bindu, whose nature it is to create, maintain, and destroy. The space within is Śiva Himself and Bindu [3] is Parama-kuṇḍali."

Also: "The circumference (Vṛtta) is the Kuṇḍalinī-Śakti, and She possesses the three Guṇas. The space within, O Beloved Maheśāni is both Śiva and Śakti." [4]

This Bindu is, according to some, Īśvara, the Cause of All. Some Paurāṇikas call Him Mahā-Viṣṇu; others call Him Brahma Puruṣa.

Cf. "There was neither day nor night, neither the firmament nor the earth, neither darkness nor any other light; there was *That*, the Brahma-Male,[5] imperceptible to hearing, and the other sources of knowledge united with Pradhāna." [6]

The Śāradā [7] says: "The eternal Śiva should be known both as Nirguṇa (attributeless) and Saguṇa (possessed of attributes). He is Nirguṇa when (considered as) dissociated from the workings of Prakṛti, but when Sakala (*i.e.*, so associated with Prakṛti) He is Saguṇa." [8]

This shows that the Bindu is Saguṇa-Brahman. We should know that Saguṇa-Brahman is in reality but one, though He is called by different names according to the inclinations of men. There is no need to go into further details.

---

[1] Caṇaka, which under its outward sheath contains two undivided halves.

[2] Apparently Nirvāṇa-kalā.

[3] That is, the circumference as opposed to the inner space.

[4] Jñānārṇava-Tantra, XXIV, 21.

[5] Prādhānikaṁ Brahma-pumān.

[6] Kālikā-Purāṇa, XXIV, v. 125.

[7] Ch. I.

[8] And, so, also, the Śāktānanda-taraṅgiṇī (Ch. I) says of the Devī that Mahā-māyā without Māyā is Nirguṇa, and with Māyā Saguṇa.

Summary of Verses 41 to 49

Above (the end) of the Suṣumnā-Nāḍī is the Lotus of a thousand petals; it is white and has its head downward turned; its filaments are red. The fifty letters of the Alphabet from A to La, which are also white, go round and round its thousand petals twenty times. On its pericarp is Haṁsaḥ, and above it is the Guru who is Parama-Śiva Himself. Above the Guru are the Sūrya-and Candra-Maṇḍalas, and above them Mahāvāyu. Over the latter is placed Brahmarandhra, and above it Mahāśaṅkhinī. In the Maṇḍala of the Moon is the lightning-like triangle within which is the sixteenth Kalā [1] of the Moon, which is as fine as the hundredth part of the lotus-fibre, and of a red colour, with its mouth downward turned. In the lap of this Kalā is the Nirvāṇa-Kalā, subtle like the thousandth part of the end of a hair, also red and with the mouth downward turned. Below Nirvāṇa-Kalā is the Fire called Nibodhikā which is a form of Avyakta-nāda.[2] Above it (Nibodhikā), and within Nirvāṇa-kalā, is Para Bindu, which is both Śiva and Śakti. The Śakti of this Para-Bindu is the Nirvāṇa-Śakti, who is Light (Tejas) and exists in the form of Haṁsah (Hamsa-rūpā), and is subtle like the ten-millionth part of the end of a hair. That Haṁsah is Jīva. Within the Bindu is the void (Śūnya) which is the Brahma-pada (place of the Brahman).

According to the view expressed in the fifth chapter of the Āgama-kalpa-druma and other works, the triangle A-Ka-Tha [3] is in the pericarp of the Sahasrāra. At its three corners are three Bindus: the lower Bindu at the apex of the triangle is Ha-kāra,[4] and is male (Puruṣa); and the two Bindus at the corners constitute the Visarga in the form Sa [5] and represent Prakrti. Haṁsah which is Puruṣa and Prakṛti thus shows itself in the form of three Bindus. In its middle is Amā-kalā, and in Her lap is Nirvāṇa-Śakti, and the vacant space within Nirvāṇa-Śakti is Para-brahman. It has been said: " Within the Maṇḍala of the moon in the white Lotus of a thousand petals shines like lightning the triangle A-Ka-Tha united with

---

[1] That is, Amā-kalā.

[2] Avyakta-nādātmaka-nibodhikākhya-vahni.

[3] That is, the letters arranged in the form of the triangle referred to in v. 4 of Pādukā-pañchaka. The Devī is Mātṛkā-mayī.

[4] *Viz.*, Haṁ representing the " Male " Bindu.

[5] That is, literally " standing Sa," or Visarga, in the form Sa. The letter Sa, or more strictly Sa without the vowel, changes into Visargah; thus, Tejas becomes Tejah, Rajas Rajah.

Ha-La-Kṣa.[1] Within it, is the excellent (Para) Bindu (Śūnya), placed below Visarga. In this region is the downward-turned sixteenth Kalā, of the colour of the rising sun, in shape like the crescent moon who discharges a stream of nectar, and within Her is Parā-Śakti, possessing the effulgence of ten million suns. She is as subtle as the thousandth part of the Lotus fibre, and is Cidātmikā.[2] Within Her is Bindu who is the Nirañjana-Puruṣa, who is beyond mind and speech and is Saccidānanda, and Visarga (who is also there) is Prakṛti. Haṁsa who is both Pum [3] and Prakṛti shines by His own effulgence."

Those who follow this view, place Sa-kāra over the Bindu, and place the Guru above Visarga [4] and Bindu which together make Haṁsah. But this cannot be right. The Nirvāṇa-Tantra speaks of the Guru as worshipping the Para Bindu-rūpa-Śakti, and as being close to Her and in the act of worshipping Her. The worshipper should always sit at a level lower than, and in front of the object of worship, and never at a higher level than, and behind the object of worship. *Cf.* Nirvāṇa [5]: "Meditate upon the Nirañjanā Devī within the Satyaloka in the Cintāmaṇi-gṛha [6] as placed on the jewelled throne or lion-seat (Siṁhāsana), and on your Guru as being near Her and worshipping Her."

The Mahākālī-Tantra, moreover, speaks explicitly of the presence of the Guru over the two letters Haṁ and Sah.[7] It is to be understood that if there be any texts which differ from, or add to, those here adopted, then they must be taken to refer to different methods and opinions.

(*This is the end of seventh section*)

---

[1] These Varṇas are inside the triangle A-Ka-Tha.

[2] Of the nature of Cit. *Cf.* definition of Māyā-Śakti in Tattva-Saṁdoha 14.

[3] The Male, Puruṣa.

[4] Lit. Generator of Visarga, for from Sa Visarga comes.

[5] Nirvāṇa-Tantra, Ch. X.

[6] The room made of Cintāmaṇi stone which grants all desires, described in the Rudra-yāmala and Brahmāṇda-Purāṇa. The Lalitā refers to it as being the place or origin of all those Mantras which bestow all desired objects (Cintita).

[7] In the Jñānārṇava-Tantra (I, v. 13) it is said: "Pārvatī, in Hakāra with Bindu (Haṁ) is Brahmā and, O Maheśvarī, the two Bindus of Visarga (Sah) are Hari and Myself. By reason of this inseparable connection men in this world speak of Hari-Hara."

Verse 50

Hūṁkāreṇaiva devīṁ yamaniyamasamabhyāsaśīlaḥ suśīlo
jñātva śrīṇāthavaktrāt-kramamiti ca mahāmokṣavartmaprakāśaṁ.
Brahmadvārasya madhye viracavati sa tāṁ śuddhabuddhisvabhāvo
Bhitvā talliṅgarūpaṁ pavanadahanayorākrameṇaiva guptaṁ

He whose nature is purified by the practice of Yama, Niyama, and the like,[1] learns from the mouth of his Guru the process which opens the way to the discovery of the great Liberation. He whose whole being is immersed in the Brahman then rouses the Devī by Hūṁ-kāra, pierces the centre of the Liṅga, the mouth of which is closed, and is therefore invisible, and by means of the Air and Fire (within him) places Her within the Brahmadvāra.[2]

Commentary

Having described the Cakras ending with the Sahasrāra, he now wishes to speak of the union of Kuṇḍalinī, and preliminary to that he refers to the mode of rousing Kuṇḍalinī.[3]

The sense conveyed by this verse is that the man who has attained success in Yoga learns from his Guru the process, which consists of contracting the heart, rousing Kuṇḍalinī by the power of the air and fire, and so forth[4]; and having learned it from the mouth of his Guru, he rouses Kuṇḍalinī, attacking Her with air and fire, and by uttering the Kūrca

[1] See Introduction.

[2] That is, within Citriṇī-Nāḍī.

[3] In the Yoga-process known as Ṣaṭcakrabheda, generally described in the Introduction, but which practically must be learned of the Guru.

[4] The Commentator Śaṁkara, citing Gorakṣa Saṁhitā, says that air makes the fire go upwards, and the fire awakens Kuṇḍalinī and She also goes upwards.

"Hūṁ" and piercing the mouth of the Svayambhu-Liṅga places Kuṇḍalinī within Brahmadvāra, or, in other words, within the mouth of the Nāḍī Citriṇī.

"*He whose nature is purified*" (Suṣīla)—*i.e.*, the man who regularly practises Yama and so forth, and has trained himself.

"*By practising Yama, Niyama,*" *etc.* (Yama-niyama-sama-bhyāsaśīla). —It must be observed that it is not merely by the practice of Yama and Niyama that perfection in the preliminary Yoga practices [1] is attained. But the Sādhaka has by practice to destroy such inclinations as lust, anger, and the like which interfere with Yoga, and cultivate others, such as controlling the inner air, steadiness of mind, and so forth, which are helpful in Yoga practice. It is because of this that in v. 54 the Author has used the word "Yamādyaih" in the plural. Practising Yama and the like is necessary, however, for those whose minds are disturbed by lust and other propensities. If, however, a man by reason of merit and good fortune acquired in a previous birth, and by his nature, is free from anger, lust, and other passions, then he is capable of real Yoga without the preliminary practices. This must be well understood.

"*From the mouth of his Guru*" (Śrī-nātha-vaktrāt).—The process cannot be learnt without the instructions of the Guru. Hence it has been said: "It can be learnt from the Guru alone, and not from ten million Śāstras."

"*Process*" (Krama).—Steps, order.

"*Which opens the way to the discovery of the great Liberation*" (Mahā-mokṣa-vartma-prakāśa).—By this is meant the 'process' by which the entrance into the channel of the Nāḍī Citriṇī is opened out. 'Way of Liberation' (Mokṣa-vartma) is the way through the channel within Citriṇī. The 'discovery' (Prakāśa) is made of this by making one's way through it.

"*He*" (Sah)—*i.e.*, the man who has distinguished himself by his success in Yoga practices.

"*Whose whole being is immersed in the Brahman*" (Śuddha-buddhi-svabhāva [2]).—Śuddha-buddhi means the Brahman, and he whose Svabhāva (own being) is in Him. This compound word may also mean 'He whose

[1] Aṅga-yoga. See Introduction, and Viśvanātha citing Gautamīya-Tantra (See *post*, p. 123.)

[2] Śaṁkara reads prabhāva, and renders the passage as "He whose power is due to the purity of the Buddhi".

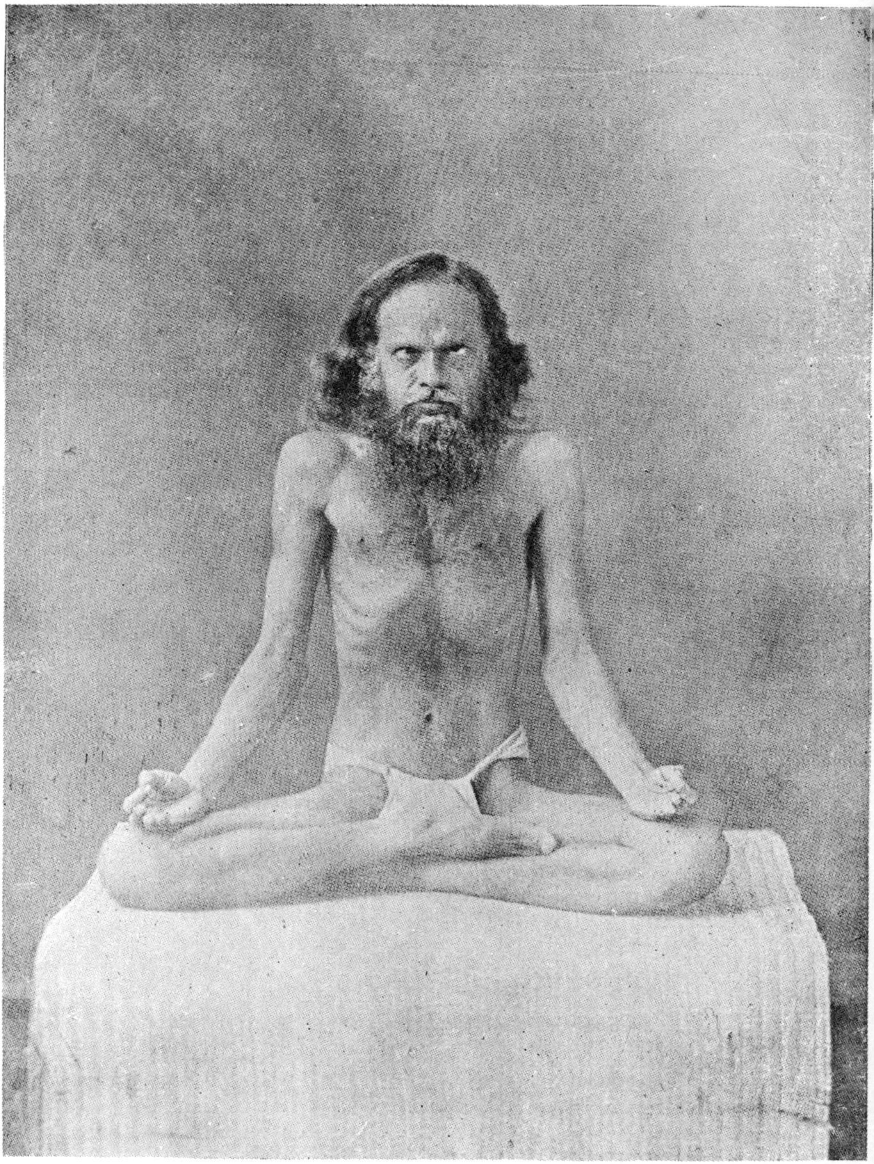

Plate XII] Uḍḍiyāṇa-Bandha in Siddhāsana [To face Page 457
2nd Stage

being (Bhāva) by reason of the purity of his mind (Śuddha-buddhi) is immersed in the Spirit (Sva=Ātmā)."

"*Rouses the Devī by Hūṁ-kāra*" (Hūṁ-kāreṇaiva Devīṁ).—The Āgama-kalpa-druma says: "Then having mentally recited Haṁsa, gently contract the anus." [1] It therefore follows that in moving Kuṇḍalinī the Haṁsa-Mantra should be uttered. The Author of the Lalitā-rahasya, following this, says that in moving Kuṇḍalinī the Mantra "Hūṁ Haṁsah" should be employed. But from the fact that the part is to be contracted after the Haṁsa-Mantra is recited, the intention appears to be that the Jīvātmā, which is of the shape of the flame of a lamp, should by the recitation of the Haṁsa-Mantra be brought from the heart to the Mūlādhāra, and then moved along with Kuṇḍalinī.

The Āgama-kalpa-druma in a subsequent passage says: "Raising and again raising the Śakti with the Ātmā from the abode of Brahmā,[2] the excellent Sādhaka should (and so forth)." This shows that She should be led away along with Ātmā or Jīvātmā. The Kālī-Kulāmṛta has: "Having led Jīva from the heart by the Haṁsa-Mantra to the Mūla Lotus,[3] and having roused the Paradevatā Kuṇḍalinī by Hūṁ-kāra." The Kaṅkāla-mālinī says: "O daughter of the King of Mountains, having drawn the Jīvātmā by the Praṇava, let the Sadhaka move Prāṇa and Gandha [4] with Kuṇḍalinī by the aid of the 'So'haṁ' Mantra, and make the Devī enter the Svādhiṣṭāna."

The wise should, from the above texts, understand that the Jīvātmā should be brought from the heart by the aid of either the Praṇava or Haṁsa Mantra, and then Kuṇḍalinī should be roused by the Kūrca-bīja alone.

"*The mouth of which is closed,*" *etc.* (Guptaṁ).—This word may be read either as an adjective qualifying Liṅga, and mean unmanifested by reason of its mouth being closed,[5] or may be read as an adverb qualifying "places" and then the word would mean "imperceptibly".

In the Āgama-kalpa-druma, Pañcama-śākhā, the mode of rousing the Kuṇḍalinī is described in detail thus: "Having seated oneself in the

---

[1] Śanair ākuñcayed gudaṁ—that is, by Aśvinī-mudrā.

[2] Brahmā is in Mūlādhāra.

[3] Mukhāṁbhuja. This may be a mis-script for Mūlaṁbuja.

[4] *i.e.*, Pṛthivī.

[5] On the top of the Liṅga is Nāda-bindu—*i.e.*, Candra-Bindu. The mouth is the Bindu which Kuṇḍalinī pierces.

Padmāsana posture, the two hands should be placed in the lap. Thereafter, having mentally recited the Haṁsa Mantra, the anus should be gently contracted. One should then repeatedly raise the air by the same way,[1] and having raised it let him pierce the Cakra. I now speak of its processes. In the Mūlādhāra Lotus is a very beautiful triangle. Inside it is Kāma [2] (lustrous) like ten million young suns; above Him (Kāma) and surrounding Svayambhu-Liṅga, is Kuṇḍalinī-Śakti." Also *cf.* As the result of excitation by the Kāmāgni and the action of the Kūrca-mantra on Her, She is seized with desire for Para-Haṁsa." [3]

The Bhūta-śuddhi [4] also says: " O Śivā, the Sādhaka should contract the chest (lit., heart), letting his breath remain there,[5] and he should control the base of the throat and other parts of the body,[6] and then suddenly opening the door by means of a key-like motion (Kuñcikā) [7] and (the fire of desire) should be kindled, O Parameśvarī, by means of the air (Pavana)." " Then the Serpent,[8] who is sleeping on the Liṅga in the Mūlādhāra and who is stung by the heat of the fire, should be awakened in the Liṅga at the mouth of the Yoni and by the heat (of her desire) be led forcibly upwards." [9] " Move the air into the Nādī according to the rules of Kuṁbhaka (retention of breath) and the method shown by the Guru. Let the Jīva thus controlled be led by the concealed passage, and by the upward breath make all the Lotuses turn their heads upwards. Having fully awakened Her, let the wise one lead Her to Bhānu (the Sun) at the summit of the Meru (*i.e.*, the Sahasrāra)."

---

[1] Tena vartmanā—that by which Kuṇḍalinī is to go.

[2] The Kāma-vāyu, or Air of Kāma.

[3] Paraṁ Haṁsābhilāṣiṇī—*i.e.*, passion is excited in Her, and She is impelled by the fire of Kāma towards the Paraṁ Haṁsa in the Sahasrāra.

[4] This passage is obscure, and cannot be traced in the only published edition of the Tantra, but is similar to certain passages in the Haṭhayoga-pradīpikā which deal with Bhūta-śuddhi. It seems to contain passages from various texts to illustrate the process of Bhūta-śuddhi. The Commentator has, however, more clearly described the process in his own words.

[5] He thus closes the passage of the upward breath.

[6] That is, the chest and the anus, thus closing the passage of the upward and downward airs.

[7] That is, the motion of the Kāma-vāyu spoken of *post.*

[8] Nāginī, one of the names of Kuṇḍalinī.

[9] That is, the Trikoṇa in the Mūlādhāra which surrounds the Svayambhu-Liṅga.

Now pay attention to the procedure established by a careful consideration of the above text [1]: The Yogī should sit in the proper posture and place his two hands with palms upwards in his lap and, steady his mind (Citta) by the Khecharī Mudrā. He should next fill the interior of his body with air and hold it in by Kuṁbhaka,[2] and contract the heart.[3] By so doing the escape of the upward breath is stopped. Then, when he feels that the air within him from the belly to the throat is tending downward through the channels in the Nādīs, he should contract the anus and stop the downward air (Apāna); then, again having raised the air, let him give the Kāma [4] within the triangle in the pericarp of the Mūlādhāra Lotus a turn from the left to the right (Vāmāvartena); by so doing the fire of Kāma there is kindled, and Kuṇḍalinī gets heated (excited) thereby. He should then pierce the mouth of the Svayaṁbhu-Liṅga, and through its aperture with the aid of the " Hūṁ " Bīja, lead Her who desires union [5] with Parama-Śiva, within the mouth of the Citriṇī-Nāḍi. This is the clear sense of texts.

---

[1] The passages in quotation marks are here cited from different books on Haṭhayoga.

[2] Retention of breath in Prāṇāyāma.

[3] Hṛdayaṁ ākuñcayet—that is, by Jālaṁdhara-Bandha, etc. See Introduction.

[4] Kāma-vāyu.

[5] Sāma-rasya, a term used on the material plane to denote sexual union.

Verse 51

Bhitvā liṅgatrayaṁ tatparamarasaśive sūkṣmadhāmṇi pradīpe
sā devī śuddhasattvā taḍidiva vilasattanturūpasvarūpā.
Brahmākhyāyāḥ sirāyāḥ sakalasarasijaṁ prāpya dedīpyate
tanmokṣākhyānandarūpaṁ ghaṭayati sahasā sūkṣmatālakṣaṇena.

The Devī who is Śuddha-sattvā[1] pierces the three Liṅgas, and, having reached all the lotuses which are known as the Brahma-nāḍī lotuses, shines therein in the fullness of Her lustre. Thereafter in Her subtle state, lustrous like lightning and fine like the lotus fibre, She goes to the gleaming flame-like Śiva, the Supreme Bliss and of a sudden produces the bliss of Liberation.

Commentary

Now he speaks of the mode of the Union of Kuṇḍalinī (with Śiva). The meaning of this verse, in brief, is that the Devī Kuṇḍalinī pierces the three Liṅgas—*viz.*, Svayambhu, Bāṇa, and Itara[2]—and by so doing makes a passage for Herself; and when she reaches the lotuses in (or appertaining to) the Nādī called Brahma-nādī She shines in the fullness of Her lustre in these lotuses. Then, when in Her subtle form, fine like the lotus fibre, She approaches Śiva, who is Supreme Bliss[3] Itself, and who is in His Bindu form in the pericarp of the Sahasrāra, She brings to the Sādhaka the Bliss of eternal Liberation[4] when that is least expected.

"*Pierces*" (Bheda) means making a passage through that which is obstructed.

---

[1] A form of embodied Caitanya. See Commentary, *post.*

[2] In the Mūlādhāra, Anāhata, and Ājñā-Cakras respectively.

[3] Paramarasa=Paramānanda.

[4] Mokṣākhyānandarūpaṁ=Nityānandarupa-muktiṁ.

"*Śuddha-sattvā.*"—Sattva, Ati-sattva, Parama-sattva, Śuddha-sattva, and Viśuddha-sattva are the five different degrees of Caitanya pervading the body.[1] Śuddha-sattvā is therefore the fourth (Turīyā) stage. By Brahmanāḍī is meant Citriṇī. The Lotuses are the six Lotuses which are strung upon Citriṇī.

"*The three Liṅgas*" (Liṅga-trayaṁ).—The three Liṅgas already described. By this we are to understand that the six Cakras and five Śivas are included. She pierces all these, which altogether make fourteen knots (Granthi).

The Śāktānanda-taraṅgiṇī speaks of "Her who goes along the Channel of Brahman [2] having pierced the fourteen knots." [3]

The Svatantra-Tantra speaks of the distinctive features of Liṅga and Śiva.

"The Devī goes to Brahman (Niṣkala) [4] after having pierced the Śivas placed in the six Cakras. As She reaches each of the different Cakras, She acquires the beauty characteristic of each and bewitches Maheśāna [5]; and having there repeatedly enjoyed Him who is filled with joy, She reaches the Eternal One (Śāśvata). He is said to be transpierced (Bhinna), as He is bewitched by Parā."

The Māyā-Tantra says: "The Devī goes along the Śakti-mārga, piercing the three Liṅgas in the Cakras in each of Her different forms [6] (Tattadrūpena), and having attained union (in the Sahasrāra) with Niṣkala (Brahman) She is satisfied." Tattadrūpeṇa—*i.e.*, in the forms Vaikharī, Madhyamā, and Paśyantī.

It has been said that [7] "The first state (Bhāva) is Vaikharī, and Madhyamā is placed in the heart; between the eyebrows is the Paśyantī state, and the Parā state is in the Bindu." [8] The meaning of the above

---

[1] Śarīrāvacchinna-Caitanya.

[2] Brahma-randhra, the channel within Citriṇī is called Brahmanāḍī and Brahma-randhra.

[3] That is, 3 Liṅgas, 6 Cakras, and the 5 Śivas—*viz.*, Brahmā and the rest—in the 5 Cakras.

[4] The supreme or Nirguṇa-Brahman.

[5] That is, the Śiva in the particular Cakra.

[6] That is, She unites, in Her passage along the Nāḍī, with each of the Liṅgas in that form of Hers which is appropriate to such union.

[7] See Commentary on v. 11, *ante*.

[8] According to v. 11, Parā is in Mūlādhāra, Paśyantī in Svādhiṣṭhāna, Madhyamā in Anāhatā and Vaikharī in the mouth. What is, however, here described is Layakrama.

quotation is that the four sound-producing (Śabdotpādikā) Śaktis—*viz.*, Parā, Paśyantī, Madhyamā, and Vaikharī—are identical with Kuṇḍalinī (Kuṇḍalinyabheda-rūpā). Hence at the time when Kuṇḍalinī starts to go to Sahasrāra She in Her form of Vaikharī bewitches Svayaṁbhū-Liṅga; She then similarly bewitches Bāna-Liṅga in the heart as Madhyamā, and Itara-Liṅga between the eyebrows as Paśyantī, and then when she reaches Para-Bindu She attains the stage of Parā (Parābhāva).

The Method of Cākra-bheda is thus described: " O Parameśvarī, let the Sādhaka carry along with Her the Lotuses which are on the Citriṇī, and which have their origin in the mud of blood and fat.[1] Let him [2] enter the channel (Nāla) [3] on the left, from below, and in this way Cakra-bheda (piercing the Cakra) is effected. After having thus pierced the six Cakras, She along with Jīva should be led as the rider guides a trained mare by the reins."

Also *cf.* " The Devī should be led by the Haṁsa-Mantra to the Sahasrāra through the points of union of the six Cakras (with the Nāḍī along the road of Suṣumnā."

" *Gleaming flame-like* " (Sūkṣma-dhāmni-pradīpe).—The gleam is the Haṁsa, which is the luminous energy (*Tejas*) of the Para Bindu, in its aspect as Nirvāṇa-Śakti (Nirvāṇa-śaktyātmaka). The Parama-Śiva shines with it.

We now describe how the joy of Liberation is brought about.

The Devī by dissolving Kuṇḍalinī in the Para-Bindu effects the Liberation of some Sādhakas through their meditation upon the identity of Śiva and Ātmā in the Bindu. She does so in the case of others by a similar process, and by their meditation on Śakti.[4] In other cases, again, this is done by the concentration of thought on the Parama-Puruṣa, and in other cases by the meditation of the Sādhaka on the bliss of union in the Bindu of Śiva and Śakti.

---

[1] Lotuses grow in the mud, and these Lotuses grow in the blood and fat of the body. The process described is Kuṇḍalinī-Yoga, or, as it is called in the Tippaṇī of Śaṁkara, Bhūta-śuddhi.

[2] As the Sādhaka, who has taken the Jīvātmā from the heart to the Mūlādhāra, and thus identifies himself with Kuṇḍalinī, it is he who enters.

[3] That is, the Nāḍī.

[4] Śaktyātmaka-cintana; or it may mean meditation on the union of Śiva and Śakti.

The Māyā-Tantra says [1]: "Those who are learned in Yoga say that it is the union of Jīva and Ātmā. According to others (*i.e.*, Śaivas) it is the experience of the identity of Śiva and Ātmā. The Āgama-vādīs proclaim that Yoga [2] is the knowledge (Jñāna) relating to Śakti. Otherwise men say that the knowledge of the Purāṇa-Puruṣa is Yoga, and others again, the Prakṛtī-vādīs, declare that the bliss of union of Śiva and Śakti is Yoga." [3] By "union of Jīva and Ātmā" is meant Samādhi. By Yoga is meant that by which oneness is attained with the Paramātmā. Having spoken of Samādhi, he then deals with the different kinds of Yoga in Dhyāna. By "bliss of union (Sāmarasya) of Śiva and Śakti" is meant the sense of enjoyment arising from the union of male and female.[4]

The Bṛhat-Śrīkrama speaks of the manner in which this is to be meditated upon: "They with the eye of knowledge [5] see the stainless Kalā, who is united with Cidānanda [6] on Nāda. He is the Mahādeva, white like pure crystal, and is the effulgent First Cause (Bimba-rūpa-nidāna),[7] and She is Parā, the lovely woman of beauteous body [8], whose limbs are listless by reason of Her great passion." [9]

By Kalā in the above is meant Kuṇḍalinī. Bimba-rūpa-nidāna qualifies Para-Śiva or Cidānanda. Cidānanda is the Bindu-rūpa Śiva or Para-Śiva.

---

[1] These verses also occur in Ch. XXV, vv. 1, 2 of Śāradā-Tilaka. By "union of Jīva and Ātmā" is meant the realization of the identity of the individual with the supreme spirit as indicated in the Mahāvākya "Tat tvam asi (That thou art)." By Purāṇa-Puruṣa, the Puruṣa in Sāṁkhya-Darśana is meant; the Vaiṣṇava understand by it Nārāyaṇa (collective humanity). By "knowledge of Śakti" is meant the Knowledge that Śakti is inseparate from Śiva.

[2] Śaktyātmaka-jñāna.

[3] Sāmarasyātmakaṁ jñānam. Tantrāntara says that Sāma-rasya is the Dhyāna of a Kulayogī.

[4] Strīpumyogāt yat saukhyaṁ sāmarasyaṁ prakīrtam. In other words, the bliss of Union of Śiva and Śakti, of which sexual union is the material type.

[5] Jñāna-cakṣuh.

[6] Cidānanda is Consciousness-Bliss.

[7] A variant reading is Bindu-rūpa-nidāna, the First Cause in the Bindu form.

[8] Vāmoru—lit., beautiful thighs, the part being selected as an example of the whole.

[9] Madālasa-vapuh.

It has also been said elsewhere: " Having united Kuṇḍalī with the Śūnya-rūpa [1] Para-Śiva, and having caused the Devī so united to drink the excellent nectar from their union, She by the same way should be brought back to the Kula cavity." [2]

" Having brought them together and meditated upon Their union,[3] let the Deha-devatā [4] be satisfied with the nectar which flows from such a union."

The Gandharva-mālikā speaks of a different process: " The Sahasrāra is the beautiful and auspicious place of Sadā-Śiva. It is free from sorrow and divinely beautiful with trees which always bear and are adorned by flowers and fruits. The Kalpa Tree [5] adds to its beauty. This tree contains all the five " elements," and is possessed of the three Guṇas. The four Vedas are its four branches. It is laden with beautiful unfading flowers which are yellow, white, black, red, green, and of variegated colour. Having meditated on the Kalpa Tree in this manner, then meditate upon the jewelled altar below it. O Beauteous One, on it is a beautiful bed adorned with various kinds of cloth and Mandāra flowers, and scented with many kinds of scents. It is there that Mahādeva constantly stays. Meditate upon Sadāśiva, who is like the purest crystal, adorned with all kinds of gems, long-armed,[6] and of enchanting beauty. He is ever gracious and smiling. In His ears are ear-rings, and a chain of gems goes round His neck. A garland of a thousand lotuses resting on His neck adorns His body. He has eight arms and three eyes like the petals of the lotus. On His two feet He wears twinkling toe-ornaments, and His body is Śabda-Brahma (Śabda-Brahma-maya). O lotus-eyed One, meditate thus on His Gross Body (Sthūla-vapuh). He is the quiescent, corpse-like [7] Deva within the Lotus who is void of all action."

Also: " Meditate upon the Devī-Kuṇḍalinī who encircles the Svayambhu-Liṅga. Lead the Devī, with the aid of the Haṁsa-Mantra

---

[1] Śūnya-rūpa. Śūnya means " the void " or space within the Bindu —the Śiva who is That, the Supreme Śiva.

[2] Kula-gahvara: the Mūlādhāra.

[3] Sāmarasya: *v. ante*.

[4] That is, the body of the Sādhaka considered as Devatā.

[5] A celestial wishing-tree which grants all fruit.

[6] Associated with the idea of strength.

[7] Śiva without Śakti is Śava (corpse): Devī-bhāgavataṁ, and v. 1 of the Ānandalaharī.

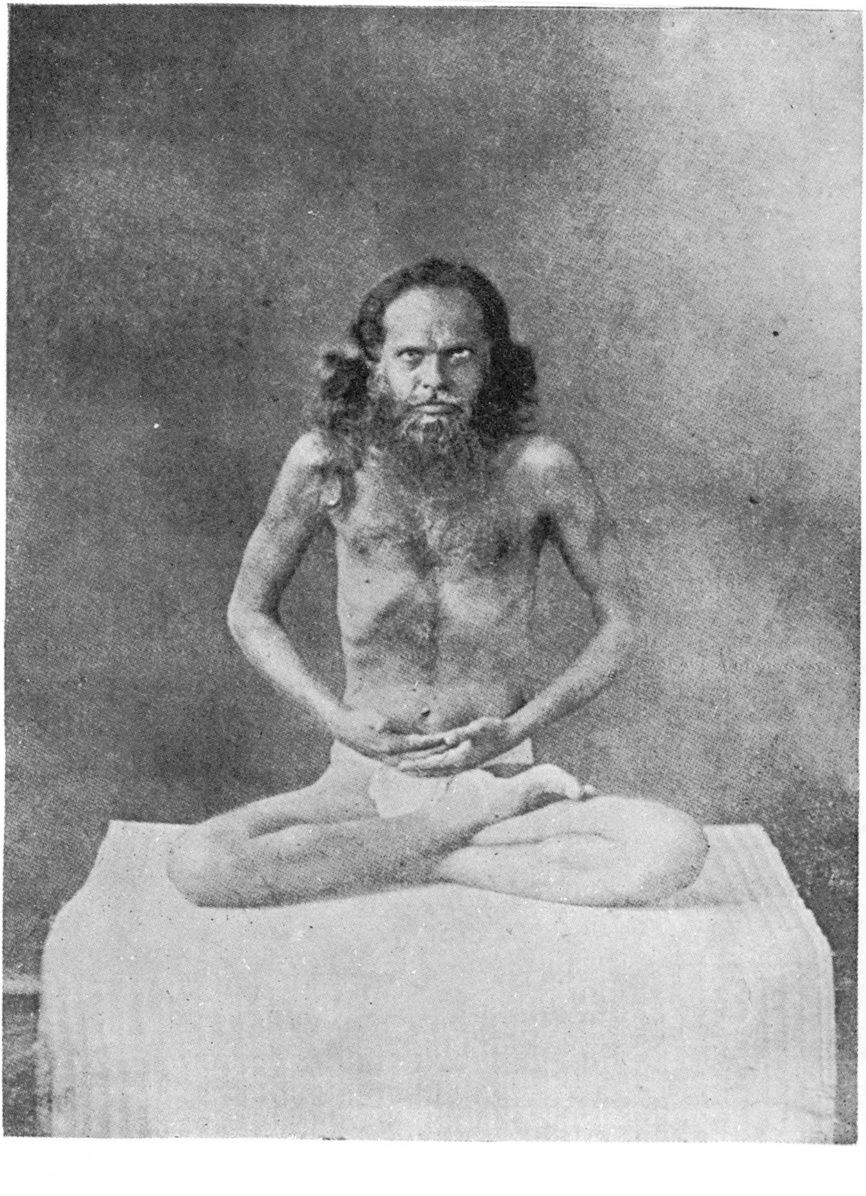

Plate XIII] Mahābandha [To face Page 465

to the Sahasrāra, where, O Parameśvarī, is the great Deva Sadāśiva. And then place there the beautiful Kuṇḍalinī, who is excited by Her desire. Kuṇḍalinī, O Beloved, then wakes up and kisses the lotus-mouth of Śiva, who is gladdened by the scent of Her lotus-like mouth, and O Deveśī, She then enjoys Sadāśiva but a very little while when immediately, O Devī, O Parameśvarī, there issues nectar. This nectar issuing from their union is of the colour of lac.[1] With this nectar, O Deveśī should the Para-Devatā [2] be satisfied. Having thus satisfied the Devatās in the six Cakras with that ambrosial stream, the wise one should by the same way bring Her back to Mūlādhāra. The mind should in this process of going and coming be dissolved there.[3] O Pārvatī, he who practises this Yoga day by day is freed from decay and death, and is liberated from the bondage of this world."

Other similar processes should be looked for in other Tantras.

[1] Red which is the colour of lac, is also that of the Rajoguṇa.

[2] Kuṇḍalinī.

[3] In the Śivasthānaṁ.

Verse 52

Nītvā tāṁ kulakuṇḍalīṁ layavaśājjīvena sārdhaṁ sudhīr
mokṣe dhāmani śuddhapadmasadane śaive pare svāmini.
Dhyāyediṣṭaphalapradāṁ bhagavatīṁ caitanyarūpāṁ parāṁ
yogīndro gurupādapadmayugalālambī samādhau yataḥ.

The wise and excellent Yogī rapt in ecstasy,[1] and devoted to the Lotus feet of his Guru, should lead Kula-Kuṇḍalī along with Jīva to Her Lord the Para-śiva in the abode of Liberation within the pure Lotus, and meditate upon Her who grants all desires as the Caitanya-rūpā-Bhagavatī.[2] When he thus leads Kula-Kuṇḍalinī, he should make all things absorb into Her.

Commentary

Having spoken of the Dhyāna-Yoga of Kuṇḍalinī, he now speaks of the Samādhi-Yoga of Kuṇḍalinī. The substance of this verse is that the wise (Sudhī) and excellent Yogī (Yogīndra) intent on the attainment of Samādhi should first of all lead Her who has been roused, who then, taking with Her Jīvā, reaches the Brahmadvāra, causing the absorption into Herself of everything as She moves along. When She who is the Iṣṭa-devatā and the giver of all good fruits is led up to Her Lord and is united with Him, the Para Bindu, She should be meditated upon as the Supreme (Parā, *i.e.*, Para-Bindu, Paraṁ-bindu-śvarūpaṁ). When She has been led to Her Lord Śiva, the Para-Bindu, and has been united with Him, She should be meditated upon as the Iṣṭa-devatā who grants good fruit.

---

[1] Samādhi. *Vide* Introduction, and *post*, Commentary.

[2] The Devī who is the Cit in all bodies.

He should there (in the Sahasrāra) dissolve the Para-Bindu in the Cidātmā,[1] which is in the void within the Bindu, and should meditate upon Her (Kuṇḍalinī) as Śuddha-caitanya-rūpā.[2] He thus realizes the identity of Jīva and Ātmā, being conscious within himself that "I am He" (So'ham); and having dissolved the Citta he remains unmoved, by reason of his full and all-pervading Knowledge.

The Revered Preceptor (Śrīmat-Ācārya)[3] has said: "The wise one should absorb the Kāraṇa[4] Ma-kāra into the Cidātmā, and realize: 'I am Cidātmā, I am eternal, pure (Śuddha), enlightened (Buddha), liberated (Mukta); I am That which alone is (Sat), without a second (Advaya); I am Supreme Bliss wherein is all bliss and Vāsudeva's very self, I am—Om.[5] Having realized that the mind (Citta) is the discriminator, he absorbs it into its witness.[6] Let not the mind (Citta) be distracted when it is absorbed into Cidātmā. Let him (the Sādhaka) rest in the fullness of his Illumination like a deep and motionless ocean."

"Ma-kāra"[7]: This is said for those who are Sādhakas of the Praṇava. By Kāraṇa is here meant Para-Bindu. By "I am Vāsudeva" (Vāsudevo'ham) the Vaiṣṇavas are alluded to (*vide ante*, vv. 44, 49).

We thus see that the worshipper of any particular Devatā should realize that Kuṇḍalinī is one with the object of his worship. In Praṇava worship, for instance, the worshipper realizes his identity with the Oṁkāra; in other forms of worship he realizes his identity with Kuṇḍalinī, who is embodied by all the Mantras of different worshippers.

The Tantrāntara says: "The King among Yogīs becomes full of Brahma-bliss by making his mind the abode of the great void which is set in the light of the Sun, Moon, and Fire."[8]

---

[1] The Brahman as Cit.

[2] Pure Cit.

[3] That is, Śaṁkarācārya.

[4] That is, the Bindu is Ma-kāra. It is the Kāraṇa or Cause of all.

[5] Cidātmāhaṁ nitya-śuddha-buddha-mukta-sadavayaḥ.
Paramānanda-saṁdoho'haṁ vāsudevo'haṁ om iti.

[6] That is, the Ātmā, of which it is said Ātmā sākṣī ceta kevalo nirguṇaśca.

[7] The Bindu is the Ma-kāra.

[8] That is, in the region of the Sahasrāra. See v. 4 of the Pādukā-pañcaka.

"*Lead Kuṇḍalī along with Jīva*" (Jīvena sārdham nitvā).—The Jīvātmā which is the Haṁsa, in form like the tapering flame of a light, should be brought to the Mūlādhāra from its place in the heart, and then led along with Kuṇḍalinī.

"*Abode of Liberation*" (Mokṣe dhāmani).—This qualifies Pure Lotus (Śuddha-padma).[1] It is here that Liberation is attained.

"*Devoted to the two Lotus feet of his Guru*" (Guru-pāda-padma-yugalālambī).—This qualifies Yogīndra (excellent yogī). The Author means that Siddhi can only be attained by the instructions of the Guru. The Sādhaka should therefore seek shelter at his feet.

"*Rapt in ecstasy*" (Samādhau yataḥ).—The Kulārṇava-Tantra (ix, 9) defines Samādhi thus: "Samādhi is that kind of contemplation[2] in which there is neither 'here' nor 'not here' which is illumination and is still like the ocean, and which is the Void Itself."[3]

Also elsewhere: "The Munis declare that the constant realization of the identity of the Jīvātmā with the Paramātmā is Samādhi, which is one of the eight limbs (Aṅga) of Yoga."[4] Patañjali defines "Yoga to be the control of the modifications (or functions) of Citta (Yogaś-citta-vṛtti-nirodhaḥ)."

Rapt (Yataḥ)—*i.e.*, he who constantly and with undivided attention practises it.

"*When he leads Kula-Kuṇḍalinī he should make all things absorb into her*" (Laya-vaśāt-nītvā).[5]—Below is shown the process of absorption:

"O Deveśī, the Laṁ-kāra[6] should next be meditated upon in the Triangle; there should also Brahmā and then Kāma-deva be contemplated. Having fixed Jīvā there with the utterance of the Praṇava, let him lead the Woman, who is longing for the satisfaction of Her passion,[7] to the place of Her husband,[8] O Queen of the Devās. O Great Queen, O beloved of my life, let him think of Ghrāṇa (Pṛthivī) and meditate on the adorable

---

[1] Śaṁkara reads it as Śukla-padma, white lotus.

[2] Dhyāna.

[3] Svarūpa-śūnya.

[4] This is from Śāradā-Tilaka, Ch. XXV, v. 26.

[5] Viśvanātha reads it as Naya-vaśāt.

[6] Bīja of Pṛthivī.

[7] Visarga-nāśa-kāminī.

[8] That is, the Bindu in Sahasrāra.

Śakti Dākinī. O Daughter of the Mountain, O Queen of the Gaṇas,[1] O Mother, all these should be led into Pṛthivī."

Also: "Then, O Great Queen, the blessed Pṛthivī should be absorbed into Gandha, and then, O Daughter of the Mountain King, the Jīvātmā should be drawn (from the heart) with the Praṇava (Mantra), and the Sādhaka should lead Prāṇa,[2] Gandha,[3] and Kuṇḍalinī into Svādhiṣṭhāna with the Mantra So'haṁ."

And also: "In its (Svādhiṣṭhāna) pericarp should Varuṇa and Hari [4] be meditated upon. And, O Beauteous One, after meditating on Rākiṇī [5] all these and Gandha (smell) should be absorbed into Rasa (taste), and Jīvātmā, Kuṇḍalinī, and Rasa, should be moved into Maṇipūra."

And again: "O thou of beautiful hips [6] (Suśroṇi), in its [7] pericarp the Sādhaka should meditate upon Fire, and also on Rudra, who is the destroyer of all, as being in company with the Śakti Lākinī and beautiful to behold. And, O Śivé, let him next meditate on the lustrous sense of vision, and absorb all these and Rasa (taste) into Rūpa (Sight), and thereafter lead Jīvātmā, Kuṇḍalinī, and Rūpa, into Anāhata."

And again: "Let him meditate in its [8] pericarp on Vāyu, who dwells in the region of Jīva, as also on the Yoni-maṇḍala, which is made beauteous by the presence of the Bāṇa-Liṅga. Let him there also meditate on Vāyu [9] as united with Rākiṇī and touch (Tvākindriya or Sparśa), and there, O Thou who purifiest, Jīvā, Kuṇḍalinī, and Rūpa, should be placed in Sparśa (Touch), and then Jīvā, Kuṇḍalinī, and Sparśa, should be placed in the Viśuddha."

And again: "Let him meditate in its [10] pericarp on the Ethereal region,[11] and on Śiva accompanied by Sākinī, and having placed Speech

---

[1] Attendant (Upadevatā) on Śiva, of whom Gaṇeśa is the Lord.

[2] *Sic* in text: *Quaere* Ghrāṇa or Prāṇa in sense of Haṁsa.

[3] *i.e.*, Gandha-Tanmātra.

[4] *i.e.*, Viṣṇu.

[5] Purāṇakariṇī—one of her names.

[6] *i.e.*, one who has a beautiful figure, the part being selected for the whole.

[7] "Its"—*i.e.*, of Maṇipūra-padma.

[8] "Its"—*i.e.*, of Anāhata-padma.

[9] Vāyu here is Īśa the Lord of Air.

[10] Viśuddha-padma.

[11] Ākāśa.

(Vāk), and Hearing (Śrotra), in Ether, let him, O Daughter of the Mountain, place all these and Sparśa in Śabda (Sound), and place Jīvā Kuṇḍalinī, and Śabda, in the Ājñā-Cakra."

The above passages are from Kaṅkālamālinī-Tantra.

"Triangle" in the above is the Triangle in the Mūlādhāra, from which the commencement is made. Laṁ-kāra should be meditated upon as within this Triangle. Leading of Jīvā with the use of the Praṇava is a variant practice. "Visarga-nāśakāmiṇī"; by Visarga is meant the agitation caused by an excess of Kāma (desire). The compound word means She who is striving to satisfy Her desire (Kāma). The bringing of Jīvā by the Haṁsa-Mantra is, according to the teaching of some, "Place of her husband" (Patyau pade): This is the Bindu, the Śiva in the Lotus of a thousand petals. Sādhaka should lead Her there.

The Bīja Laṁ, Brahmā, Kāmadeva, Ḍākinī-Śakti, and the sense of smell (Ghrāṇendriya)—all these are absorbed into Pṛthivī, and Pṛthivī is absorbed into the Gandha-tattva. Jīvātmā, Kuṇḍalinī, and Gandha-tattva, are drawn upward by the Praṇava, and brought into the Svādhiṣṭhāna by the So'haṁ Mantra. This is the process to be applied right through. After leading Jīvā, Kuṇḍalinī, and Śabda-tattva, into Ājñā-Cakra, Śabda-tattva should be absorbed into Ahaṁkāra which is there, and Ahaṁkāra into Mahat-tattva, and Mahat-tattva into Sūkṣma-prakṛti, whose name is Hiraṇya-garbha, and Prakṛti again into Para-Bindu.

The Mantra-tantra-prakāśa says: "Let Vyoma (Ether) be absorbed into Ahaṁkāra, and the latter with Śabda into Mahat, and Mahat again, into the unmanifest (Avyakta), supreme (Para), Cause (Kāraṇa), of all the Śakti. Let the Sādhaka think attentively that all things beginning with Pṛthivī are absorbed into Viṣṇu,[1] the Cause who is Sat, Cit, and Ānanda."

That is, Mahat, which is all Śaktis (Sarva-Śakti), should be absorbed into Sūkṣma-prakṛti, who is known by the name of Hiraṇya-garbha, and that Prakṛti should be absorbed into Para, by which is meant the Cause in the form of Para-Bindu. In this connection the Ācārya has laid down the rule that the gross should be dissolved into the subtle.[2] *Cf.*: "It should be attentively considered and practised that the gross is absorbed into the subtle, and all into Cidātmā." The absorption of all things, beginning

[1] Viṣṇu is specified by this particular Tantra, but it may be any other Devatā who is the Iṣṭa-devatā of the Sādhaka.

[2] *Vide*, v. 40 and Commentary under it.

with Pṛthivī and ending with Anāhata,[1] takes place in the aforesaid manner; that being so, the feet and the sense of Smell (Ghrāṇendriya) and all pertaining to Pṛthivī are dissolved in the place of Pṛthivī as they inhere in Pṛthivī.

Similarly, the hands, the sense of Taste (Rasanendriya), and all that pertains to Water, are dissolved in the region of Water. In the region of Fire (Vahni-sthāna) are dissolved the anus, the sense of Vision (Cakṣurindriya), and all that pertains to Fire. In the region of Air (Vāyusthāna) the genitals, the sense of Touch (Tvākindriya), and all that pertains to Vāyu, are dissolved. In the place of Ākāśa are dissolved the sense of Speech (Vāk) and hearing (Śrotrendriya) and all that pertains to Ākāśa (Ether).

In the Ājñā-Cakra the dissolution of Ahaṁkāra, Mahat, Sūkṣma-prakṛti, and so forth, takes place, each dissolving into its own immediate cause. The letters of the alphabet should then be absorbed in the reverse order (Viloma), beginning with Kṣa-kāra and ending with Akāra. By "all things" it is meant that "Bindu," "Bodhinī" and so forth, which have been shown above to be causal bodies (Kāraṇa Śarīra), should be dissolved in a reversed order (Vilomena) into the Primordial Cause (Ādi-kāraṇa)—the Para-Bindu. Thus the Brahman alone remains.

The process is thus described: "The Sādhaka, having thus made his determination (Saṁkalpa), should dissolve [2] the letters of the Alphabet in the Nyāsa-sthāna.[3] The dissolution of Kṣa is in La, and La in Ha; Ha, again, is dissolved into Sa, and Sa into Ṣa, and thus it goes on till A is reached. This should be very carefully done."

Also [4]: "Dissolve the two letters into Bindu, and dissolve Bindu into Kalā. Dissolve Kalā in Nāda, and dissolve Nāda in Nādānta;[5] and this into Unmanī, and Unmanī into Viṣṇu-vaktra [6]; Viṣṇu-vaktra should

---

[1] This seems an error, for the last Mahābhūta Ākāśa is dissolved in Viśuddha.

[2] Saṁharet.

[3] The places where the Varṇas have been placed in Mātṛkā-Nyāsa.

[4] Here is shown the Anuloma process. The two letters are Ha and Kṣa.

[5] *i.e.*, that which is beyond Nāda. See Introduction.

[6] Puṁ-Bindu; *v. post.*

be dissolved into Guru-vaktra.[1] Let the excellent Sādhaka then realize that all the letters are dissolved in Parama-Śiva."

By Viṣṇu-vaktra is meant Puṁ-Bindu. "The Sūrya-Bindu is called the Face, and below are Moon and Fire." "Bindu is said to be the Male, and Visarga is Prakṛti." [2]

All these authorities imply the same thing, and go to prove that it is the "mouth of Viṣṇu" (Viṣṇu-vaktra) where dissolution should take place. The following from Keśavācārya [3] also leads to the same conclusion: "Lead Her (Unmanī) into the Male, which is the Bindu; lead Bindu into Parātmā, and Parātmā into Kāla-tattva, and this latter into Śakti, and Śakti into Cidātmā, which is the Supreme (Kevala), the tranquil (Śānta), and effulgent."

We have seen that each dissolves into its own immediate cause. Nādānta is therefore dissolved in Vyāpikā-Śakti, the Vyāpikā-Śakti in Unmanī and Unmanī in Samānī [4] and Samānī in Viṣṇu-vaktra. When the letters have been thus dissolved, all the six Cakras are dissolved, as the petals of the Lotuses consist of letters.[5]

The Viśvasāra-Tantra says: "The petals of the Lotuses are the letters of the Alphabet, beginning with A." [6] The Sammohana-Tantra [7] describes the dissolution [8] of the Lotuses and the petals thus: "Dissolve the letters from Va to Sa of the petals in Brahmā,[9] and dissolve Brahmā in the Lotus of six petals which contains the letters Ba to La, and which is

---

[1] That is, the mouth of the Supreme Bindu (cited from Śāradā-Tilaka, Ch. V, vv. 134-135). Also *cf.* Śāradā, Ch. XII, 123, and Kulārṇava, IV, 76.

[2] *Cf.* Śāradā, Ch. XXV, v. 51. Also Nityā-Ṣoḍaśikā, I, 201, and Kāma-Kalāvilāsa.

[3] Also called Keśava-Bhāratī—a great Vaiṣṇava teacher who initiated Śrī-Caitanya the greatest among latter-day Vaiṣṇavas, into Saṁnyāsa or the path of Renunciation.

[4] *Sic.* This is in conflict with other texts, according to which Unmanī is above Samānī.

[5] Padma-dalānāṁ varṇa-mayatvāt.

[6] Ādivarṇātmakaṁ patraṁ padmanām pārikīrtitaṁ.

[7] Ch. IV. The passage cited also occurs in Śāradā-Tilaka, Ch. V, vv. 129-134.

[8] Vilaya.

[9] That is, Mūlādhāra where Brahmā or Kamalāsana is.

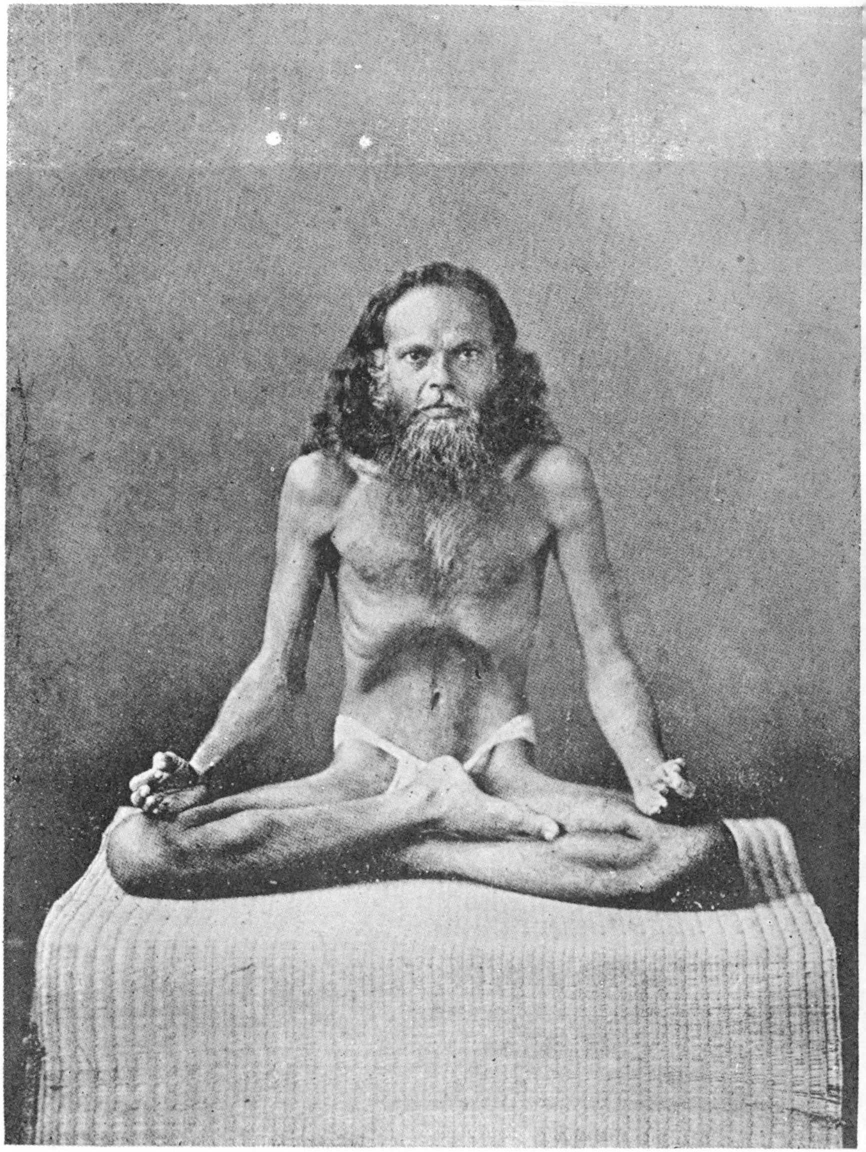

Plate XIV] Mūlābandha in Siddhāsana [To face Page 473

called Svādhiṣṭhāna. Do this as the Guru directs." And so forth. And ending with:

"The wise one should then dissolve it (Viśuddha) in the (Lotus of) two petals which contains the two letters Ha and Kṣa, and dissolve the two letters which are in the latter lotus into Bindu, and dissolve Bindu into Kalā."[1]

We thus see that the four letters in the Mūlādhāra are dissolved therein and Mūlādhāra is dissolved in Svādhiṣṭhāna. Proceeding in this way till the Ājñā-Cakra is reached, the letters Ha and Kṣa which are there are also dissolved at this place. Then the Lotus itself is dissolved into Bindu, Bindu into Bodhinī, and proceeding in this way as already shown everything is dissolved, into Para-Bindu. When the Ājñā-Cakra is dissolved, all that it contains in its pericarp—Hākinī, Itara-Liṅga, Praṇava—are unable to exist without support, and therefore after the dissolution into Prakṛti these also are dissolved into Para-Bindu.

[1] That is, the Bindu of the Ājñā-Cakra is dissolved into Kuṇḍalinī.

Verse 53

Lākṣābhaṁ paramāmṛtaṁ paraśivātpītvā punaḥ kuṇḍalī
nityānandamahodayāt kulapathānmūle viśetsundarī.
Taddivyāmṛtadhārayā sthiramatiḥ saṁtarpayeddaivataṁ
yogī yogaparaṁparāviditayā brahmāṇḍabhāṇḍasthitaṁ.

The beautiful Kuṇḍalī drinks the excellent red[1] nectar issuing from Para-Śiva, and returns from there where shines Eternal and Transcendent Bliss[2] in all its glory along the path of Kula,[3] and again enters the Mūlādhāra. The Yogī who has gained steadiness of mind makes offering (Tarpaṇa) to the Iṣṭa-devatā and to the Devatās in the six centres (Cakra), Ḍākinī and others, with that stream of celestial nectar which is in the vessel[4] of Brahmāṇḍa, the knowledge whereof he has gained through the tradition of the Gurus.

Commentary

He now speaks of what should be done after all the different kinds of Yoga described have been understood. The meaning of this verse is that the beautiful Kuṇḍalī drinks the excellent nectar issuing from Para-Śiva, and having emerged from the place of Eternal and Transcendental Bliss, She passes along the path of Kula and re-enters Mūlādhāra. The Yogī, after having understood the different matters mentioned (Tat-tad-dhyānā-nantaram), should think of the inseparate union[5] of

[1] Śaṁkara says it is so coloured because it is mixed with the menstrual fluid, which is symbolic, like the rest of his erotic imagery. Red is the colour of the Rajo-Guṇa.

[2] Brahman is Eternity and Bliss.

[3] The Channel in the Citriṇī-nādī.

[4] The vessel is Kuṇḍalinī.

[5] Sāmarasya.

Śiva and Śakti, and with the excellent nectar produced from the bliss of such union with Para-Śiva make offering (Tarpaṇa) to Kuṇḍalinī.

"*Path of Kula*" (Kula-patha).—The path of Brahman, the channel in Citriṇī.

Kuṇḍalī drinks the nectar with which Tarpaṇa is made to her. The following authority says: "Having effected their union and having made (Her drink)," etc. It follows, therefore, that She is made to drink. The nectar is red like the colour of lac.

"*From there where shines Eternal and Transcendent Bliss*" (Nityānanda-mahodayāt)—that is She, returns from the place where eternal and transcendental Bliss is enjoyed—*i.e.*, where the Brahman is clearly realized.

"*Again enters Mūlādhāra*" (Mūle Viśet),—She has to be brought back in the same way as She was led upward. As She passed through the different Liṅga and Cakras in their order (Cakra-bheda-krameṇa) when going upward, so does She when returning to the Mūlādhāra.

The Revered Great Preceptor says: "Kuṇḍalinī,[1] Thou sprinklest all things with the stream of Nectar which flows from the tips of Thy two feet; and as Thou returneth to Thy own place Thou vivifiest and makest visible all things that were aforetime invisible, and on reaching Thy abode Thou dost resume Thy snake-like coil and sleep." [2]

"As Thou returnest Thou vivifiest and makest visible." This describes the return of Kuṇḍalī to Her own place. As She returns She infuses Rasa [3] into the various things She had previously absorbed into Herself when going upward, and by the infusion of Rasa, She makes them all visible and manifest. Her passage was Laya-krama,[4] and Her return Sṛṣṭi-krama.[5] Hence it has been said: "Kuṇḍalī, who is Bliss,[6] the Queen of the Surās,[7] goes back in the same way to the Ādhāra [8] Lotus."

---

[1] Kuhara is a cavity; Kuhariṇī would then be She whose abode is a cavity—the cavity of the Mūlādhāra.

[2] Cited from the celebrated Ānandalaharī-Stotra, Wave of Bliss Hymn, attributed to Śaṁkarācārya. See "Wave of Bliss," a translation, by A. Avalon.

[3] Rasa: sap, sap of life—that is, She re-vitalizes them.

[4] See v. 52 and next note.

[5] That is, She recreates or revives as She returns to her own abode; just as She "destroys" or absorbs all things on Her upward progress.

[6] Mudrā-kārā—that is Ānanda-rūpiṇī; for Mudrā=Ānanda-dāyinī. Mudrā is derived from Mud=ānanda (bliss)+Rāti=dadāti (gives): Mudrā therefore means that which gives bliss.

[7] Sura=Deva. Here the different Devas in the Cakras.

[8] *i.e.*, Mūlādhāra.

The Bhūta-śuddhi-prakaraṇa has the following: "Let the Tattvas Pṛthivī, etc., in their order, as also Jīva and Kuṇḍalinī, be led back from Paramātmā and each placed in its respective position." She is then particularly described: "She is lustrous when first She goes, and She is ambrosial [1] when She returns."

"*Stream of celestial nectar*" (Divyāmṛtadhārā).—This is the excellent nectar which, as has already been shown, is produced by the union [2] of Śiva and Śakti, and runs in a stream from the Brahma-randhra to the Mūlādhāra. It is for this reason that the Author says in v. 3 that "the Brahma-dvāra which shines in Her mouth is the entrance to the place sprinkled by ambrosia."

"*Knowledge whereof he has gained through the tradition of the Gurus*" (Yoga-paramparā-viditayā).—This qualifies "Stream of Nectar". It means that the knowledge is gained from instructions (in Yoga practice) handed down traditionally through the succession of Gurus.

"*Which is in the vessel of Brahmāṇḍa*" (Brahmāṇḍa-bhāṇḍa-sthitaṁ).—This qualifies Amṛta (nectar).[3] The vessel or support (Bhāṇḍa) on which the Brahmāṇḍa (Universe) rests is Kuṇḍalinī. Kuṇḍalinī is the Bhāṇḍa as She is the Source (Yoni) of all.

By Daivatam [4] is meant the Iṣṭadevatā and Ḍākinī and others in the six Cakras. It has been said: "O Deveśī, with this nectar should offering (Tarpaṇa) be made to the Para-devatā, and then having done Tarpaṇa to the Devatās in the six Cakras," and so forth.

---

[1] Because ambrosia (Amṛta) gives life.

[2] Sāmarasya.

[3] Viśvanātha reads this as an adjective qualifying Daivatam, and this seems more in consonance with the text. The Brahmāṇḍa is compared to a Bhāṇḍa, and the Devatās are in that. The offering is then made with that stream of nectar to the Devatās who are in the Universe. Or, according to Kālīcaraṇa, offering is made to the Devatās of the Amṛtā which Kuṇḍalī has drunk.

[4] Daivatam is the collective form of Devatās.

Verse 54

Jñātvaitatkramamuttamaṁ yatamanā yogī yamādyair-yutaḥ
śrīdīkṣāgurupādapadmayuglāmodapravāhodayāt.
Samsāre na hi janyate na hi kadā saṁkṣīyate saṁkṣaye
nityānandaparaṁparāpramuditaḥ śāntaḥ satāmagraṇīḥ.

The Yogī who has after practice of Yama, Niyama, and the like,[1] learnt this excellent method from the two Lotus Feet of the auspicious Dīkṣā-guru,[2] which are the source of uninterrupted joy, and whose mind (Manas) is controlled, is never born again in this world (Samsāra). For him there is no dissolution even at the time of Final Dissolution.[3] Gladdened by constant realization of that which is the source of Eternal Bliss,[4] he becomes full of peace and foremost among all Yogīs.[5]

Commentary

He here speaks of the good to be gained by knowing the method of Yoga practice.

"*From the lotus feet of his auspicious Dīkṣā-guru, which are the source of uninterrupted joy*" (Śri-dīkṣā-guru-pāda-padma-yugalā-moda-pravāhodayāt).—Amoda means joy or bliss; and by Pravāha is meant uninterrupted and continuous connection. Āmoda pravāha therefore means Nityānanda, or "Eternal Bliss". Bliss such as this comes from the Lotus feet of the Guru, which also lead to knowledge of Yoga practice.

---

[1] See Introduction.

[2] The Guru who has given him initiation.

[3] Saṁkṣaya=Pralaya.

[4] Nityānanda=Brahman.

[5] Satām—lit., "of the Good".

The Dīkṣā-guru is here spoken of as he is the first to initiate, and also by reason of his pre-eminence. But in his absence refuge may be sought with other Gurus. It has therefore been said: " As a bee desirous of honey goes from one flower to another, so does the disciple desirous of knowledge (Jñāna) go from one Guru to another." [1]

" *Gladdened by constant realization of that which is the source of Eternal Bliss* " (Nityānanda-paramparā-pramudita)—*i.e.*, who is united with the Stream of Eternal Bliss.

"*Foremost among the good*" (Satām agraṇiḥ)—*i.e.*, he is counted to be foremost among the good who are the Yogīs.

---

[1] This is from Ch. XII, of Niruttara-Tantra. This verse also occurs in Kulārṇava (Tāntrik Texts, Vol. V), Ch. XIII, 132.

Verse 55

Yo'dhīte niśi saṁdhyayorathe divā yogī svabhāvasthito
mokṣajñānanidānametadamalaṁ śuddhaṁ ca guptaṁ paraṁ.
Śrīmacchrīgurupādapadmayugalālambī yatāntarmanā-
stasyavaśyamabhīṣṭadaivatapade ceto narīnṛtyate.

If the Yogī who is devoted to the Lotus Feet of his Guru, with heart unperturbed and concentrated mind, reads this work which is the supreme source of the knowledge of Liberation, and which is faultless, pure, and most secret, then of a very surety his mind[1] dances at the Feet of his Iṣṭa-devatā.

Commentary

He here speaks of the good to be gained by the study of the verses relating to the six Cakras.

"*Heart unperturbed*" (Svabhāva-sthitah).—*i.e.*, engrossed in his own true spiritual being.

"*Concentrated mind*" (Yatāntarmanāh)—*i.e.*, he who by practice of Yoga has steadied and concentrated his mind on the inner spirit (Antarātmā).

The rest is clear.

Here ends the Eighth Section of the Explanation of the Verses descriptive of the Six Cakras, forming part of the Śrī-tattva-cintāmaṇī, composed by Śrī-Pūrṇānandayati.

---

[1] Cetas or Citta.

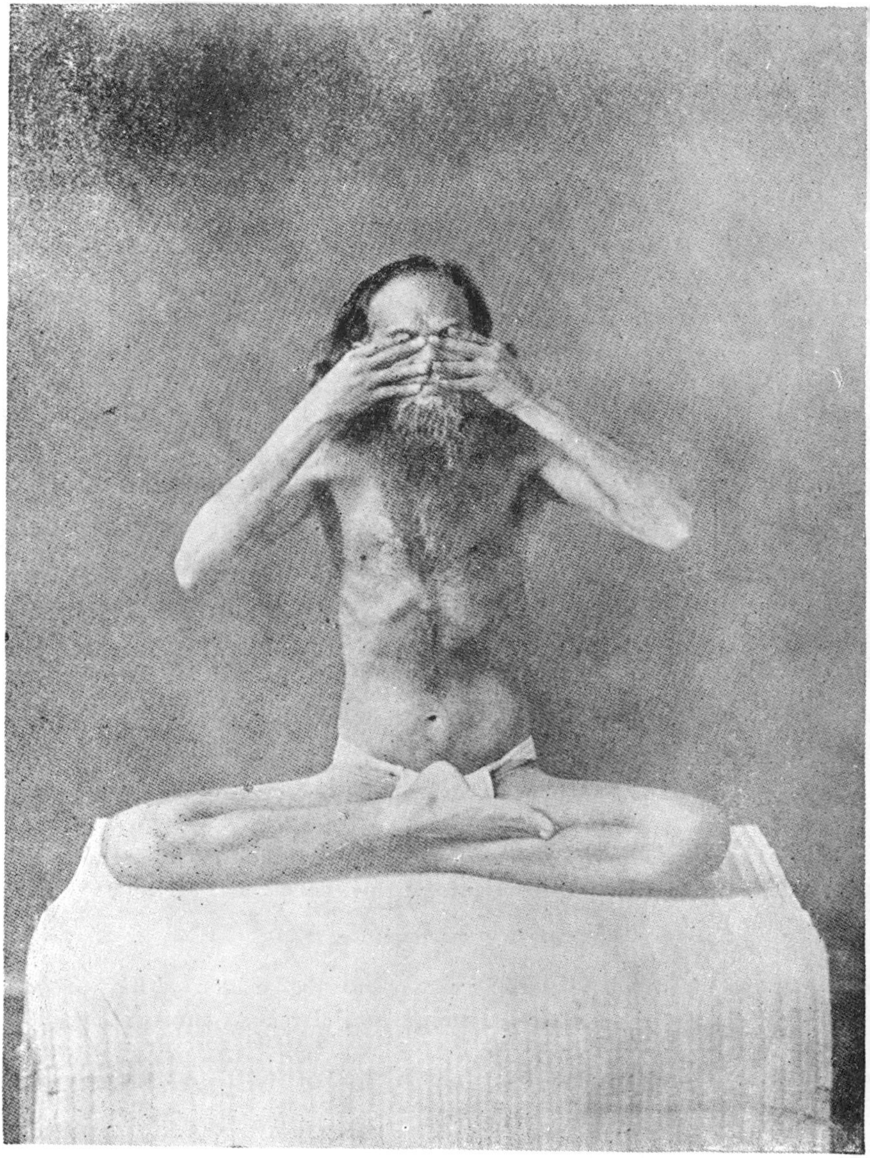

Plate XV] Yonimudrā in Siddhāsana [To face Page 481

THE FIVEFOLD FOOTSTOOL[1] (PĀDUKĀ-PAÑCAKA)

Introductory Verse[2]

I MEDITATE on the Guru in the Lotus of a thousand petals, which is radiant like the cool rays of the full moon, whose lotus hands make the gestures which grant blessing and dispel fear. His raiment, garland, and perfumes, are ever fresh and pure. His countenance is benign. He is in the Haṁsa in the head. He is the Haṁsa Himself.

[1] The meaning of this is explained in v. 7, *post*.

[2] This verse is inserted as it was found in a manuscript belonging to the late Acalānanda-Svāmī, now in the possession of the Varendra Anusaṁdhāna Samiti.

Verse 1

Brahmarandhra-sarasīruhodare
nityalagnamavadātamadbhutaṁ
Kuṇḍalivivarakāṇḍamaṇḍitaṁ
dvādaśārṇasarasīruhaṁ bhaje.

I adore the wonderful White Lotus of twelve letters [1] which is within the womb (Udare) of, and inseparable from, the pericarp of the Lotus in which is the Brahma-randhra, and which is adorned by the channel of Kuṇḍalī. [2]

Commentary

The hymn Pādukā-pañcaka, composed by Him of Five Faces,[3] destroys all demerit.[4] Kālīcaraṇa by his Ṭīkā called Amalā (Stainless) makes patent its beauty.

Sadāśiva, the Liberator of the three Worlds, being desirous of speaking of Gurudhyāna-Yoga [5] in the form of a hymn (Stotra), first of all describes the place of the Guru.

The verb Bhaje is First Person Singular, Ātmanepada, emphasizing that Śiva Himself adores or worships. He says, " I do adore or worship." By saying so He expresses the necessity that all worshippers (Upāsakas) of the Mantras revealed by Him should adore this wonderful twelve-petalled Lotus. He thus shows the necessity of His worship.

---

[1] Dvādaśārṇa—that is, twelve petals. The petals of the lotus are not independent of the letters thereon.

[2] That is, the Citriṇī-Nādī. The lotus rests on the upper end of Citriṇī.

[3] Śiva. See as to the five faces the citation from the Liṅgārcana-Tantra, v. 7, *post*. There is also a concealed sixth face, " like the colour caused by deadly poison," known as Nīlakaṇṭha.

[4] Aghas—sin and sorrow, pain and penalty.

[5] Yoga with the Supreme known as the Guru.

The meaning of this verse in brief is this: I adore the twelve-petalled Lotus which is within the pericarp of the Sahasrāra.

"*Wonderful*" (Adbhuta).—It excites our wonder by reason of its being pervaded by the lustre (Tejas) of Brahman, and for other reasons.

"*Lotus of twelve letters*" (Dvādaśārṇa-sarasīruha)—*i.e.*, the Lotus which contains twelve letters. The twelve letters, according to those learned in the Tantras, are the twelve letters which make the Gurumantra; they are स, ह, ख, फ्रें, ह, स, क्ष, म, ल, व, र, यूं—Sa, ha, kha, phreṁ, ha, sa, kṣa, ma, la, va, ra, yūṁ. Some say that by Dvādaśārṇa is meant the twelfth vowel, which is the Vāg-bhava-bīja.[1] But that cannot be. If it were so, the authority quoted below would be tautologous: "(Meditate on) your Guru who is Śiva as being on the lustrous (Haṁsapīṭha, the substance of which is Mantra—Mantra-maya), which is in the pericarp of the Lotus of twelve letters, near the region of the Moon[2] in the pericarp, and which is adorned by the letters Ha, La, and Kṣa, which are within the triangle A-Ka-Tha. The lotus of twelve letters is in the pericarp (of the Sahasrāra)."

The above passage speaks of the Mantramaya-pīṭha. The Mantra substance of this Pīṭha is the Guru-mantra in the form of Vāg-bhava-bīja.[3] There would therefore be a repetition of the same Mantra.[4] "Dvādaśārṇa" is made up by Bahuvrīhi-Samāsa—that in which there are Dvādaśa (twelve) Arṇas (letters). This lotus has therefore twelve petals, on which are the twelve letters.

It is true that the letters are not here specified, and there has been nothing said as to where they are placed; but the Guru-Gītā says[5] that "the letters Haṁ and Sa surround (that is, as petals) the Lotus," wherein the Guru should be meditated. This leads us to the conclusion that the letters Haṁ and Saḥ are repeated six times, thus making twelve, and so the number of petals becomes clearly twelve, as each petal contains one letter. This is a fit subject of consideration for the wise.

---

[1] *i.e.*, Bīja of Sarasvatī—Aiṁ.

[2] Candra-maṇḍala, by the Commentator (reading the locative as Sāmīpye saptamī, *i.e.*, locative case indicative of Proximity).

[3] Aiṁ.

[4] That is, if we understand that the body of both the Pīṭha and the petals is Aiṁ. The Vāgbhava-Bīja Aim is the Guru-Bīja also.

[5] This verse is quoted in full under v. 6, *post*.

"*Inseparable from*" (Nitya-lagnaṁ).—That is, it is connected with the Sahasrāra in such a way that the one cannot be thought of without thinking of the other.

"*Which is within the womb of and inseparable from the pericarp of the Lotus in which is the Brahmarandhra*" (Brahmarandhra-sarasīruhodara).—That is, the Sahasrāra, the thousand-petalled lotus in which is the Brahmarandhra; within its womb, that is to say, within it (Tanmadhye), that is, within its pericarp (Tat-karṇikāyāṁ).

The Kaṅkāla-Mālinī, in describing the Lotus of a thousand petals, thus speaks of the place of the Brahma-randhra: "In its (Sahasrāra) pericarp, O Deveśī, is Antarātmā, and above it is the Guru; above him is the Sūrya Maṇḍala and Candra Maṇḍala and Mahā-vāyu, and above it is Brahma-randhra."

Some say that by Udara (belly or interior) is meant within the triangle in the pericarp. That is not right. The word Udara here means "interior" or "centre". The interior of the Lotus contains its pericarp but the text does not mean the interior of the triangle in the pericarp, because the triangle is not here mentioned. The Śyāmā-saparyā quotes the following explicitly:

"The Lotus of twelve petals (or Letters) is within the pericarp of the white Lotus of a thousand petals, which has its head turned downward, and the filaments of which are of the colour of the rising sun, and which is adorned by all the letters of the alphabet." Here the statement 'within the pericarp' is explicit.

"*Adorned by the channel of Kuṇḍalī*" (Kuṇḍalī-vivara-kāṇḍa-maṇḍitaṁ).—The Vivara (Channel) is that by which Kuṇḍalinī goes to Śiva in the Sahasrāra. The Citriṇī contains within it this passage or channel. Citriṇī is the tube (stalk), as it were, through which the passage runs, and Citriṇī adorns and is adorned by this Lotus. As a Lotus rests on its stalk, so does the twelve-petalled Lotus rest on Citriṇī and is made beautiful by its stalk.

Verse 2

Tasya kandalitakarṇikāpuṭe
kḷptarekhamakathādirekhayā.
Koṇalakṣitahalakṣamaṇḍali-
bhāvalaksyamabalālayaṁ bhaje.

I adore the Abode of Śakti in the place where the two pericarps come together. It is formed by the lines [1] A, Ka, and Tha; and the letters Ha, La, and Kṣa, which are visible in each of its corners, give it the character of a Maṇḍala.[2]

Commentary

The Guru should be meditated upon as in the triangle A-Ka-Tha within the pericarp of the Lotus before-mentioned. He now wishes to describe the triangle so that an adequate conception of it may be formed.

"*The abode of Śakti*" (Abalālayaṁ). By Abalā is meant Śakti. Here She is Kāma-kalā triangular in form, and the three Śaktis, Vāmā, Jyeṣṭā, and Raudrī, are lines of the triangle. These three lines or Śaktis emanate from the three Bindus.[3] Kāma-kalā is the abode of Śakti.

The Yāmala speaks of the identity of Kāma-kalā with this abode. The passage begins, "I now speak of Kāma-kalā," and proceeding says: [4] "She is the three Bindus. She is the three Śaktis. She is the threefold Manifestation. She is everlasting. That is, Kāma-kalā is composed of the three Śaktis spoken of (Triśakti-rūpā). He next speaks of the attributes of Abalālaya (abode of Śakti).

---

[1] A-Ka-Thādi—*i.e.*, the lines formed by the letters A to Ah, Ka to Ta and Tha to Sa. These letters placed as three lines form the three sides of the triangle.

[2] *i.e.*, the diagram where the Divinity is summoned and worshipped.

[3] Bindu-trayāṅkurabhūtā—that is, they have the three Bindus as their sprouting shoot. (See Kāmakalāvilāsa.)

[4] Tribinduh sā trimūrtih sā triśaktih sā sanātanī.

"*The place where the two pericarps come together*" (Kandalita-Karṇikā-puṭe).—Kaṇḍala ordinarily means a quarrel in which one attacks the other with words. Here its significance is merely that the pericarp of one (the twelve-petalled lotus) is included within that of the other (Sahasrāra).

Place (Puṭa), *i.e.*, the place where the triangle is "*formed by the lines A, Ka, and Tha*" (Kḷpta-rekhaṁ a-ka-thādi-rekhayā). The sixteen vowels beginning with A form the line Vāmā, the sixteen letters beginning with Ka form the line Jyeṣṭā, and the sixteen letters beginning with Tha form the line Raudrī. The Abode of Śakti is formed by these three lines.

The Bṛhat Śrī-krama, in dealing with Kāma-kalā, says: "From the Bindu as the sprouting root (Aṅkura) She has assumed the form of letters." [1]

"*The letters Ha, La, and Kṣa, which are visible in its corners, give it the character of a Maṇḍala*" (Koṇa-lakṣita-hala-kṣa-maṇḍalī-bhāva-lakṣyaṁ).—In its corners—*i.e.*, in the inner corners of the aforesaid triangle. The three corners of the triangle are at the apex,[2] the right and the left. The letters Ha, La, and Kṣa, which are visible there, give the place the character of a Maṇḍala.

One cannot form an adequate conception (Dhyāna) of this triangle without knowing it in all its particulars, and that is why other authorities are quoted. This triangle should be so drawn that if one were to walk round it would always be on one's left.

The Śāktānanda-taraṅgiṇī says: "Write the triangle A-Ka-Tha so that walking outside it is always on one's left.[3]

Kālī Ūrdhvāmnāya: "The Tri-bindu [4] is the Supreme Tattva, and embodies within itself Brahmā, Viṣṇu, and Śiva (Brahmaviṣṇu-śivāt-makam). The triangle composed of the letters has emanated from the Bindu." Also: "The letters A to Visarga make the line Brahmā which is the line of Prajāpati; the letters Ka to Ta make the most supreme (Parātparā) line of Viṣṇu. The letters Tha to Sa make the line of Śiva. The three lines emanate from the three Bindus."

---

[1] Varṇāvayava-rūpiṇī. Bindu appears in the form of letters by germinating as a sprout. The letters are sprouts from Bindu: that is, the Universe is evolved from Bindu.

[2] The triangle, it should be remembered, has its apex downward.

[3] Vāmāvartena vilikhet. The drawing is made in the direction which is the reverse to that of the hands of a watch.

[4] *i.e.*, the three Bindus considered as one and also separately.

Tantra-jīvana: "The lines Rajas, Sattva, and Tamas, surround the Yoni-Maṇḍala." Also: "Above is the line of Sattva; the line of Rajas is on the left, and the line of Tamas is on one's right." [1]

By a careful consideration of the above authorities, the conclusion is irresistible that the letters A-Ka-Tha go in the direction above-mentioned.

The Svatantra-Tantra says: "The lines A-Ka-Tha surround the letters Ha, La and Kṣa." It therefore places the letters Ha, La, Kṣa within the triangle.

It is needless to discuss the matter at greater length.

---

[1] That is, on the left and right of the Yoni or the right and left of the spectator.

VERSE 3

Tatpuṭe paṭutaḍitkaḍārima-
spardhamānamaṇipāṭalaprabhaṁ.
Cintayāmi hṛdi Cinmayaṁ vapur-
nādabindumaṇipīṭhamaṇḍalaṁ.

IN my heart I meditate on the Jewelled Altar (Maṇipīṭha), and on Nāda and Bindu as within the triangle aforespoken. The pale red [1] glory of the gems in this altar shames the brilliance of the lightning flash. Its substance is Cit.

COMMENTARY

The place of the Guru is on the jewelled altar within the triangle. He therefore describes the jewelled altar (Maṇipīṭha).

"*In my heart*" (Hṛdi), *i.e.*, in my Mind (Manasi).

"*On the Jewelled Altar and on Nāda and Bindu*" (Nāda-bindu-mani-pīṭha-maṇḍalaṁ).—The compound word may be formed in two ways: Maṇi-pīṭha-maṇḍalam along with Nāda and Bindu (Nāda-bindubhyam saha), or Nāda and Bindu and Maṇi-pīṭha-maṇḍalam—*i.e.*, all these three. Some interpret this to mean that the Maṇḍala Maṇipīṭha is composed of Nāda and Bindu. But that cannot be. Nāda is white, and Bindu is red; and the pale red glory whereby the Maṇi-pīṭha shames the lustre of the lightning flash is neither red nor white.

The Śāradā-Tilaka says: "This Bindu is Śiva and Śakti,[2] and divides itself into three different parts; its divisions are called Bindu, Nāda, and Bīja." If this be interpreted to mean, as it ought to be, that Bindu is Para-Śakti-maya, and Bīja, Nāda, and Bindu, are respectively Fire, Moon and Sun, then Nāda being the Moon is white, and Bindu being the Sun is red. Pūrṇānanda also speaks [3] of Nāda as being white like Baladeva etc.

---

[1] Pāṭala.

[2] Para-Śakti-maya=Śiva-Śakti-maya.

[3] V. 35, Ṣaṭ-cakra-nirūpaṇa, *ante*.

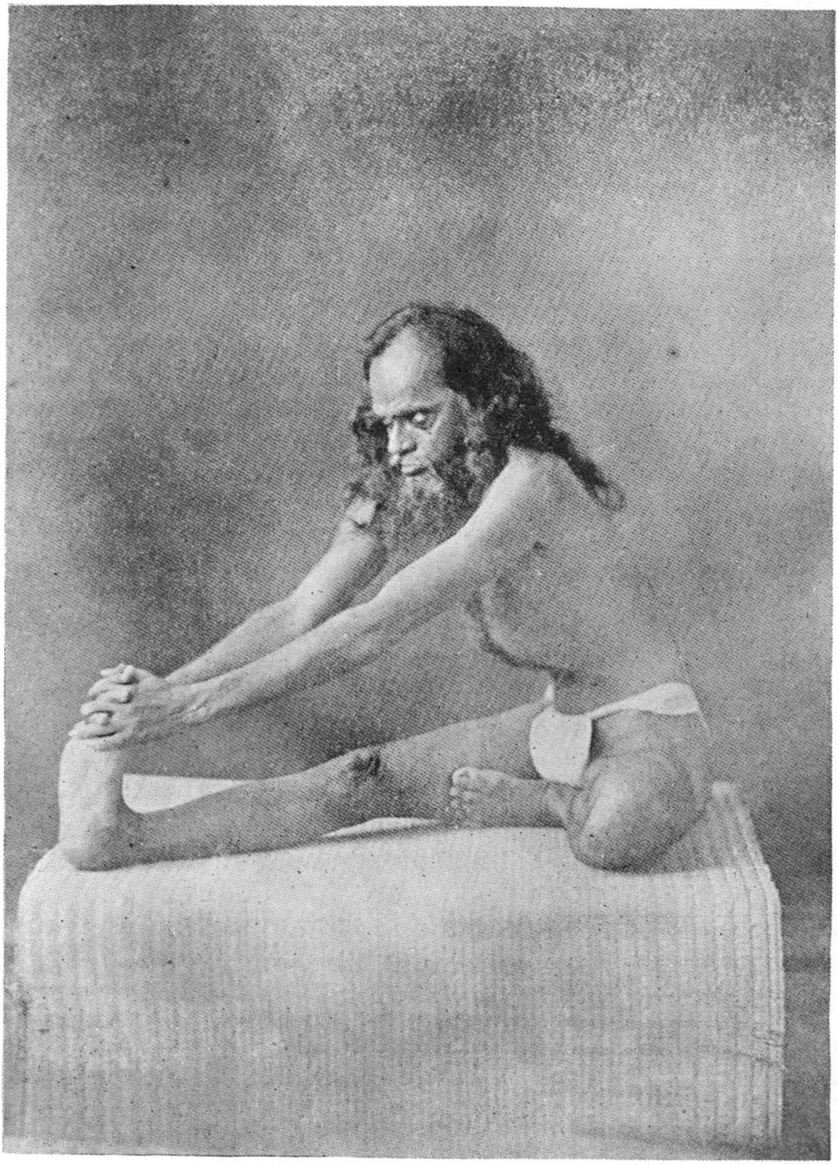

Plate XVI] Mahāmudrā [To face Page 489

The Bṛhat-Śrī-krama also says: "There was the imperishable Bindu, lustrous (red) like the young Sun."

Now, as one is white and the other red, they can never be the pale red gem. The meaning given by us is therefore correct. The solution is that Nāda is below, and Bindu above, and Maṇi-pīṭha in between the two —thus should one meditate. This has been clearly shown in the Guru-dhyāna in Kaṅkāla-mālinī-Tantra: "Meditate on the excellent Antarātma [1] in the (region of the) Lotus of a thousand petals, and above it (Antarātmā) meditate on the resplendent throne [2] between Nāda and Bindu, and on this throne (meditate) upon the eternal Guru, white like a mountain of silver."

"*The pale red glory of the gems in this altar shames the brilliance of lightning*" (Paṭu-taḍit-kaḍārima-sparddhamāna-maṇi-pāṭala-prabhaṁ).—This qualifies Maṇi-pīṭha-maṇḍalam. To be "paṭu" is to be able to fully do one's work. Now, lightning wants to display itself. Here the idea is that the pale red lustre of the gems in the Pīṭha shames the uninterrupted brilliance of the reddish-yellow (Piṅgala) lightning flash. It is of a pale red colour inasmuch as the Maṇi-pīṭha is covered all over with gems.

"*Its substance is Cit*" (Cinmayaṁ vapuḥ).—The Cinmaya or Jñāna-maya body. The body of Nāda, Bindu and Maṇi-pīṭha is Cinmaya or Jñāna-maya.[3] Others interpret it to mean "I meditate on the Cinmaya body of the twelfth vowel,[4] the Bīja of Sarasvatī, which is the Guru-mantra." But that is wrong. The Guru is white, and his Bīja is also white; to attribute to it a pale red lustre would be incongruous.

---

[1] This Antarātmā is Haṁsa. Unless the words in the text, "in the lotus of a thousand petals," be read Sāmīpye saptamī, the view here expressed differs from that adopted by Kālīcaraṇa, that Haṁsa is in the twelve-petalled lotus.

[2] Siṁhāsana—lit., lion seat, the seat of the honoured one, the King's seat.

[3] That is, their substance is pure Cit not in association with Māyā.

[4] The Bīja of Sarasvatī or Vāgbhava-Bīja is Aiṁ. Ai is the twelfth vowel.

Verse 4

Ūrdhvamasya hūtabhukśikhātrayaṃ
tadvilāsaparibṛṁhaṇāspadaṁ.
Viśvaghasmaramahoccidotkaṭaṁ
vyāmṛśāmi yugamādihaṁsayoḥ.

I INTENTLY meditate on the three lines above it (Maṇipīṭha), beginning with the line of Fire, and on the brilliance of Maṇipītha, which is heightened by the lustre of those lines. I also meditate on the primordial Haṁsa,[1] which is the all-powerful Great Light in which the Universe is absorbed.[2]

Commentary

On Haṁsa-pīṭha, which is within the triangle on Maṇi-pīṭha, between Nāda and Bindu, is the place of the Guru. He now wishes to describe Haṁsa and the triangle in order that a clear conception of these two may be gained.

The meaning of this verse is, shortly this: I meditate on the primordial Haṁsa,[3] I meditate on the three lines, beginning with the line of Fire, above the place of Maṇi-pīṭha and also on the glory of the Maṇi-pīṭha itself illumined as it is by the light of the three lines of Fire and others. The verb " I meditate " occurs once in this verse, and governs three nouns in the objective case.

" *I intently meditate* " (Vyāmṛṣāmi).—That is, I think with mind undisturbed, excluding all subjects likely to interfere with my thoughts.

" *Above it* " (Ūrdhvam asya)—that is, above Maṇi-pīṭha.

" *The three lines beginning with the line of Fire* " (Huta-bhuk-śikhā-trayaṁ).—This compound word is made up according to the rule known

[1] That is, the Parama-haṁsa which is both Prakṛti and Puruṣa.

[2] Lit., " Light which devours the Universe."

[3] *i.e.*, the union of Haṁ and Saḥ whereby the Haṁsa is formed.

as Śāka-pārthiva, by which the word Ādi, which comes in between two words is dropped. Ādi means " and others ". The Line of Fire,[1] which is called the Line Vāmā, emanates from Vahni Bindu in the South, and goes to the North-East Corner; and the Line of Moon emanates from Candra-Bindu in the North-East Corner, and goes towards the North-West Corner: this is the line Jyeṣṭhā. The Line of Sun emanates from Sūrya Bindu in the North-West Corner, and reaches Vahni Bindu: this is the Line Raudrī. The triangle which is formed by the three lines uniting the three Bindus is Kāma-kalā (Kāma-kalā-rūpaṁ).

The Bṛhat-Śrī-krama says: " She whose form is letters is coiled up in the Bindu and comes out thereof as a sprouting seed from the South. From there [2] She goes to the Īśāna corner (N.-E.). She who thus goes is the Śakti Vāmā. This is Citkalā Parā and the line of Fire. The Śakti which has thus gone to the Īśāna corner then goes in a straight line (that is, to the N.-W.). This line is the line of Jyeṣṭhā. This, O Parameśvarī, is Tripurā, the Sovereign Mistress. Again turning left [3] She returns to the place of sprouting. She is Raudrī, who by Her Union with Icchā and Nāda makes the Śṛṅgāta." [4]

The Māheśvarī-saṁhitā says: " Sūrya, Candra and Vahni are the three Bindus, and Brahmā, Viṣṇu and Śaṁbhu are the three lines."

The Prema-yoga-taraṅgiṇī, in describing the Sahasrāra, quotes an authority which is here cited, clearly showing that the place of the Guru is within this triangle. " Within it is the excellent lightning-like triangle. Within the triangle are two imperishable Bindus in the form of Visarga. Within it, in the void, is Śiva, known by the name of Parama." [5]

---

[1] Here Fire is the origin of life, and is therefore associated with Brahmā. Moon is associated with Viṣṇu. And the Sun spoken of here stands for the twelve suns (Āditya) which rise to burn the world at dissolution (Pralaya).

[2] Yasmāt is according to the reading given in the original. The same passage is quoted elsewhere reading yāmyāt (from the south) in place of yasmāt.

[3] Reading vakrībhūtā punar vāme for vyaktībhūya punar vāme.

[4] According to another reading, " By the union of Icchā and Jñāna, Raudrī makes the Śṛṅgāta." The passage above quoted shows that the Kāma-kalā is a subtle form of Kuṇḍalinī, more subtle than the A-Ka-Tha triangle. *Cf.* Ānandalaharī, v. 21, where the Sūkṣma-dhyāna of Kuṇḍalinī is given.

[5] *i.e.*, Parama-Śiva.

Śaṁkarācārya also has shown this clearly in his Ānandalaharī. The Author of the Lalitā-rahasya also speaks of the Guru as seated on Visarga. Visarga is the two Bindus, Candra and Sūrya, at the upper angles of the (down-turned) triangle.

"*On the primordial Haṁsa*" (Ādi-hamsayor-yugam).—Literally interpreted it would mean the union of[1] the primordial Haṁ and Saḥ. By Ādi (first) is implied the Parama-haṁsa, which is also known as Antarātmā, and not the Jīvātmā, which resembles the flame of a lamp. The Haṁsa here is the combination of Prakṛti and Puruṣa.

In Āgama-kalpadruma-pañcaśākhā it is said: "Haṁkāra is Bindu, and Visarga is Saḥ. Bindu is Puruṣa, and Visarga is Prakṛti. Haṁsa is the union of Pum (Male) and Prakṛti (Female). The world is pervaded by this Haṁsa."

Some interpret "*Asya Ūrdhvaṁ*" to mean "above Maṇi-pīṭha," and say that the verse means: "I meditate on the union of the two who constitute the primordial Haṁsa above Maṇi-pīṭha." This is wrong. The Kaṅkāla-mālinī speaks of the Maṇi-pīṭha as above Haṁsa and between Nāda and Bindu. So how can these be below Haṁsa? This is impossible. This also shows the impossibility of the reading adopted by some—namely, *Huta-bhuk-śikhā-sakham*[2] in place of *Huta-bhuk-śikhā-trayam.* If this reading were accepted, then the words *Ūrdhvaṁ asya* (above it) have no meaning. The interpretation "I meditate on the union of," as given above, may, however, be understood in the following sense. We have seen that the Kaṅkāla-mālinī speaks of the Haṁsa as below the Maṇi-pīṭha, which is between Nāda and Bindu. The interpretation mentioned is in great conflict with the view of Kaṅkāla-mālinī. But if Huta-bhuk-śikhā-trayam be read as qualifying Haṁsa, then the difficulty may be removed. Then the meaning would be: "Below Maṇi-pīṭha is Haṁsa, and above it is the triangular Kāma-kalā which is formed by the Haṁsa."[3]

[1] *i.e.*, Haṁ and Saḥ. The union of the two makes Haṁsaḥ. This is the beginning and end of creation. The outgoing breath (Niśvāsa) Haṁ of the Supreme is the duration of the life of Brahmā the Creator (*cf.* Tavāyur mama niśvāsah—Prapañcasāra-Tantra, Ch. I) and Saḥ is the indrawing breath by which creation returns to Prakṛti.

[2] Huta-bhuk-śikhā-sakha—the friend of the flame of Fire. By this is meant Vāyu (air). As there is no Vāyu in this region, therefore Vāyu cannot be above the triangle or above Maṇi-pīṭha.

[3] Tasya pariṇatasya. Apparently the sense is that the three Bindus, or Haṁsa are below, but that the triangle which they collectively form, or the Kāma-kalā, is above, and in this sense the Haṁsa is both above and below Maṇi-pīṭha.

" *Which is the all-powerful Great Light in which the Universe is absorbed* " (Viśva-ghasmara-mahoccidotkaṭam).—" Bhakṣ " and " Ghas " mean the same thing. The root " Ghas " means " to devour," and the roots " Cid," " Hlād," and " Dīp," all mean " to shine ". The Great Light (Mahoccit) which is the Devourer (Ghasmara) of the Universe: By that is meant that It is all-powerful (Utkaṭa). Utkaṭa, which literally means very high, here means very powerful.

Verse 5

Tatra nāthacaraṇā ravindayoḥ
kuṅkumāsavaparīmarandayoḥ.
Dvandvamindumakarandaśītalaṁ
mānasaṁ smarati maṅgalāspadaṁ.

THE mind there contemplates the two Lotuses which are the Feet of the Guru, and of which the ruby-coloured nectar is the honey. These two Feet are cool like the nectar of the Moon, and are the place of all auspiciousness.

Commentary

Having described the place where the two Lotus Feet of the Guru should be meditated upon, he now speaks of the (Sādhaka's) union therewith by meditation (Dhyāna) on them, in this and the following verse.

"*There*" (Tatra)—*i.e.*, in the triangle on the Maṇi-pīṭha. The meaning of this verse, in short, is: "The mind there, within the triangle on the Maṇi-pīṭha, contemplates upon the Lotus Feet of the Guru."

"*Of which the ruby-coloured nectar is the honey*" (Kuṅkumāsava-parīmarandayoḥ).—This qualifies "the lotuses". Kuṅkuma means red, the colour of lac. The excellent nectar which is of the colour of lac is the honey of the Lotus Feet of the Guru. Some read "Jharī" for "Parī"; the meaning would then be: "from which flows like honey the ruby-coloured nectar."

"*Cool like the nectar of the Moon*" (Indu-makaranda-śītalaṁ)—*i.e.*, they are cool as the nectar-like beams of the Moon. As the beams of the Moon counteract heat, so does devotion to the Feet of the Guru overcome sorrow and suffering.

"*Place of all auspiciousness*" (Maṅgalāspadam).—It is the place where one gets all one desires. The sense is that by devout concentration on the feet of the Guru all success is attained.

Verse 6

Niṣaktamaṇipādukāniyamitāghakolāhalaṁ
sphuratkisalayāruṇaṁ nakhasamullasaccandrakaṁ.
Parāmṛtasarovaroditasarojasadrociṣaṁ
bhajāmi śirasi sthitaṁ gurupadāravinddvayaṁ.

I adore in my head the two Lotus Feet of the Guru. The jewelled footstool on which they rest removes all sin. They are red like young leaves. Their nails resemble the moon shining in all her glory. Theirs is the beautiful lustre of lotuses growing in a lake of nectar.

Commentary

He says here: "I adore the two Lotus Feet of the Guru, resting on the footstool already described in my head." By adoration here meditation is meant.

"*The jewelled footstool on which they rest removes all sin*" (Niṣaktamaṇi-pādukā-niyamitagha-kolāhalaṁ).—That is, all the multitude of sins are removed by devotion to the jewelled footstool which serves as the resting-place of His Feet. Or it may be interpreted thus: "The footstool which is studded with gems—that is, the Maṇi-pīṭha-maṇḍala which is the footstool—removes all the multitude of sins. By meditating on the Feet of the Guru as resting on this stool all sins are destroyed." Or it may be thus interpreted: "The five footstools with which are inseparably connected the gems (by which are meant the Cintāmaṇi-like feet of the Guru) destroy all the multitude of sins." By meditating first on the fivefold footstool, and then on the feet of the Guru as resting thereon, sin is removed. As the removal of sins is effected by meditation on the fivefold footstool, it is the cause which effects such removal.

"*They are like young leaves*" (Sphurat-kisalayāruṇaṁ).—That is, the feet of the Guru possess the red colour of newly opened leaves. The leaves of the Mango and Kenduka[1] tree when newly opened are of a red colour, and comparison is made with them.

"*Their nails resemble the moon shining in all her glory*" (Nakha-samullasat-candrakaṁ)—*i.e.*, the toe-nails are like so many beautifully shining moons.

"*Theirs is the beautiful lustre of lotuses growing in a lake of nectar*" (Parāmṛta-sarovarodita-saroja-sadrociṣaṁ).—That is, they have the clear lustre of lotuses growing in a lake of nectar. He means to say that the excellent nectar drops constantly from the Lotus Feet of the Guru. Purṇānanda has said the same thing in v. 43 of the Ṣaṭ-cakra-nirūpaṇaṁ. The excellent nectar is the lake on which the Feet show like lotuses. It has been said that the place of the Guru is between the pericarps of the two Lotuses afore-mentioned. Now, a question may be raised as to whether it is in the pericarp of the twelve-petalled lotus below, or in that of the Sahasrāra above. To solve this the following passages are quoted:

Bṛhat-Śrīkrama: "Then meditate upon the Lotus which with its head downward is above all, and which drops nectar on the Śakti of the Guru in the other Lotus."

Yāmala: "The Lotus of a thousand petals is like a canopy;[2] it is above all, and drops red nectar."

Gurugītā: "In your own Guru meditate on the Supreme Guru as having two arms in the Lotus whose petals have the letters Haṁ and Saḥ and as surrounded by all the causes[3] of the universe. Although He manifests in all in varying degrees, He is without and beyond the Universe. On His will there are no limitations.[4] From Him emanates the Light of Liberation. He is the visible embodiment of the letters of the word[5] Guru."

The Śyāmā-saparyā quotes the following: "The Lotus Sahasrāra downward turned, in the head, is white. Its filaments are of the colour of the rising sun; all the letters of the Alphabet are on its petals. In the

---

[1] *Diospyros glutinosa.*

[2] Which is an emblem of supremacy.

[3] *i.e.*, the Avāntara-kāraṇa-śarīras. See Ṣaṭ-cakra-nirūpaṇa, vv. 39 *et seq.*

[4] Svacchandaṁ ātmecchayā=By His own will He is free.

[5] *Cf.* Mantrārṇā devatā prokta devatā guru-rūpiṇī.

The word Guru signifies many beneficent qualities. (See Kulārṇava, Tāntrik Texts, Vol. V, Ch. XVII.)

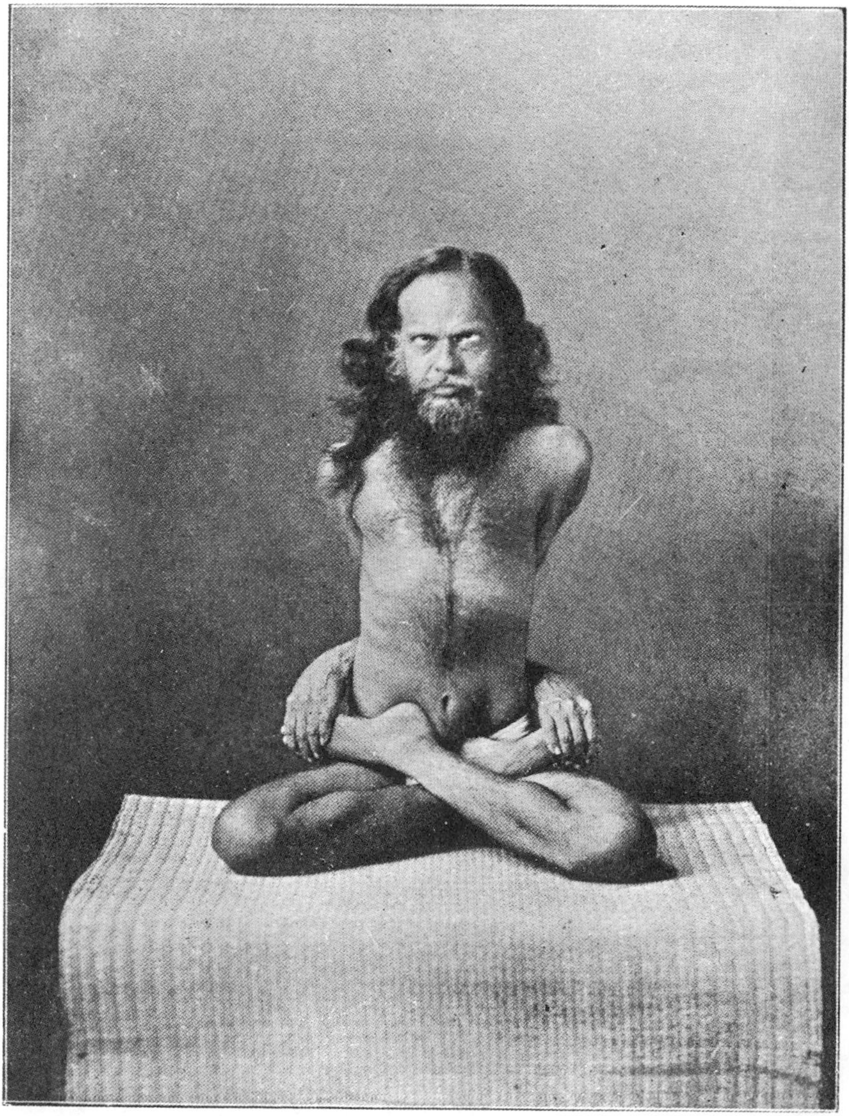

Plate XVII] **Baddha**-Padmāsana [To face Page 497

pericarp of the Sahasrāra is Candra Maṇḍala, and below the pericarp is the lustrous lotus of twelve petals which contains the triangle A-Ka-Tha, marked out by the letters Ha, La and Kṣa. Meditate there on your Guru who is Śiva, seated on the Haṁsa-pīṭha which is composed of Mantras."

The above and similar passages indicate that the place of the Guru is in the pericarp of the Lotus of twelve petals.

The Kaṅkāla-Mālinī says: "Meditate on the excellent Antarātma in the Lotus [1] of a thousand petals, and on the shining throne which is between Nāda and Bindu, and (on the throne) meditate constantly upon your own Guru, who is like a Mountain of Silver," etc.

The Yāmala says: [2] "(Meditate on your Guru) in the Lotus of a thousand petals. His cool beauty is like that of the full moon, and His Lotus hands are lifted up to grant boons and to dispel fear."

The Puraścaraṇa-rasollāsa (Ch. VII) has the following dialogue: "Śrī Mahādeva said: 'There in the pericarp of the wonderful everlasting Lotus of a thousand petals meditate always on your own Guru.' Śrī-Pārvatī said: 'The head of the Great Lotus of a thousand petals, O Lord, is always downward turned; then say, O Deva, how can the Guru constantly dwell there?' Śrī-Mahādeva said: 'Well hast thou asked, O Beloved. Now listen whilst I speak to Thee. The great Lotus Sahasrāra has a thousand petals, and is the abode of Sadā-Śiva and is full of eternal bliss. It is full of all kinds of delightful fragrance, and is the place of spontaneous bliss.[3] The head of this Lotus is always downward, but the pericarp is always turned upward,[4] and united with Kuṇḍalinī is always in the form of a triangle.'

The Bālā-vilāsa Tantra has the following: "Śrī-Dakṣiṇāmūrti said: 'As you awake in the morning meditate on your Guru in the White Lotus of a thousand petals, the head of which great Lotus is downward turned, and which is decorated with all the letters of the Alphabet. Within it is the triangle known by the name of A-Ka-Tha, which is decked by the

---

[1] Or in the region of the lotus of a thousand petals.

[2] The Commentator does not say from which of the different Yamalas he has quoted this and the passage in the first group.

[3] Sahajānanda—that is, the bliss springs up itself. This bliss is Svabhāva.

[4] That is, apparently, if we regard that portion of the pericarp which is attached to the lotus as its head. The triangle is A-Ka-Tha.

letters Ha, La and Kṣa. He of the smiling countenance is on the Haṁsa-pīṭha,[1] which is in the region of the Candra-Maṇḍala within it (the Sahasrāra).' Śrī-Devī said: 'O Lord, how does the Guru stay when its head is turned downwards?' Śrī-Dakṣiṇāmūrti said: 'The Candra-Maṇḍala in the pericarp of the Lotus of a thousand petals is turned upward; the Haṁsa is there, and there is the Guru's place.' "

These and similar passages speak of the place of the Guru as in the pericarp of the Lotus of a thousand petals.

As there are two distinct methods, one should follow the instruction of the Guru and adopt one of the two in his Sādhana (Anuṣṭāna). For it has been laid down in the Kulārṇava-Tantra (Ch. XI): "Beloved Vedas and Tantras handed down to us by tradition, as also Mantras and usages, become fruitful if communicated to us by the Guru, and not otherwise."

---

[1] Kāma-kalā.

Verse 7

Pādukāpañcakastotraṁ pañcavaktrādvinirgataṁ.
Ṣadāmnāyaphalaprāptaṁ prapañce cātidurlabhaṁ.

This hymn of praise of the Fivefold Footstool was uttered by Him of Five Faces. By (the recitation and hearing of) it is attained that good which is gained by (thc rccitation and hearing of) all the hymns in praise of Śiva. Such fruit is only attainable by great labour in the Wandering (Saṁsāra).

Commentary

He now speaks of the good gained by reciting and listening to this Stotra.

"*Hymn of praise of the fivefold Footstool*" (Pāduka-pancakastotram).—Paduka means a footstool (Pada-rakṣanā-dhāra). The five of these are: (1) The (twelve-petalled) Lotus; (2) the triangle A-Ka-Tha in its pericarp (3) the region of the Nāda, Bindu, and Maṇi-pīṭha in it; (4) the Haṁsa below; and (5) the triangle on the Maṇi-pīṭha. Or they may be counted thus: (1) The Lotus (*i.e.*, twelve-petalled); (2) the triangle (A-Ka-Tha); (3) Nāda-Bindu; (4) the Maṇi-pīṭha Maṇḍala; (5) the Haṁsa—which is above it and taken collectively form the triangular Kāma-kalā.[1]

---

[1] These two accounts appear to agree as to the position of the following in the order stated—*viz.*, twelve-petalled Lotus with A-Ka-Tha triangle in which are Maṇi-pīṭha, with Bindu above and Nāda below. There remains then to be considered the position of Haṁsa and the Kāma-kalā which they form. Both are one and the same, the first being the three Bindus, and the second the triangle; they make (Kāma-kalā), from which emanates (and in this sense forms part of it) the lower A-Ka-Tha triangle (for this Varṇa-maya). In the second classification, the three Bindus and the triangle (Kāma-kalā) which they form are treated as one, and placed above the Maṇi-pīṭha. In the first classification, apparently with a view to gain accordance with the Kaṅkāla-mālinī-Tantra cited under v. 4, the Haṁsa and the triangle which they form are taken separately, the first being placed below and the other above Maṇi-pīṭha.

Stotra is a hymn of praise. This hymn, including the verse which speaks of the benefit to be gained by listening to it, is one of seven verses.

"*Uttered by Him of Five Faces*" (Pañca-vaktrād vinirgatam).—The Five faces of Śiva as given in the Liṅgārcana Tantra are: "On the West [1] (*i.e.*, back) is Sadyo-jāta; on the North (*i.e.*, left) is Vāma-deva; on the South (right) is Aghora; and on the East (front) is Tat-puruṣa. Īśāna should be known as being in the middle. They should thus be meditated upon in a devout spirit." Vinirgata means uttered (*lit.*, come out)—that is, uttered by these Five Faces.

"*By it is attained that good*" (Ṣaḍāmnāya-phala-prāptam).—This literally means: "by it is obtained the fruit of what has been spoken by the Six Mouths." The Six Faces are the five given above and a sixth concealed one which is below, called Tāmasa. This is alluded to in Ṣaḍvaktra-nyāsa in the Śiva-Tantra thus: "Om Haṁ Hrīṁ Auṁ Hrīṁ Tāmasāya Svāhā"; as also in the meditation (Dhyāna) there given, thus: "The lower face, Nīla-kaṇṭa, is of the colour caused by the deadly poison Kāla-kūṭa." [2]

Ṣaḍāmnāya is what has been spoken by these Faces—that is, all the hymns of praise to Śiva. By the fruit of this is meant the benefit gained by reciting or listening to all these Mantras, and practising the appropriate Sādhana. This is what is gained through this hymn.

"*It is attainable by great labour in this Wandering*" (Prapañce cātidurlabhaṁ).—By Prapañca is meant this Saṁsāra (Wandering or World), comprising the Universe from all effects up to Brahmā, and which is shown by Māyā. It is difficult of attainment (Durlabha), as it is the result of manifold merit acquired by the practice of laborious endeavour (Tapas) in previous births.

End of the Commentary (Ṭippaṇī) of the Name of Amalā (Stainless), written by Śrī-Kalīcāraṇa on the Pādukā-pañcaka-Stotra.

[1] The direction one faces is the East.

[2] The poison churned out of the ocean and drunk by Śiva. The word [illegible]ns the secret emissary of Death.

APPENDIX I

INDEX OF HALF VERSES

APPENDIX II

INDEX OF AUTHORS

APPENDIX III

INDEX OF WORKS

APPENDIX IV

INDEX OF WORDS

Śā

Ṣa

Sa

Ha

A CATALOGUE OF SELECTED DOVER BOOKS IN ALL FIELDS OF INTEREST

A CATALOGUE OF SELECTED DOVER BOOKS IN ALL FIELDS OF INTEREST

VISUAL ILLUSIONS: THEIR CAUSES, CHARACTERISTICS, AND APPLICATIONS, Matthew Luckiesh. Thorough description and discussion of optical illusion, geometric and perspective, particularly; size and shape distortions, illusions of color, of motion; natural illusions; use of illusion in art and magic, industry, etc. Most useful today with op art, also for classical art. Scores of effects illustrated. Introduction by William H. Ittleson. 100 illustrations. xxi + 252pp.
21530-X Paperbound $2.00

A HANDBOOK OF ANATOMY FOR ART STUDENTS, Arthur Thomson. Thorough, virtually exhaustive coverage of skeletal structure, musculature, etc. Full text, supplemented by anatomical diagrams and drawings and by photographs of undraped figures. Unique in its comparison of male and female forms, pointing out differences of contour, texture, form. 211 figures, 40 drawings, 86 photographs. xx + 459pp. 5⅜ x 8⅜. 21163-0 Paperbound $3.50

150 MASTERPIECES OF DRAWING, Selected by Anthony Toney. Full page reproductions of drawings from the early 16th to the end of the 18th century, all beautifully reproduced: Rembrandt, Michelangelo, Dürer, Fragonard, Urs, Graf, Wouwerman, many others. First-rate browsing book, model book for artists. xviii + 150pp. 8⅜ x 11¼. 21032-4 Paperbound $3.50

THE LATER WORK OF AUBREY BEARDSLEY, Aubrey Beardsley. Exotic, erotic, ironic masterpieces in full maturity: Comedy Ballet, Venus and Tannhauser, Pierrot, Lysistrata, Rape of the Lock, Savoy material, Ali Baba, Volpone, etc. This material revolutionized the art world, and is still powerful, fresh, brilliant. With *The Early Work,* all Beardsley's finest work. 174 plates, 2 in color. xiv + 176pp. 8⅛ x 11.
21817-1 Paperbound $3.75

DRAWINGS OF REMBRANDT, Rembrandt van Rijn. Complete reproduction of fabulously rare edition by Lippmann and Hofstede de Groot, completely reedited, updated, improved by Prof. Seymour Slive, Fogg Museum. Portraits, Biblical sketches, landscapes, Oriental types, nudes, episodes from classical mythology—All Rembrandt's fertile genius. Also selection of drawings by his pupils and followers. "Stunning volumes," *Saturday Review.* 550 illustrations. lxxviii + 552pp. 9⅛ x 12¼. 21485-0, 21486-9 Two volumes, Paperbound $10.00

THE DISASTERS OF WAR, Francisco Goya. One of the masterpieces of Western civilization—83 etchings that record Goya's shattering, bitter reaction to the Napoleonic war that swept through Spain after the insurrection of 1808 and to war in general. Reprint of the first edition, with three additional plates from Boston's Museum of Fine Arts. All plates facsimile size. Introduction by Philip Hofer, Fogg Museum. v + 97pp. 9⅜ x 8¼. 21872-4 Paperbound $2.50

GRAPHIC WORKS OF ODILON REDON. Largest collection of Redon's graphic works ever assembled: 172 lithographs, 28 etchings and engravings, 9 drawings. These include some of his most famous works. All the plates from *Odilon Redon: oeuvre graphique complet,* plus additional plates. New introduction and caption translations by Alfred Werner. 209 illustrations. xxvii + 209pp. 9⅛ x 12¼.
21966-8 Paperbound $5.00

ALPHABETS AND ORNAMENTS, Ernst Lehner. Well-known pictorial source for decorative alphabets, script examples, cartouches, frames, decorative title pages, calligraphic initials, borders, similar material. 14th to 19th century, mostly European. Useful in almost any graphic arts designing, varied styles. 750 illustrations. 256pp. 7 x 10. 21905-4 Paperbound $4.00

PAINTING: A CREATIVE APPROACH, Norman Colquhoun. For the beginner simple guide provides an instructive approach to painting: major stumbling blocks for beginner; overcoming them, technical points; paints and pigments; oil painting; watercolor and other media and color. New section on "plastic" paints. Glossary. Formerly *Paint Your Own Pictures*. 221pp. 22000-1 Paperbound $1.75

THE ENJOYMENT AND USE OF COLOR, Walter Sargent. Explanation of the relations between colors themselves and between colors in nature and art, including hundreds of little-known facts about color values, intensities, effects of high and low illumination, complementary colors. Many practical hints for painters, references to great masters. 7 color plates, 29 illustrations. x + 274pp.
20944-X Paperbound $2.75

THE NOTEBOOKS OF LEONARDO DA VINCI, compiled and edited by Jean Paul Richter. 1566 extracts from original manuscripts reveal the full range of Leonardo's versatile genius: all his writings on painting, sculpture, architecture, anatomy, astronomy, geography, topography, physiology, mining, music, etc., in both Italian and English, with 186 plates of manuscript pages and more than 500 additional drawings. Includes studies for the Last Supper, the lost Sforza monument, and other works. Total of xlvii + 866pp. 7⅞ x 10¾.
22572-0, 22573-9 Two volumes, Paperbound $11.00

MONTGOMERY WARD CATALOGUE OF 1895. Tea gowns, yards of flannel and pillow-case lace, stereoscopes, books of gospel hymns, the New Improved Singer Sewing Machine, side saddles, milk skimmers, straight-edged razors, high-button shoes, spittoons, and on and on . . . listing some 25,000 items, practically all illustrated. Essential to the shoppers of the 1890's, it is our truest record of the spirit of the period. Unaltered reprint of Issue No. 57, Spring and Summer 1895. Introduction by Boris Emmet. Innumerable illustrations. xiii + 624pp. 8½ x 11⅝.
22377-9 Paperbound $6.95

THE CRYSTAL PALACE EXHIBITION ILLUSTRATED CATALOGUE (LONDON, 1851). One of the wonders of the modern world—the Crystal Palace Exhibition in which all the nations of the civilized world exhibited their achievements in the arts and sciences—presented in an equally important illustrated catalogue. More than 1700 items pictured with accompanying text—ceramics, textiles, cast-iron work, carpets, pianos, sleds, razors, wall-papers, billiard tables, beehives, silverware and hundreds of other artifacts—represent the focal point of Victorian culture in the Western World. Probably the largest collection of Victorian decorative art ever assembled—indispensable for antiquarians and designers. Unabridged republication of the Art-Journal Catalogue of the Great Exhibition of 1851, with all terminal essays. New introduction by John Gloag, F.S.A. xxxiv + 426pp. 9 x 12.
22503-8 Paperbound $5.00

A HISTORY OF COSTUME, Carl Köhler. Definitive history, based on surviving pieces of clothing primarily, and paintings, statues, etc. secondarily. Highly readable text, supplemented by 594 illustrations of costumes of the ancient Mediterranean peoples, Greece and Rome, the Teutonic prehistoric period; costumes of the Middle Ages, Renaissance, Baroque, 18th and 19th centuries. Clear, measured patterns are provided for many clothing articles. Approach is practical throughout. Enlarged by Emma von Sichart. 464pp. 21030-8 Paperbound $3.50

ORIENTAL RUGS, ANTIQUE AND MODERN, Walter A. Hawley. A complete and authoritative treatise on the Oriental rug—where they are made, by whom and how, designs and symbols, characteristics in detail of the six major groups, how to distinguish them and how to buy them. Detailed technical data is provided on periods, weaves, warps, wefts, textures, sides, ends and knots, although no technical background is required for an understanding. 11 color plates, 80 halftones, 4 maps. vi + 320pp. 6⅛ x 9⅛. 22366-3 Paperbound $5.00

TEN BOOKS ON ARCHITECTURE, Vitruvius. By any standards the most important book on architecture ever written. Early Roman discussion of aesthetics of building, construction methods, orders, sites, and every other aspect of architecture has inspired, instructed architecture for about 2,000 years. Stands behind Palladio, Michelangelo, Bramante, Wren, countless others. Definitive Morris H. Morgan translation. 68 illustrations. xii + 331pp. 20645-9 Paperbound $3.00

THE FOUR BOOKS OF ARCHITECTURE, Andrea Palladio. Translated into every major Western European language in the two centuries following its publication in 1570, this has been one of the most influential books in the history of architecture. Complete reprint of the 1738 Isaac Ware edition. New introduction by Adolf Placzek, Columbia Univ. 216 plates. xxii + 110pp. of text. 9½ x 12¾. 21308-0 Clothbound $12.50

STICKS AND STONES: A STUDY OF AMERICAN ARCHITECTURE AND CIVILIZATION, Lewis Mumford.One of the great classics of American cultural history. American architecture from the medieval-inspired earliest forms to the early 20th century; evolution of structure and style, and reciprocal influences on environment. 21 photographic illustrations. 238pp. 20202-X Paperbound $2.00

THE AMERICAN BUILDER'S COMPANION, Asher Benjamin. The most widely used early 19th century architectural style and source book, for colonial up into Greek Revival periods. Extensive development of geometry of carpentering, construction of sashes, frames, doors, stairs; plans and elevations of domestic and other buildings. Hundreds of thousands of houses were built according to this book, now invaluable to historians, architects, restorers, etc. 1827 edition. 59 plates. 114pp. 7⅞ x 10¾. 22236-5 Paperbound $3.50

DUTCH HOUSES IN THE HUDSON VALLEY BEFORE 1776, Helen Wilkinson Reynolds. The standard survey of the Dutch colonial house and outbuildings, with constructional features, decoration, and local history associated with individual homesteads. Introduction by Franklin D. Roosevelt. Map. 150 illustrations. 469pp. 6⅝ x 9¼. 21469-9 Paperbound $5.00

THE ARCHITECTURE OF COUNTRY HOUSES, Andrew J. Downing. Together with Vaux's *Villas and Cottages* this is the basic book for Hudson River Gothic architecture of the middle Victorian period. Full, sound discussions of general aspects of housing, architecture, style, decoration, furnishing, together with scores of detailed house plans, illustrations of specific buildings, accompanied by full text. Perhaps the most influential single American architectural book. 1850 edition. Introduction by J. Stewart Johnson. 321 figures, 34 architectural designs. xvi + 560pp.
22003-6 Paperbound $4.00

LOST EXAMPLES OF COLONIAL ARCHITECTURE, John Mead Howells. Full-page photographs of buildings that have disappeared or been so altered as to be denatured, including many designed by major early American architects. 245 plates. xvii + 248pp. 7⅞ x 10¾. 21143-6 Paperbound $3.50

DOMESTIC ARCHITECTURE OF THE AMERICAN COLONIES AND OF THE EARLY REPUBLIC, Fiske Kimball. Foremost architect and restorer of Williamsburg and Monticello covers nearly 200 homes between 1620-1825. Architectural details, construction, style features, special fixtures, floor plans, etc. Generally considered finest work in its area. 219 illustrations of houses, doorways, windows, capital mantels. xx + 314pp. 7⅞ x 10¾. 21743-4 Paperbound $4.00

EARLY AMERICAN ROOMS: 1650-1858, edited by Russell Hawes Kettell. Tour of 12 rooms, each representative of a different era in American history and each furnished, decorated, designed and occupied in the style of the era. 72 plans and elevations, 8-page color section, etc., show fabrics, wall papers, arrangements, etc. Full descriptive text. xvii + 200pp. of text. 8⅜ x 11¼.
21633-0 Paperbound $5.00

THE FITZWILLIAM VIRGINAL BOOK, edited by J. Fuller Maitland and W. B. Squire. Full modern printing of famous early 17th-century ms. volume of 300 works by Morley, Byrd, Bull, Gibbons, etc. For piano or other modern keyboard instrument; easy to read format. xxxvi + 938pp. 8⅜ x 11.
21068-5, 21069-3 Two volumes, Paperbound $10.00

KEYBOARD MUSIC, Johann Sebastian Bach. Bach Gesellschaft edition. A rich selection of Bach's masterpieces for the harpsichord: the six English Suites, six French Suites, the six Partitas (Clavierübung part I), the Goldberg Variations (Clavierübung part IV), the fifteen Two-Part Inventions and the fifteen Three-Part Sinfonias. Clearly reproduced on large sheets with ample margins; eminently playable. vi + 312pp. 8⅛ x 11. 22360-4 Paperbound $5.00

THE MUSIC OF BACH: AN INTRODUCTION, Charles Sanford Terry. A fine, nontechnical introduction to Bach's music, both instrumental and vocal. Covers organ music, chamber music, passion music, other types. Analyzes themes, developments, innovations. x + 114pp. 21075-8 Paperbound $1.50

BEETHOVEN AND HIS NINE SYMPHONIES, Sir George Grove. Noted British musicologist provides best history, analysis, commentary on symphonies. Very thorough, rigorously accurate; necessary to both advanced student and amateur music lover. 436 musical passages. vii + 407 pp. 20334-4 Paperbound $2.75

JOHANN SEBASTIAN BACH, Philipp Spitta. One of the great classics of musicology, this definitive analysis of Bach's music (and life) has never been surpassed. Lucid, nontechnical analyses of hundreds of pieces (30 pages devoted to St. Matthew Passion, 26 to B Minor Mass). Also includes major analysis of 18th-century music. 450 musical examples. 40-page musical supplement. Total of xx + 1799pp.
(EUK) 22278-0, 22279-9 Two volumes, Clothbound $17.50

MOZART AND HIS PIANO CONCERTOS, Cuthbert Girdlestone. The only full-length study of an important area of Mozart's creativity. Provides detailed analyses of all 23 concertos, traces inspirational sources. 417 musical examples. Second edition. 509pp. 21271-8 Paperbound $3.50

THE PERFECT WAGNERITE: A COMMENTARY ON THE NIBLUNG'S RING, George Bernard Shaw. Brilliant and still relevant criticism in remarkable essays on Wagner's Ring cycle, Shaw's ideas on political and social ideology behind the plots, role of Leitmotifs, vocal requisites, etc. Prefaces. xxi + 136pp.
(USO) 21707-8 Paperbound $1.75

DON GIOVANNI, W. A. Mozart. Complete libretto, modern English translation; biographies of composer and librettist; accounts of early performances and critical reaction. Lavishly illustrated. All the material you need to understand and appreciate this great work. Dover Opera Guide and Libretto Series; translated and introduced by Ellen Bleiler. 92 illustrations. 209pp.
21134-7 Paperbound $2.00

BASIC ELECTRICITY, U. S. Bureau of Naval Personel. Originally a training course, best non-technical coverage of basic theory of electricity and its applications. Fundamental concepts, batteries, circuits, conductors and wiring techniques, AC and DC, inductance and capacitance, generators, motors, transformers, magnetic amplifiers, synchros, servomechanisms, etc. Also covers blue-prints, electrical diagrams, etc. Many questions, with answers. 349 illustrations. x + 448pp. 6½ x 9¼.
20973-3 Paperbound $3.50

REPRODUCTION OF SOUND, Edgar Villchur. Thorough coverage for laymen of high fidelity systems, reproducing systems in general, needles, amplifiers, preamps, loudspeakers, feedback, explaining physical background. "A rare talent for making technicalities vividly comprehensible," R. Darrell, *High Fidelity*. 69 figures. iv + 92pp. 21515-6 Paperbound $1.35

HEAR ME TALKIN' TO YA: THE STORY OF JAZZ AS TOLD BY THE MEN WHO MADE IT, Nat Shapiro and Nat Hentoff. Louis Armstrong, Fats Waller, Jo Jones, Clarence Williams, Billy Holiday, Duke Ellington, Jelly Roll Morton and dozens of other jazz greats tell how it was in Chicago's South Side, New Orleans, depression Harlem and the modern West Coast as jazz was born and grew. xvi + 429pp.
21726-4 Paperbound $3.00

FABLES OF AESOP, translated by Sir Roger L'Estrange. A reproduction of the very rare 1931 Paris edition; a selection of the most interesting fables, together with 50 imaginative drawings by Alexander Calder. v + 128pp. 6½x9¼.
21780-9 Paperbound $1.50

LAST AND FIRST MEN AND STAR MAKER, TWO SCIENCE FICTION NOVELS, Olaf Stapledon. Greatest future histories in science fiction. In the first, human intelligence is the "hero," through strange paths of evolution, interplanetary invasions, incredible technologies, near extinctions and reemergences. Star Maker describes the quest of a band of star rovers for intelligence itself, through time and space: weird inhuman civilizations, crustacean minds, symbiotic worlds, etc. Complete, unabridged. v + 438pp. (USO) 21962-3 Paperbound $2.50

THREE PROPHETIC NOVELS, H. G. WELLS. Stages of a consistently planned future for mankind. *When the Sleeper Wakes,* and *A Story of the Days to Come,* anticipate *Brave New World* and *1984,* in the 21st Century; *The Time Machine,* only complete version in print, shows farther future and the end of mankind. All show Wells's greatest gifts as storyteller and novelist. Edited by E. F. Bleiler. x + 335pp. (USO) 20605-X Paperbound $2.50

THE DEVIL'S DICTIONARY, Ambrose Bierce. America's own Oscar Wilde—Ambrose Bierce—offers his barbed iconoclastic wisdom in over 1,000 definitions hailed by H. L. Mencken as "some of the most gorgeous witticisms in the English language." 145pp. 20487-1 Paperbound $1.25

MAX AND MORITZ, Wilhelm Busch. Great children's classic, father of comic strip, of two bad boys, Max and Moritz. Also Ker and Plunk (Plisch und Plumm), Cat and Mouse, Deceitful Henry, Ice-Peter, The Boy and the Pipe, and five other pieces. Original German, with English translation. Edited by H. Arthur Klein; translations by various hands and H. Arthur Klein. vi + 216pp.
20181-3 Paperbound $2.00

PIGS IS PIGS AND OTHER FAVORITES, Ellis Parker Butler. The title story is one of the best humor short stories, as Mike Flannery obfuscates biology and English. Also included, That Pup of Murchison's, The Great American Pie Company, and Perkins of Portland. 14 illustrations. v + 109pp. 21532-6 Paperbound $1.25

THE PETERKIN PAPERS, Lucretia P. Hale. It takes genius to be as stupidly mad as the Peterkins, as they decide to become wise, celebrate the "Fourth," keep a cow, and otherwise strain the resources of the Lady from Philadelphia. Basic book of American humor. 153 illustrations. 219pp. 20794-3 Paperbound $2.00

PERRAULT'S FAIRY TALES, translated by A. E. Johnson and S. R. Littlewood, with 34 full-page illustrations by Gustave Doré. All the original Perrault stories—Cinderella, Sleeping Beauty, Bluebeard, Little Red Riding Hood, Puss in Boots, Tom Thumb, etc.—with their witty verse morals and the magnificent illustrations of Doré. One of the five or six great books of European fairy tales. viii + 117pp. 8⅛ x 11. 22311-6 Paperbound $2.00

OLD HUNGARIAN FAIRY TALES, Baroness Orczy. Favorites translated and adapted by author of the *Scarlet Pimpernel.* Eight fairy tales include "The Suitors of Princess Fire-Fly," "The Twin Hunchbacks," "Mr. Cuttlefish's Love Story," and "The Enchanted Cat." This little volume of magic and adventure will captivate children as it has for generations. 90 drawings by Montagu Barstow. 96pp.
(USO) 22293-4 Paperbound $1.95

THE RED FAIRY BOOK, Andrew Lang. Lang's color fairy books have long been children's favorites. This volume includes Rapunzel, Jack and the Bean-stalk and 35 other stories, familiar and unfamiliar. 4 plates, 93 illustrations x + 367pp.
21673-X Paperbound $2.50

THE BLUE FAIRY BOOK, Andrew Lang. Lang's tales come from all countries and all times. Here are 37 tales from Grimm, the Arabian Nights, Greek Mythology, and other fascinating sources. 8 plates, 130 illustrations. xi + 390pp.
21437-0 Paperbound $2.75

HOUSEHOLD STORIES BY THE BROTHERS GRIMM. Classic English-language edition of the well-known tales — Rumpelstiltskin, Snow White, Hansel and Gretel, The Twelve Brothers, Faithful John, Rapunzel, Tom Thumb (52 stories in all). Translated into simple, straightforward English by Lucy Crane. Ornamented with headpieces, vignettes, elaborate decorative initials and a dozen full-page illustrations by Walter Crane. x + 269pp. 21080-4 Paperbound **$2.00**

THE MERRY ADVENTURES OF ROBIN HOOD, Howard Pyle. The finest modern versions of the traditional ballads and tales about the great English outlaw. Howard Pyle's complete prose version, with every word, every illustration of the first edition. Do not confuse this facsimile of the original (1883) with modern editions that change text or illustrations. 23 plates plus many page decorations. xxii + 296pp.
22043-5 Paperbound $2.75

THE STORY OF KING ARTHUR AND HIS KNIGHTS, Howard Pyle. The finest children's version of the life of King Arthur; brilliantly retold by Pyle, with 48 of his most imaginative illustrations. xviii + 313pp. 6⅛ x 9¼.
21445-1 Paperbound $2.50

THE WONDERFUL WIZARD OF OZ, L. Frank Baum. America's finest children's book in facsimile of first edition with all Denslow illustrations in full color. The edition a child should have. Introduction by Martin Gardner. 23 color plates, scores of drawings. iv + 267pp. 20691-2 Paperbound $2.50

THE MARVELOUS LAND OF OZ, L. Frank Baum. The second Oz book, every bit as imaginative as the Wizard. The hero is a boy named Tip, but the Scarecrow and the Tin Woodman are back, as is the Oz magic. 16 color plates, 120 drawings by John R. Neill. 287pp. 20692-0 Paperbound $2.50

THE MAGICAL MONARCH OF MO, L. Frank Baum. Remarkable adventures in a land even stranger than Oz. The best of Baum's books not in the Oz series. 15 color plates and dozens of drawings by Frank Verbeck. xviii + 237pp.
21892-9 Paperbound $2.25

THE BAD CHILD'S BOOK OF BEASTS, MORE BEASTS FOR WORSE CHILDREN, A MORAL ALPHABET, Hilaire Belloc. Three complete humor classics in one volume. Be kind to the frog, and do not call him names . . . and 28 other whimsical animals. Familiar favorites and some not so well known. Illustrated by Basil Blackwell. 156pp. (USO) 20749-8 Paperbound $1.50

East O' the Sun and West O' the Moon, George W. Dasent. Considered the best of all translations of these Norwegian folk tales, this collection has been enjoyed by generations of children (and folklorists too). Includes True and Untrue, Why the Sea is Salt, East O' the Sun and West O' the Moon, Why the Bear is Stumpy-Tailed, Boots and the Troll, The Cock and the Hen, Rich Peter the Pedlar, and 52 more. The only edition with all 59 tales. 77 illustrations by Erik Werenskiold and Theodor Kittelsen. xv + 418pp. 22521-6 Paperbound $3.50

Goops and How to be Them, Gelett Burgess. Classic of tongue-in-cheek humor, masquerading as etiquette book. 87 verses, twice as many cartoons, show mischievous Goops as they demonstrate to children virtues of table manners, neatness, courtesy, etc. Favorite for generations. viii + 88pp. 6½ x 9¼.
22233-0 Paperbound $1.50

Alice's Adventures Under Ground, Lewis Carroll. The first version, quite different from the final *Alice in Wonderland,* printed out by Carroll himself with his own illustrations. Complete facsimile of the "million dollar" manuscript Carroll gave to Alice Liddell in 1864. Introduction by Martin Gardner. viii + 96pp. Title and dedication pages in color. 21482-6 Paperbound $1.25

The Brownies, Their Book, Palmer Cox. Small as mice, cunning as foxes, exuberant and full of mischief, the Brownies go to the zoo, toy shop, seashore, circus, etc., in 24 verse adventures and 266 illustrations. Long a favorite, since their first appearance in St. Nicholas Magazine. xi + 144pp. 6⅝ x 9¼.
21265-3 Paperbound $1.75

Songs of Childhood, Walter De La Mare. Published (under the pseudonym Walter Ramal) when De La Mare was only 29, this charming collection has long been a favorite children's book. A facsimile of the first edition in paper, the 47 poems capture the simplicity of the nursery rhyme and the ballad, including such lyrics as I Met Eve, Tartary, The Silver Penny. vii + 106pp. (USO) 21972-0 Paperbound $2.00

The Complete Nonsense of Edward Lear, Edward Lear. The finest 19th-century humorist-cartoonist in full: all nonsense limericks, zany alphabets, Owl and Pussycat, songs, nonsense botany, and more than 500 illustrations by Lear himself. Edited by Holbrook Jackson. xxix + 287pp. (USO) 20167-8 Paperbound $2.00

Billy Whiskers: The Autobiography of a Goat, Frances Trego Montgomery. A favorite of children since the early 20th century, here are the escapades of that rambunctious, irresistible and mischievous goat—Billy Whiskers. Much in the spirit of *Peck's Bad Boy,* this is a book that children never tire of reading or hearing. All the original familiar illustrations by W. H. Fry are included: 6 color plates, 18 black and white drawings. 159pp. 22345-0 Paperbound $2.00

Mother Goose Melodies. Faithful republication of the fabulously rare Munroe and Francis "copyright 1833" Boston edition—the most important Mother Goose collection, usually referred to as the "original." Familiar rhymes plus many rare ones, with wonderful old woodcut illustrations. Edited by E. F. Bleiler. 128pp. 4½ x 6⅜. 22577-1 Paperbound $1.00

TWO LITTLE SAVAGES; BEING THE ADVENTURES OF TWO BOYS WHO LIVED AS INDIANS AND WHAT THEY LEARNED, Ernest Thompson Seton. Great classic of nature and boyhood provides a vast range of woodlore in most palatable form, a genuinely entertaining story. Two farm boys build a teepee in woods and live in it for a month, working out Indian solutions to living problems, star lore, birds and animals, plants, etc. 293 illustrations. vii + 286pp.

20985-7 Paperbound $2.50

PETER PIPER'S PRACTICAL PRINCIPLES OF PLAIN & PERFECT PRONUNCIATION. Alliterative jingles and tongue-twisters of surprising charm, that made their first appearance in America about 1830. Republished in full with the spirited woodcut illustrations from this earliest American edition. 32pp. 4½ x 6⅜.

22560-7 Paperbound $1.00

SCIENCE EXPERIMENTS AND AMUSEMENTS FOR CHILDREN, Charles Vivian. 73 easy experiments, requiring only materials found at home or easily available, such as candles, coins, steel wool, etc.; illustrate basic phenomena like vacuum, simple chemical reaction, etc. All safe. Modern, well-planned. Formerly *Science Games for Children.* 102 photos, numerous drawings. 96pp. 6⅛ x 9¼.

21856-2 Paperbound $1.25

AN INTRODUCTION TO CHESS MOVES AND TACTICS SIMPLY EXPLAINED, Leonard Barden. Informal intermediate introduction, quite strong in explaining reasons for moves. Covers basic material, tactics, important openings, traps, positional play in middle game, end game. Attempts to isolate patterns and recurrent configurations. Formerly *Chess.* 58 figures. 102pp. (USO) 21210-6 Paperbound $1.25

LASKER'S MANUAL OF CHESS, Dr. Emanuel Lasker. Lasker was not only one of the five great World Champions, he was also one of the ablest expositors, theorists, and analysts. In many ways, his Manual, permeated with his philosophy of battle, filled with keen insights, is one of the greatest works ever written on chess. Filled with analyzed games by the great players. A single-volume library that will profit almost any chess player, beginner or master. 308 diagrams. xli x 349pp.

20640-8 Paperbound $2.75

THE MASTER BOOK OF MATHEMATICAL RECREATIONS, Fred Schuh. In opinion of many the finest work ever prepared on mathematical puzzles, stunts, recreations; exhaustively thorough explanations of mathematics involved, analysis of effects, citation of puzzles and games. Mathematics involved is elementary. Translated bv F. Göbel. 194 figures. xxiv + 430pp. 22134-2 Paperbound $3.50

MATHEMATICS, MAGIC AND MYSTERY, Martin Gardner. Puzzle editor for Scientific American explains mathematics behind various mystifying tricks: card tricks, stage "mind reading," coin and match tricks, counting out games, geometric dissections, etc. Probability sets, theory of numbers clearly explained. Also provides more than 400 tricks, guaranteed to work, that you can do. 135 illustrations. xii + 176pp.

20335-2 Paperbound $1.75